Textbook of
BIOMECHANICS AND KINESIOLOGY

(Detailed Analysis of Musculoskeletal Structure and Function)

Textbook of
BIOMECHANICS AND KINESIOLOGY

(Detailed Analysis of Musculoskeletal Structure and Function)

Pavan Kumar G
Principal and Professor
Cauvery College of Physiotherapy
Mysuru, Karnataka, India

Ilona Gracie De Souza
HOD
Department of Movement Science
Cauvery College of Physiotherapy
Mysuru, Karnataka, India

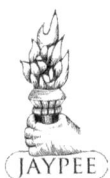

JAYPEE BROTHERS MEDICAL PUBLISHERS
The Health Sciences Publisher
New Delhi | London

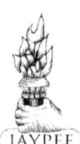 **Jaypee Brothers Medical Publishers (P) Ltd.**

Headquarters
Jaypee Brothers Medical Publishers (P) Ltd
EMCA House
23/23-B, Ansari Road, Daryaganj
New Delhi - 110 002, India
Landline: +91-11-23272143, +91-11-23272703
+91-11-23282021, +91-11-23245672
Email: jaypee@jaypeebrothers.com

Corporate Office
Jaypee Brothers Medical Publishers (P) Ltd
4838/24, Ansari Road, Daryaganj
New Delhi 110 002, India
Phone: +91-11-43574357
Fax: +91-11-43574314
Email: jaypee@jaypeebrothers.com

Overseas Office
J.P. Medical Ltd
83 Victoria Street, London
SW1H 0HW (UK)
Phone: +44 20 3170 8910
Email: info@jpmedpub.com

EU GPSR Authorised Representative
Logos Europe, 9 rue Nicolas Poussin
17000, La Rochelle, France
Phone: +33 (0) 6 67 93 73 78
E-mail: Contact@logoseurope.eu

Website: www.jaypeebrothers.com
Website: www.jaypeedigital.com

© 2022, Jaypee Brothers Medical Publishers

The views and opinions expressed in this book are solely those of the original contributor(s)/author(s) and do not necessarily represent those of editor(s) of the book.

All rights reserved. No part of this publication may be reproduced, stored or transmitted in any form or by any means, electronic, mechanical, photocopying, recording or otherwise, without the prior permission in writing of the publishers.

All brand names and product names used in this book are trade names, service marks, trademarks or registered trademarks of their respective owners. The publisher is not associated with any product or vendor mentioned in this book.

Medical knowledge and practice change constantly. This book is designed to provide accurate, authoritative information about the subject matter in question. However, readers are advised to check the most current information available on procedures included and check information from the manufacturer of each product to be administered, to verify the recommended dose, formula, method and duration of administration, adverse effects and contraindications. It is the responsibility of the practitioner to take all appropriate safety precautions. Neither the publisher nor the author(s)/editor(s) assume any liability for any injury and/or damage to persons or property arising from or related to use of material in this book.

This book is sold on the understanding that the publisher is not engaged in providing professional medical services. If such advice or services are required, the services of a competent medical professional should be sought.

Every effort has been made where necessary to contact holders of copyright to obtain permission to reproduce copyright material. If any have been inadvertently overlooked, the publisher will be pleased to make the necessary arrangements at the first opportunity.

Inquiries for bulk sales may be solicited at: jaypee@jaypeebrothers.com

Textbook of Biomechanics and Kinesiology

First Edition: **2022**
ISBN: 978-93-5465-234-9

Dedicated to

Our students

Preface

The central point of this *Textbook of Biomechanics and Kinesiology* is to have a strong foundation in biomechanics that can help to manipulate the minds of young physiotherapist. This textbook provides high quality material in a precise yet comprehensive form. Every effort has been made to make concepts clear by giving anatomical and mechanical examples. With the vast educational books on biomechanics published in and around the world, we took up the challenge to simplify biomechanics for our budding students with the key motive in mind, to help the students understand the concepts clearly, to retain and apply it in clinical practice. The textbook not only provides the theoretical aspects but also adds a section of analytical biomechanics, that comprises of numerous chapters that can be incorporated into clinical practice and research. The textbook incorporates diagrams which are student friendly and can be drawn easily. Most readers at this point in time are not exposed to clinical practice, thus failing to appreciate the biomechanical relevance that's described in this textbook. In their later years at the university, the readers will find a clear relation between biomechanics and many clinical conditions and interventions. The writings of this book was undertaken with the conviction that a systematic presentation of biomechanical aspects would be of distinct value and use to the future physiotherapist.

Intensive writings will definitely have some flaws. No one can be perfect and there could have still been some shortcomings left in our book inspite of the great care taken by us and the editorial team of publishers. I shall appreciate constructive criticism and suggestions to improve the textbook further in its future editions.

Pavan Kumar G
Ilona Gracie De Souza

Acknowledgments

Textbook of Biomechanics and Kinesiology is the brainchild of a conversation between two professional researchers thinking back to the struggles of their younger selves and looking forward to helping generations of young men still to come. It took an immense amount of work and it would not exist without the invaluable contributions of a number of incredibly thoughtful and supportive people.

We would like to take this opportunity to thank Dr GR Chandrashekar, Honorable Chairman of Cauvery Group of Institutions and Dr Sarala Chandrashekar, Managing Director of Cauvery Group of Institutions, Mysuru, Karnataka, India, for their constant encouragement and support. We would also like to express my gratitude to the Dean of Cauvery Group of Institutions for his kind cooperation and encouragement.

We are highly grateful to our parents for their constant love and support. Last but not the least, we thank all the faculty members, librarians and non-teaching staff for their time to time help in writing this textbook.

We are also thankful to the whole team of M/s Jaypee Brothers Medical Publishers (P) Ltd, New Delhi, India, who helped and guided us, Shri Jitendar P Vij (Group Chairman), Mr Ankit Vij (Managing Director), Mr MS Mani (Group President), Dr Madhu Choudhary (Publishing Head–Education), Ms Pooja Bhandari (Production Head), Ms Sunita Katla (Executive Assistant to Group Chairman and Publishing Manager), Ms Samina Khan (Executive Assistant to Publishing Head–Education), Dr Sneha Kashyap and Dr Aditya Tayal (Development Editors), Mr Rajesh Sharma (Production Coordinator), Ms Seema Dogra (Cover Visualizer), Ms Geeta Barik (Proofreader), Mr Akshay Thakur (Typesetter), Mr Ratan Lal (Graphic Designer) and their team members, for bringing out the first edition of this textbook. Without their cooperation, we could not have completed this project.

Contents

Section 1: Fundamentals — 1

1. **Basic Physics with Biomechanical Perspective** — 3
   - Force 3
   - Force Systems 5
   - Force Couple 7
   - Composition of Forces 8
   - Resolution of Forces 9
   - Human Motion 10
   - Angular Motion 12
   - Newton's Law of Motion 12
   - Torque (Moment of Force or Moment) 13
   - Practical Application of Torque 14
   - Friction 14
   - Gravity 15
   - Equilibrium 18
   - Work, Energy, and Power 19
   - Energy 19
   - Power 20
   - Springs 20
   - Levers 21
   - Levers in Human Body 22
   - Elasticity 23
   - Pulleys 27
   - The Patella as an Anatomic Pulley 27

2. **Joint Structure and Function** — 29
   - Classification of Joints 29
   - Joint Motion 33
   - Concave Convex Rule 33
   - Joint Stability 34
   - Effect of Disease on the Joints 36
   - Effects of Injury on the Joints 37
   - Effects of Immobilization on the Joints (Stress Deprivation) 37
   - Effects of Exercise 37

3. **Connective Tissue Structure and Function** — 39
   - Collagen 40
   - Specific Connective Tissue Structures 40
   - General Properties of Connective Tissue 45

4. **Muscle Structure and Function** — 48
   - Types of Muscles 48
   - Structure and Function of Skeletal Muscle 49
   - Generation of Cross-bridge Interaction 52
   - Skeletal Muscle and Exercise 52
   - Muscle Function 57
   - Classification of Muscle 58
   - Effect of Immobilization, Injury, and Aging 60

Section 2: Joint Segments in Detail — 63

5. **Temporomandibular Joint** — 65
   - Osteology 65
   - Arthrology 66
   - Stabilization 67
   - Capsule and Ligaments 68
   - Osteokinematics and Arthrokinematics 70
   - Arthrokinematics 72
   - Kinetics 72
   - Pathomechanics/TMJ Disorders 73

6. **Shoulder Joint** — 75
   - Joints at the Shoulder Complex 75
   - Stabilization 76

- Kinematics 79
- Kinetics 80
- Pathomechanics 82
- Scapulothoracic Joint 83
- Acromioclavicular Joint 85
- Sternoclavicular Joint 88

7. **Elbow Complex** 91
   - Humeroulnar Joint and Humeroradial Joint (True Elbow Joint) 91
   - Kinematics 93
   - Kinetics 94
   - Superior Radioulnar Joint 94
   - Kinematics 95
   - Kinetics 96
   - Special Feature of Elbow 96
   - Pathomechanics 96

8. **Wrist and Hand Complex** 98
   - The Wrist Complex 98
   - Osteology 99
   - Arthrology 99
   - Joints of Wrist 99
   - Wrist Ligaments 102
   - Kinematics of Wrist 104
   - Kinetics 106
   - Pathomechanics 108
   - The Hand Complex 110
   - Arches of Hand 110
   - Joints of the Hand 112
   - Kinematics and Kinetics 113
   - Prehension 118

9. **Hip Joint** 121
   - Hip Segment and the Parts 121
   - Stability 122
   - Kinematics 124
   - Pathomechanics 130
   - Angles in the Hip Segment 130
   - Hip Joint Forces and Muscle Function in Stance 133

10. **Knee Joint** 136
    - Structure of Tibiofemoral Joint 136
    - Menisci 138
    - Joint Capsule 139
    - Ligaments 140
    - Tibiofemoral Joint Function 143
    - Role of Cruciate Ligaments and Menisci in Flexion and Extension 146
    - Muscles 148
    - Patellofemoral Joint 151

11. **Ankle and Foot Complex** 154
    - Joint Structure of Ankle and Foot Complex 154
    - Forces in the Ankle Joint Complex 157
    - Pronation and Supination Twist 158
    - Metatarsophalangeal Joint 159
    - The Metatarsal Break 159
    - Interphalangeal Joint 160
    - Plantar Fascia 160
    - Arches of Foot 160

12. **Vertebral Column** 163

    Cervical Spine 165
    - Parts 165
    - Structure 165
    - Joints 166
    - Kinetics 167

    Thorax and Chest Wall 167
    - General Structure and Function 167
    - Ribs 170
    - Articulations of the Rib Cage 171
    - Kinematics of Rib Cage and Manubriosternum 173
    - Muscles Associated with Rib Cage 173
    - Developmental Aspects of Structure and Function 176

    Lumbar Segment 176
    - Types of Vertebra and its Structure 176
    - The Joints in the Lumbar Segment 178
    - Stability of the Lumbar Spine 179
    - Kinematics 181
    - Arthrokinematics 183
    - Kinetics 184
    - Lumbopelvic Rhythm 184
    - Thoracolumbar Fascia 186
    - Lumbosacral Joint 187

- Pathomechanics *187*
- Muscles of Trunk Region *189*

Sacroiliac Joint **189**
- Stability *190*
- Joint Structure *190*
- Kinematics *191*
- Kinetics *192*
- Pathomechanics *192*
- Symphysis Pubis *192*
- Sacrococcygeal Joint *193*

Section 3: Analytical Biomechanics 195

13. **Posture** 197
    - Definition *197*
    - Static and Dynamic Posture *197*
    - Active Posture *199*
    - Inactive Posture *199*
    - Postural Control *200*
    - Muscle Synergies *201*
    - Kinetics and Kinematics of Posture *202*
    - Optimal Posture *203*
    - Analysis of Sitting Postures *213*
    - Different Technique/Instruments Used for Measurement of Posture *216*
    - Appropriate Clothing *217*
    - Evaluation of Posture *217*
    - Pathomechanics/Faulty Posture *218*
    - Musculoskeletal Changes During Pregnancy *220*

14. **Gait** 224
    - Stance Phase *225*
    - Swing Phase *226*
    - Parameters that Describe Gait Patterns *227*
    - Determinants of Gait Cycle During Ambulation *229*
    - Kinematics of Gait *231*
    - Kinetics of Gait *231*
    - Gait Analysis in Relation to Hip Joint *232*
    - Pathological Gait *234*
    - Treadmill Gait *236*
    - Stair Climbing Gait *236*
    - Gait Laboratory *237*
    - Gait Analysis Systems *238*

15. **Movement Analysis in Activities of Daily Living** 243
    - Squatting *243*
    - Movement Analysis of Lifting *247*
    - Movement Analysis of Sit-to-stand *249*
    - Sitting *253*
    - Movement Analysis of Breathing *260*

16. **Movement Analysis in Sporting Activities** 263
    - Throwing and Striking *263*
    - Jumping *266*
    - Biomechanics of Running *266*
    - Jogging *271*
    - Kabaddi *271*
    - Biomechanical Analysis of Gymnastics *273*
    - Kicking *276*
    - Push Ups *277*
    - Pull Ups *277*
    - Swimming *278*
    - Cycling *278*
    - Wicket Keeping *280*
    - Biomechanics in Dance *280*

17. **Goniometry** 283
    - Definition *283*
    - Principles of Goniometry *283*
    - Types *284*
    - Measuring of ROM in Upper Extremity *287*
    - Measuring of ROM in Lower Extremity *292*

18. **Walking Aids** 298
    - Indications *298*
    - Classification of Walking Aids *298*
    - Canes *301*
    - Walker *302*

19. **Orthotics and Prosthetics** 304
    - General Classification *304*
    - Common Internal Fixators *305*
    - Biomechanical Principle of Orthosis *305*
    - Spinal Orthosis *305*
    - Upper Extremity Orthosis (Splint) *307*
    - Lower Extremity Orthosis *307*
20. **Ergonomics** 310
    - Ergonomics of Desk Job *310*
    - Prevention *311*
    - Ergonomic Chair *312*
    - Precautions While Sitting *313*
    - Ergonomics of Sitting *314*
    - Ergonomics of Driving *314*
    - Ergonomics of Standing Job *315*
    - Ergonomics of Lying Down/Sleeping *315*
21. **Starting and Derived Positions for Exercise** 316
    - Standing *316*
    - Kneeling *321*
    - Sitting *322*
    - Lying *324*
    - Hanging *325*

Index 329

Introduction to Biomechanics and Kinesiology

WHAT IS BIOMECHANICS?

It is defined as a branch of science that deals with the structure and mechanical function of biological system. It involves analysis of forces and its effects in the human body leading to its clinical implications.

It is also defined as mechanics applied to human body.

MECHANICS

It is a branch of physics that deals with the study of force and effects, which is also defined as interrelation of force matter and motion. Mechanics is of two types:
1. Statics
2. Dynamics

Statics	Dynamics
• It is a branch of mechanics that deals with object in its state of rest or in equilibrium	• It is a branch of mechanics that deals with the object in state of acceleration or in motion
• Sum of all forces acting on the object is equal to zero	• Dynamics is of two types: 1. Kinematics 2. Kinetics
For example, a person standing or sitting	For example, a person running or walking

APPLICATIONS OF BIOMECHANICS

Biomechanics is incorporated into various forms of therapy, such as physical therapy, occupational therapy, medicine, namely—orthopedics, forensic medicine, sports medicine, rehabilitation medicine, and occupational medicine. Application of biomechanics in industrial setup (ergonomics) and bioengineering has led to early detection and early intervention in the industry. Kinesiology is termed as movement science.

KINESIOLOGY

Kinesiology is originated from the Greek word "kinesis" meaning to move and "ology" is to study. However, it can be defined in a broader sense as the in-depth study of human motion. It focuses on anatomic and biomechanical interactions within the musculoskeletal system.

Basic Terminologies

Anatomical position: It is the basic and fundamental position of the body.
Components of anatomical position include:
- Body in erect position
- Head and face directing forward
- Spine erect
- Shoulders at same level

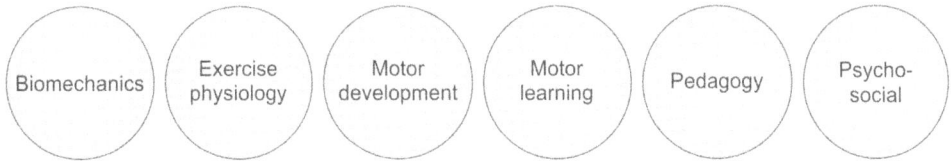

Kinesiology

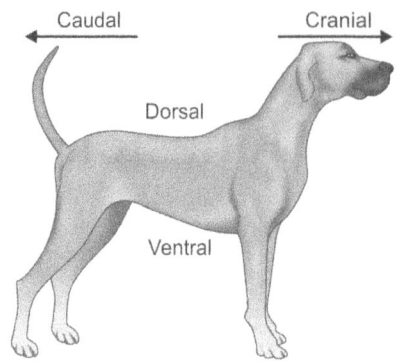

Basic terminologies

- Arms at the side and parallel to the trunk
- Anterior superior iliac spine (ASIS) are at same level
- Palms facing forward
- Legs together
- Knees straight and parallel to each other
- Feet flat and directed forward

Related to directions:
- **Anterior/ventral:** Forward
- **Posterior/dorsal:** Backward
- **Medial:** Toward midline
- **Lateral:** Away from midline
- **Superior or cranial:** Toward the head
- **Inferior or caudal:** Away from the head
- **Proximal:** Toward the trunk
- **Distal:** Away from trunk

- **Ipsilateral:** On same side
- **Contralateral:** On opposite side
- **Axial:** At or toward axis of the body (includes head, neck, and trunk)
- **Appendicular:** Away from axis of the body (includes the limb)
- **Plantar:** Bottom side of the foot
- **Dorsal:** Upper side of the foot

Related to movements:
- **Flexion:** Angle between two segments decreases
- **Extension:** Angle between two segments increases
- **Abduction:** Movement away from the midline
- **Adduction:** Movement toward the midline
- **Medial/internal rotation:** Joint rotation in a medial direction
- **Lateral/external rotation:** Joint rotation laterally
- **Circumduction:** Circular motion produced combining all movements.
- **Hyperextension:** Increase in angle beyond normal range
- **Dorsiflexion:** Pointing toes upward.
- **Plantar flexion:** Pointing toes downward.
- **Elevation:** Moving superiorly
- **Depression:** Moving inferiorly
- **Inversion:** Movement of the foot with the sole facing medially

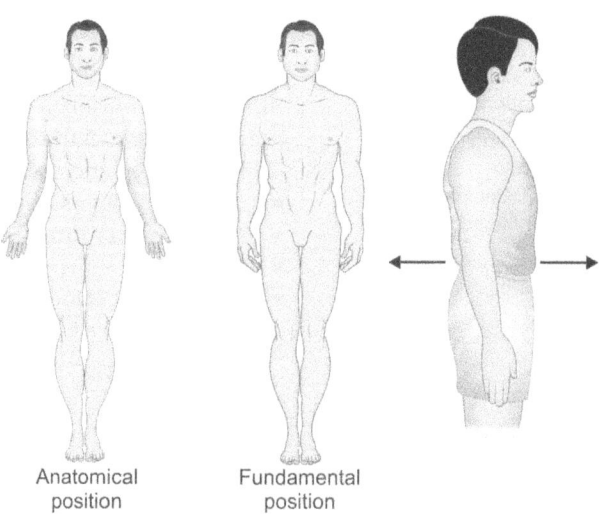

Anatomical position

Introduction to Biomechanics and Kinesiology

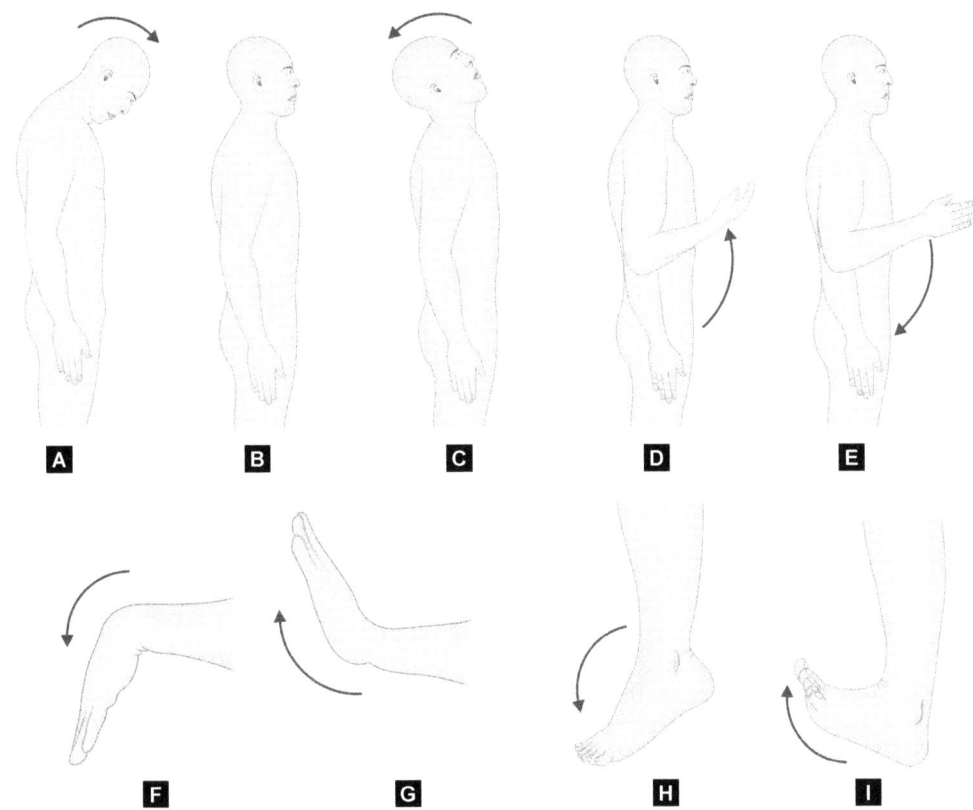

Examples of basic terminologies. (A) Cervical flexion; (B) Neutral cervical spine; (C) Cervical extension; (D) Elbow flexion; (E) Elbow extension; (F) Wrist flexion; (G) Wrist extension; (H) Ankle plantar flexion; (I) Ankle dorsiflexion

- **Eversion:** Movement of the foot with the sole facing laterally
- **Radial deviation:** Moving toward radial styloid process
- **Ulnar deviation:** Moving toward ulnar styloid process
- **Pronation:** Rotation of palm downward
- **Supination:** Rotation of palm upward

AXIS AND PLANES

Planes

It is a flat surface along which movement takes place. It is always perpendicular to the axis.

The human body is divided into three imaginary planes, namely:

1. **Sagittal plane/anterior posterior plane:** Vertical plane that partition the human body into *right* and *left*.
2. **Frontal plane/coronal plane:** Vertical plane that partition the human body into *anterior* and *posterior* parts.
3. **Transverse plane/horizontal plane:** Body is divided into *cranial* and *caudal* parts.

Axis

A straight line that passes perpendicular through a plane is termed as "axis." Movements occur around this axis. The three axes of motion are:

1. **Sagittal axis:** It is a horizontal axis that runs from anterior to posterior.
2. **Frontal axis:** It is a horizontal axis passing from right to left.
3. **Vertical axis:** It is a vertical axis from superiorly to inferiorly.

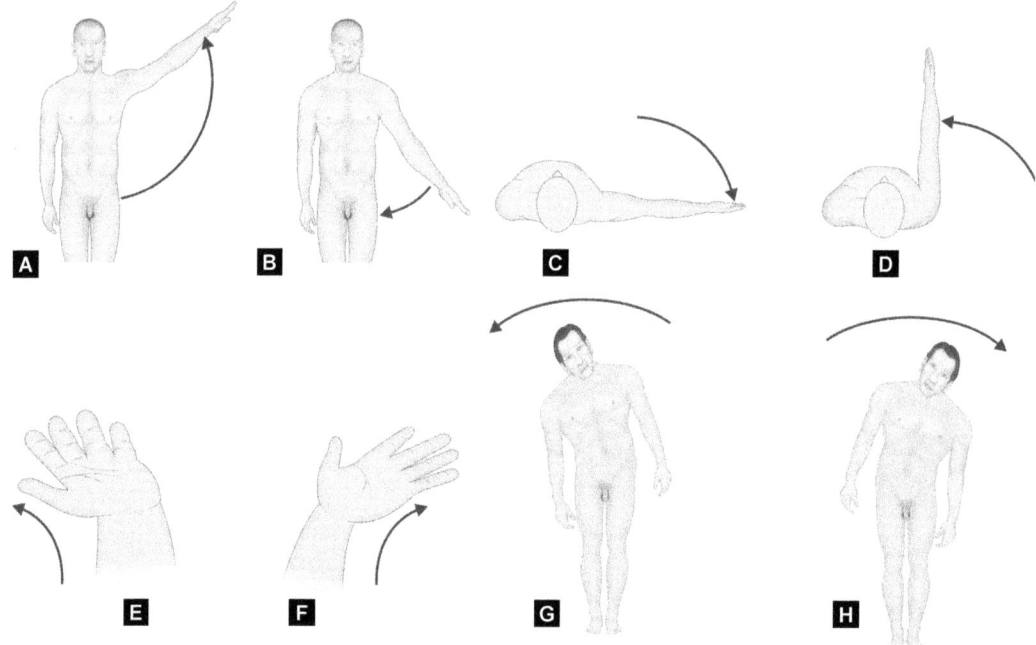

Examples of basic terminologies. (A) Shoulder abduction; (B) Shoulder adduction; (C) Shoulder horizontal abduction; (D) Shoulder horizontal adduction; (E) Wrist radial deviation; (F) Wrist ulnar deviation; (G) Trunk right lateral flexion; (H) Trunk left lateral flexion

Plane movements:

Plane	Motion	Axis
Sagittal	Flexion/extension	Frontal
Frontal	• Abduction/adduction • Side flexion • Inversion/eversion	Sagittal
Transverse	• Internal rotation/external rotation • Horizontal abduction/adduction • Supination/pronation	Vertical

KINEMATICS

It is the branch of mechanics that explains motion of the human body without reference to forces. For example:
- Shoulder flexion range of motion is "X" degrees.
- Hip flexion happens in sagittal plane.
- Elbow extension happens around frontal axis.

There are two types of motion.
1. **Osteokinematics:** Osteokinematics is the study of the movement of the bony segment which is visible. For example:
   - Elbow joint flexion: 120°
   - Shoulder abduction: 180°
2. **Arthrokinematics:** This refers to the movement at the joint surface, where one surface remains intact and the other surface moves over it.
   Fundamental movement: Joint surfaces
   - *Roll*
     ◆ Throughout the motion, multiple points maintain contact.
     ◆ Here one surface rolls over another surface.
     ◆ Mechanical, e.g., when a tire rolls over the road.
     ◆ Anatomical, e.g., during knee flexion and extension
   - *Slide:* In this, the contact point of one surface slides over the successive contact points of the other contact surface.

Introduction to Biomechanics and Kinesiology

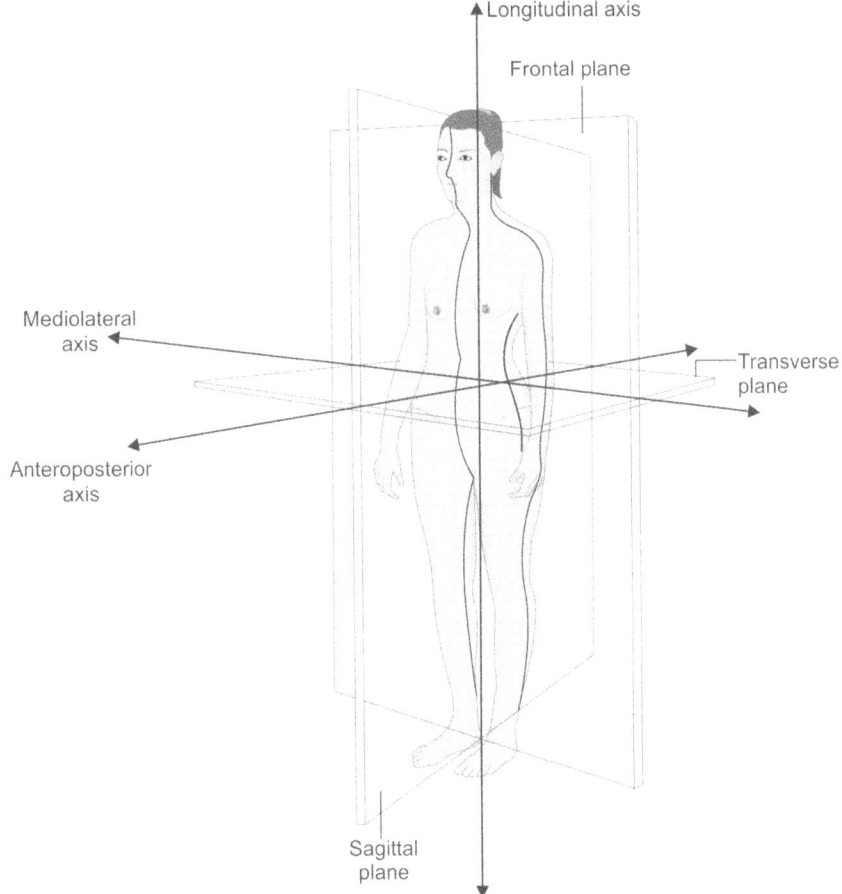

Anatomical planes and axis

- Here one surface rolls over another surface.
- It is also called as linear or translatory motion.
- *Spin:* In this, the contact point of one surface rotates over a contact point of the other surface.

KINETIC CHAIN CONCEPT

Kinetic link model is a biomechanical model that is helpful in analyzing sport activities. Human body is linked wherein the segments are interdependent and work in a proximal to distal fashion. Model highlights the contribution of entire body rather than focusing on individual segments. Muscle activation is believed to occur in a proximal-to-distal sequence in order to elicit efficient normal motion. This proximal-to-distal sequencing should be kept in mind when attempting to restore function via a rehabilitation protocol.

- The joints which are in series in the human body are not independent but are interlinked to each other. This forms a chain like system called as kinetic chain where one bony segment affects the other.
- The extremity can either be in open kinetic chain (OKC) or closed kinetic chain (CKC) depending on which end of the kinetic chain is free. If the distal end is free and proximal end is fixed it is called as OKC and vice versa for CKC. OKC allows movement of the distal joint without causing movement to the adjacent joints. Core stabilization and proximal

stabilization are important for eliciting motion in distal segments. Examples of upper extremity in open chain are shoulder shrug and biceps curls. Example of lower extremity in OKC is a person walking. Performing exercises in open kinetic chains helps to focus on individual muscle groups and on a particular joint.
- An extremity is said to be in a closed kinetic chain when the distal segment is fixed and the proximal segment is moving. Movement of one segment would produce substantial movement of adjacent segments. While performing activities in closed kinematic chain example push-ups, dip, squat or dead lift, leads to multiple joint activity and involves use of numerous muscle groups simultaneously.
- When incorporating conditioning exercises, open versus closed kinetic chain exercises should be taken into consideration.

1. **Identify the bones and joints:**

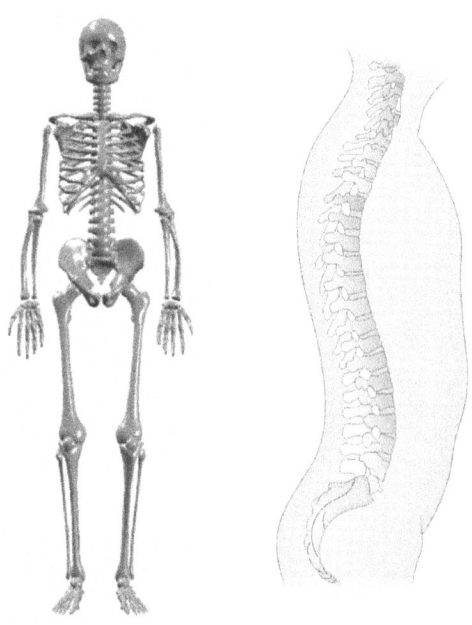

SECTION 1

Fundamentals

Section Outline

- Basic Physics with Biomechanical Perspective
- Joint Structure and Function
- Connective Tissue Structure and Function
- Muscle Structure and Function

CHAPTER 1

Basic Physics with Biomechanical Perspective

Chapter Outline

- Force: Classification, measurement, types
- Force systems
- Force couple
- Composition of forces
- Human motion: Types of motion
- Newton's law of motion
- Torque
- Friction
- Gravity
- Line of gravity
- Base of support
- Center of gravity
- Equilibrium
- Work, energy, power
- Springs
- Levers
- Elasticity-stress, strain

INTRODUCTION

This chapter is concerned with application of physical principles and methods to the human body. The concepts of force, motion, gravity, work, energy, power, and elasticity are overviewed. This chapter is useful in understanding the physical processes in human body.

FORCE

Force is that agent, which when applied to a body changes or tends to change the state of rest or uniform motion of the body.

Force is the push or pull of body that causes motion.

Force can be explained on the basis of the following terminologies:

- **Magnitude:** It defines the amount of force applied to a body.
  For example, 40 pounds, 60 pounds, etc.
- **Direction:** Direction is the way in which the force is applied to a body.
  It is either perpendicular or inclined to the surface.
  For example, toward east, west, north or south.
- **Point of application:** It is the exact location at which the force is applied to a body.
- **Line of action of force:** It is the imaginary line that extends from the point of application along with the point of deviation.
- **Representation of force:**
  - A force is represented by an arrow of specific length.
  - An arrow indicates direction.
  - Length of arrow indicates magnitude.
  - Tail of arrow indicates point of application.

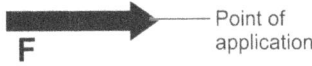

Classification of Force

Generally, a force can be classified as:

- **Based on contact:**
  - *Contact force:* Contact forces are the forces that are produced via, contact either by pushing or pulling of a body. For example, pushing a desk across, kicking a ball, etc.
  - *Noncontact force:* Noncontact forces are those produced without contact of a body.
    For example, attraction and repulsion of electrically charged particles.
- **Based on production:**
  - *External force:* External forces are those which exert a push or pull on a body and are produced outside the body.
    - Types:
      - Gravitational
      - GRF
      - Frictional
      - Impedance
  - *Internal force:* Internal forces are produced inside the body.
    For example, contraction of muscle produces tension which acts on the point of attachment and causes movement of bone at joint surfaces.

Measurement of Force

Forces can be measured using various units:
- **MKS system:**
  - The unit of meter kilogram second system is newton.
  - One newton is defined as the force applied to a body of mass 1 kg, produces an acceleration of 1 m/sec².
- **CKS system:**
  - The unit of centimeter second kilogram system is dyne.
  - One dyne is defined as force applied to a body of mass 1 g produces an acceleration of 1 cm/sec².
- **FPS system:**
  - The unit of foot pound second system is pound (lb).
  - One lb is defined as force applied to a body of mass 1 pound, produces an acceleration of 1 ft/sec².

Types of Forces

- **Tensile force (Fig. 1.1A):** Tensile force is an external force acting on a body causing elongation of the body. The line of action of forces is always opposite to each other. Mechanical, e.g., when a child sits on a swing, tension force acts along the chains of the swing. Anatomical, e.g., when capsule of a joint is stretched, tension force acts along the joint surfaces.
- **Compressive force (Fig. 1.1B):** Compression force is an external force acting on a body causing shortening of the body. Line of action of force is always toward each other. Compression forces are always opposite to tensile forces. Mechanical, e.g., compression of a sponge occurs, when a stone is placed on a sponge. Anatomical, e.g., in standing position, compression force act on hip, knee, and ankle joint. When both palms are placed together, compression force acts on both the palms.
- **Bending force (Fig. 1.2):** Bending force is an external force acting on a body causing the body to bend. Mechanical, e.g., when a pipe is subjected to bending forces, it causes curving of the pipe. Anatomical, e.g., during forward bending of trunk, tension force develops on the posterior side, while compression force develops on the anterior side. Bending occurs because of the three points force system acting on the object or four points force system acting on the object.
- **Shear force (Figs. 1.3A and B):** Shear force is an external force acting on a body, causing the body to slide over the surface on which it is placed. Mechanical, e.g., using a scissor for cutting paper, the two handles put force in different directions on the pin that holds the two parts together. The force applied to the pin is called shear force.

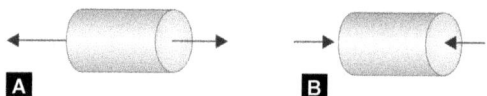

Figs. 1.1A and B: (A) Tensile stress; (B) Compressive stress

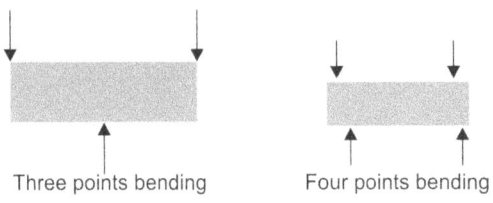

Fig. 1.2: Bending force

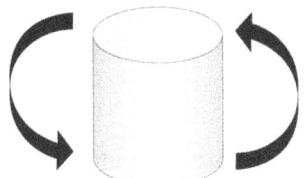

Fig. 1.5: Torsional force

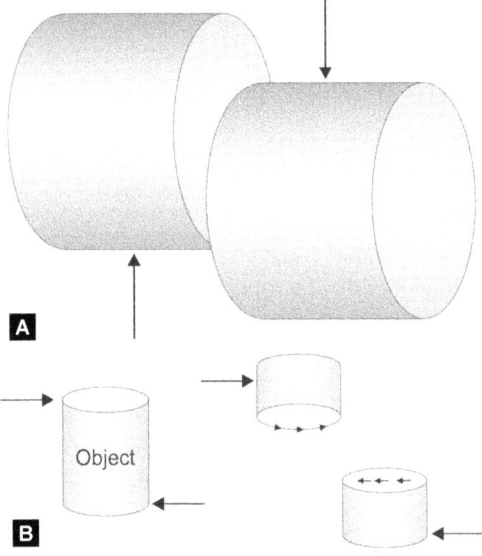

Fig. 1.3A and B: Shear force

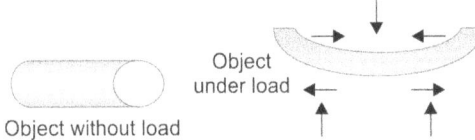

Fig. 1.4: Depicts combination of compressive and tensile forces that results in bending forces

Anatomical, e.g., when person sits from standing position, the femoral condyles slide over the tibial plateaus.

Figure 1.4 depicts combination of compressive and tensile forces that results in bending forces.

- **Torsion force (Fig. 1.5):** Torsion force is an external force acting on a body, causing the body to twist along its long axis. Mechanical, e.g., whenever we turn a key in a lock, the handle of the key is in torsion—when opening a lid of the bottle. Anatomical, e.g., during pronation and supination of forearm, torsion force is developed by pronators and supinators.

FORCE SYSTEMS

A force system is defined as summation of all the forces influencing a particular body.
There are four types of force systems:
1. Coplanar force system
2. Colinear force system
3. Concurrent force system
4. Parallel force system

Coplanar Force System

In coplanar force system, all forces act in the same plane either in the same or opposite direction.

Mechanical, e.g., coplanar force system can be applied to a lever which has a fixed axis along its length (**Fig. 1.6**).

- If two forces of equal magnitude act on lever, the lever is maintained in a state of equilibrium.

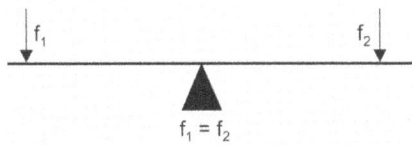

Fig 1.6: Coplanar force system

- If two unequal forces act on lever, the lever moves with respect to the greater force in downward direction while the lighter forces move upward, e.g., see-saw.

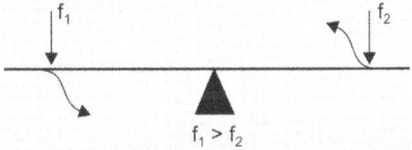

- Anatomical/clinical, e.g., when right and left rectus abdominis muscle contract together, they cause forward flexion of the trunk.

Example: Pushing a wheelchair
- If two forces of equal magnitude act on a wheelchair, the resultant force will be in linear direction along with movement of wheelchair.

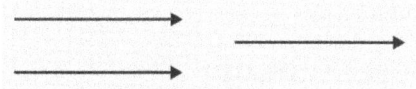

- If one force is greater than another, the resultant force moves away from the greater force (unequal force causes rotational movements).

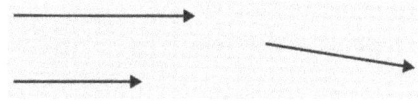

Colinear Force System

It is a specialized form of force system where forces act in the same line along the same plane.
- When greater number of colinear forces act on a body in same direction a pulling or pushing effect is seen.

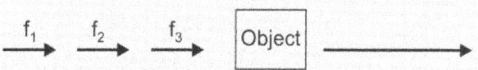

- When colinear forces act toward each other, the body undergoes compression.

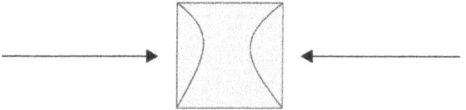

- When colinear forces act away from each other, the body undergoes distraction and tension.

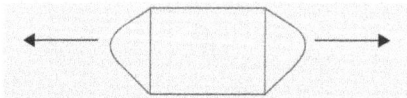

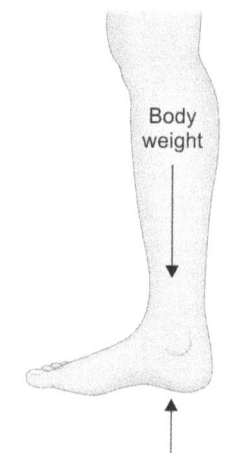

Fig. 1.7: Ground reaction force

Mechanical, e.g., two people standing at the opposite ends of a rope and pulling it.
Anatomical, e.g.,
- In standing position, the joint usually undergoes tension and compression.
  Here, the body weight forms the downward force while the ground reaction force signifies the upward force (**Fig. 1.7**).
- In upper extremity, tension force acts on the shoulder joint.
  Here, the weight of the upper extremity forms the downward force while the muscles of scapula form the upward force.
  Any imbalance in these forces causes dislocation of shoulder joint.

Concurrent Force System

In the concurrent force system (**Fig. 1.8**), the force acting have same point of application but different line of action.
- Mechanical, e.g., a box pulled by two people at the level of center of gravity (COG).

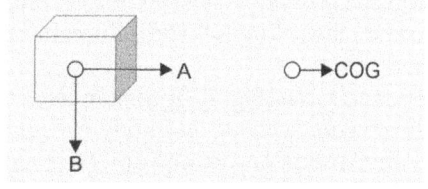

- Anatomical, e.g., action of deltoid muscle at shoulder joint. Deltoid muscle consists

Chapter 1 | Basic Physics with Biomechanical Perspective

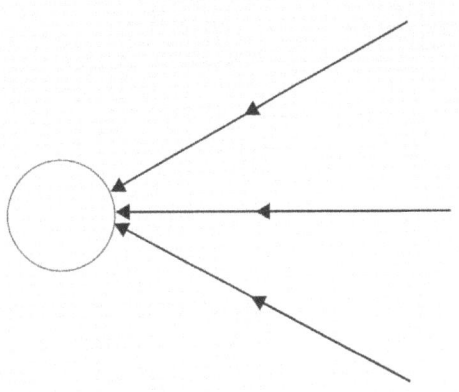

Fig. 1.8: Concurrent force system

of three fibers, i.e., anterior, middle, and posterior fibers. Anterior fiber causes flexion, middle fiber causes abduction, and posterior fiber causes extension at the shoulder joint, respectively. However, when the anterior and posterior fiber contract together, they causes abduction of the shoulder. Their common point of application is at the deltoid tuberosity **(Fig. 1.9)**.

- Another example of concurrent force system is the action of the quadriceps at the knee joint. Quadriceps is made up of rectus femoris, vastus medialis, vastus intermedius, and vastus lateralis meeting at the common point on the patella **(Fig. 1.10)**.

Parallel Force System

In parallel force system, the line of action of the forces is always parallel to each other and lies in the same plane. They never converge at a joint.

- A parallel force system exists when two or more forces act at some distance from each other.

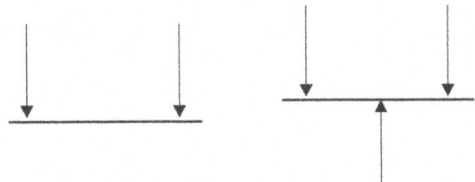

- Mechanical, e.g., common balance, see-saw.
- Anatomical, e.g., coordinated action of tibialis anterior and gastrocnemius **(Fig. 1.11)**.

FORCE COUPLE

A specialized example of parallel force system occurs when two forces of equal magnitude act at a distance in opposite direction producing a force couple.

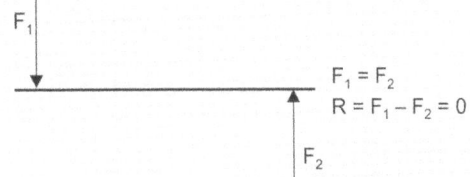

$F_1 = F_2$
$R = F_1 - F_2 = 0$

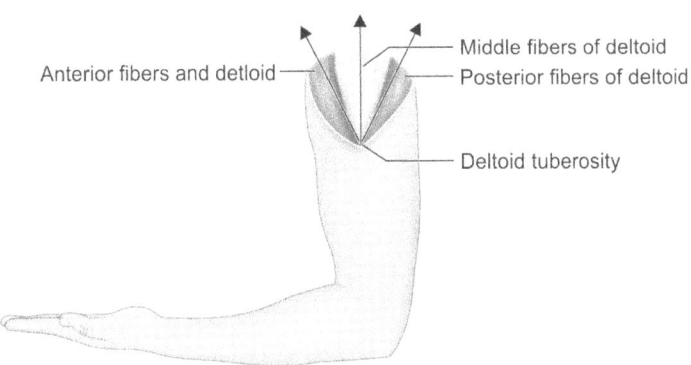

Fig. 1.9: Concurrent force system in upper extremity

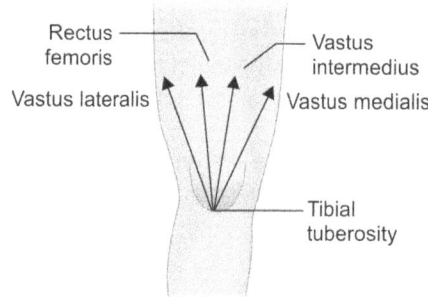

Fig. 1.10: Concurrent force system in right leg

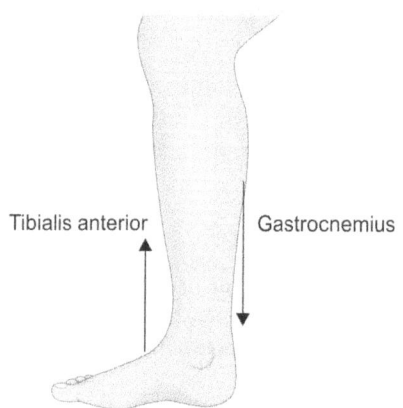

Fig. 1.11: Parallel force system

As the forces are equal and opposite, the body turns without linear displacement or oscillation.

- $F_R = 0$ but

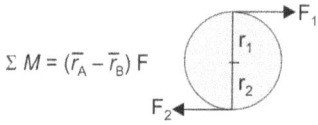

$\Sigma M = (\bar{r}_A - \bar{r}_B) F$

- Mechanical, e.g., closing or opening a water tap, steering a wheel.
- While steering toward right side, a downward force is produced by the right hand. At the same time, an upward force is produced by the left hand. The resultant force produced is zero but the wheel turns around its axis.
- Anatomical, e.g., during shoulder abduction, force couple causes lateral

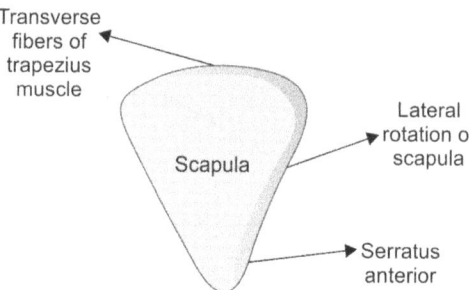

Fig. 1.12: Anatomical example of force couple

rotation of the scapula (**Fig. 1.12**).

COMPOSITION OF FORCES

- It is a process of combining all the given forces to calculate a resultant force.
- If the resultant force calculated is zero, then the body is said to be in a state of equilibrium.
- When the forces acting on a body are in the same direction, the resultant force is calculated by adding all the given forces.

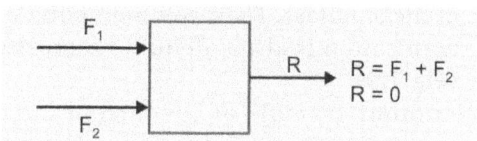

- When the forces acting on a body are in opposite direction, the resultant force is calculated by subtraction of one force from another.

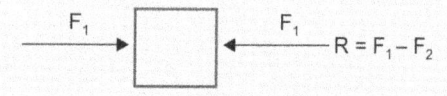

 - Practically, as forces are multidirectional, it cannot be calculated by methods of simple addition or subtraction.
 - In such cases, resultant force is calculated using graphical methods.
 - Following graphical methods are used:
- **Triangle method:** The triangle method states that *"If two forces act on two sides of a triangle, then the resultant force is represented by third side of the triangle taken in opposite order."*

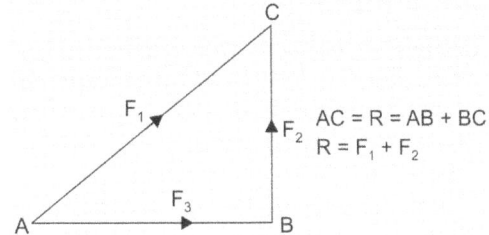

- **Parallelogram method:**
  - It states that *"If two forces are represented by adjacent sides of a parallelogram, then the resultant force is represented by the diagonal of the parallelogram drawn from the same point."*

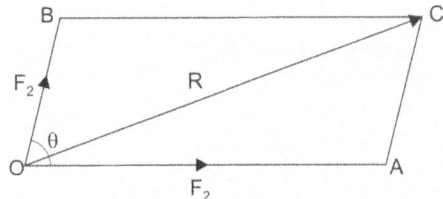

$$R = \sqrt{f1^2 + f2^2 + 2f1.f2\cos\theta}$$

  - Mechanical, e.g., when a wooden box is pulled from both the sides, the box moves in the direction of the diagonal of the parallelogram (resultant force).

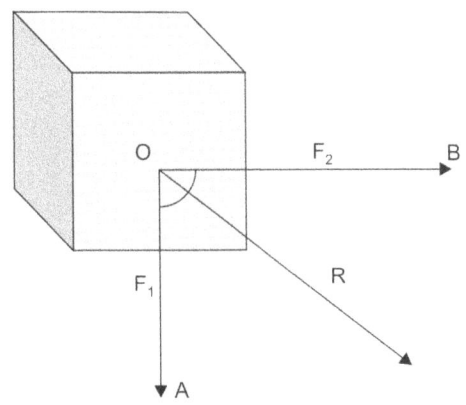

- **Anatomical:** The action of right upper trapezius and left upper trapezius, acting together will result in the resultant force of neck extension **(Fig. 1.13)**.
- **Polygon method:** This method is used when more than two forces act on a body.

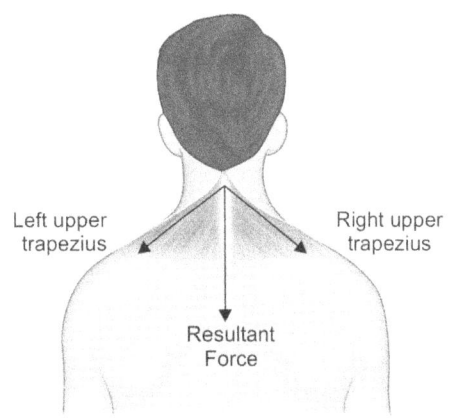

Fig. 1.13: Composition of force of upper trapezius

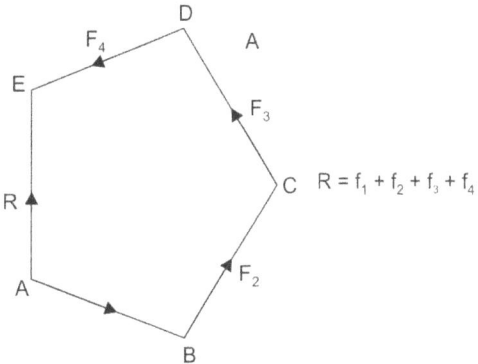

RESOLUTION OF FORCES

Forces Acting on Human Body

It is a process by which a single force or a resultant force is replaced by two perpendicular components.

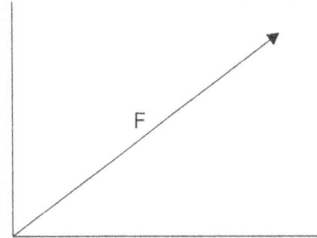

The two components are:
1. **Vertical component:** Vertical component is also called as rotatory component. It causes rotation and is always perpendicular to the bone.

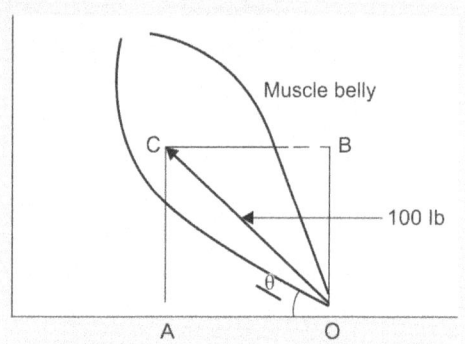

Fig. 1.14: Resolution of forces into its components

2. **Horizontal component:** Horizontal component is also called as stabilizing component. It causes either tension or compression and acts along the long axis of the bone.

For example, a muscle is pulling a bone with magnitude of 100 lb (pound) and at an angle of 60° to the long axis of the bone. Find out the value for vertical and horizontal component.

$$OC = 100 \text{ lb}$$
$$OC = R$$
OB - Vertical component
OA - Horizontal component
Angle or $\theta = 60°$

$$\sin 60° = \frac{AC}{OC} = \frac{OB}{100 lb}$$

$$= \frac{\sqrt{3}}{2} = \frac{OB}{100 lb}$$

$$OB = 50\sqrt{3} \text{ lb}$$

$$\cos 60° = \frac{OA}{OC} = \frac{OA}{100 lb}$$

$$\frac{1}{2} = \frac{OA}{100 lb}$$

$$OA = 50 \text{ lb}$$

HUMAN MOTION

Motion

Motion is an action of an object with respect to a reference point.

Types of Motion

Classification based on path of motion

- **Translatory motion (linear motion, translation):** A motion in which all parts of the moving body move toward the same direction.
  Here, the body moves in one direction or follows a linear path.
  For example,
  - Walking on a straight bar
  - Elevation, depression, protraction, and retraction of scapula
  - Pushing or pulling of bone at joint surfaces
- **Linear (or rectilinear) motion:** A motion in which all parts of a moving body move in the same direction and the path follows a straight line.

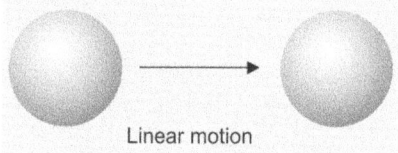
Linear motion

- **Curvilinear motion:** A motion in which the net motion of a moving body move toward the same direction although the path follows a curved line, e.g., the path of the center of mass of the body during level walking.

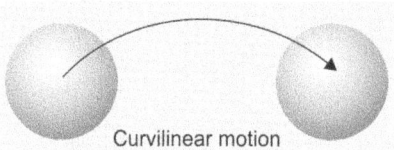
Curvilinear motion

  - Curvilinear motion is the combination of linear and circular motions. For example,
  - Curvilinear motion is commonly found in almost all joints.
- **Circular motion:** When a body moves in a circular path around a fixed point, the body is in angular motion. For example,
  - Movement of fan
  - The movement of major joints in upper and lower extremity (hip, knee, ankle, elbow, wrist joints).

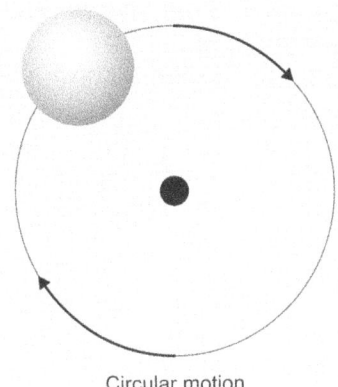
Circular motion

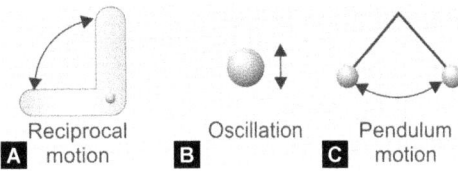

Figs. 1.16A to C: Human motion classification based on repetition of motion. (A) Reciprocal motion; (B) Oscillation; (C) Pendulum motion

- **Rotary motion (angular motion, rotation):** A motion in which the object acts as a radius and all parts of the moving object rotate in the same angular direction and follow a circular path about a pivot point.
- **Angular motion:** The rotary motion with one side of the moving object fixed, e.g., rotation of a limb.
- **Spin:** The rotary motion with the axis of rotation around the center of mass.

Figure 1.15 shows difference between angular motion and spin.

Classification based on repetition of motion
- **Single motion:** Movement performed only once
- **Reciprocal motion:** Same movement pattern that is done many times in a given time reciprocal motion **(Fig. 1.16A)**.
- **Oscillation:** Repeated motions in a small amplitude **(Fig. 1.16B)**.
- **Pendulum motion:** Repeated motions like a pendulum **(Fig. 1.16C)**.

Classification based on degree of freedom
Degree of freedom (DOF): A minimum number of kinematic variables required to specified all positions and orientations of the segments in a body system, i.e.,
- The number of planes in which the segments move
- The number of the primary axes which the segments possess, e.g.,
  - The joint that moves in one plane possesses one axis and has one degree of freedom.
  - For the glenohumeral joint, there are three angular degrees of freedom and three linear degrees of freedom.

Classification based on relative segment kinematics
Kinematic chain: A series of connected segment links
- **Open kinematic chain motion (Fig. 1.17A):** The joint motion where the distal segment moves free in space, e.g., raising lower leg or throwing a ball.
- **Closed kinematic chain motion (Fig. 1.17B):** The joint motion where the distal segment is fixed, e.g., standing up or squatting down.

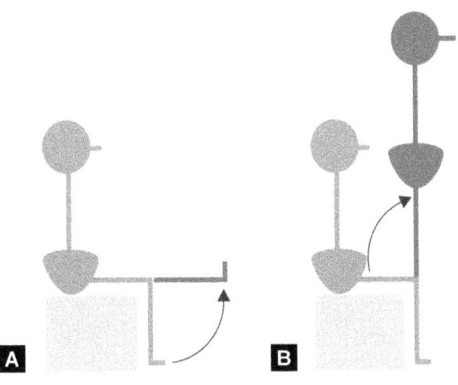

Figs. 1.17A and B: (A) Open kinematic chain; (B) Closed kinetic chain

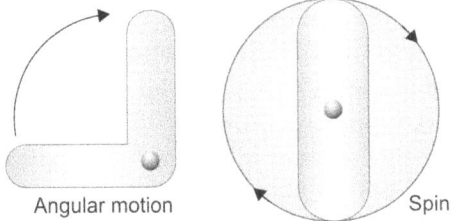

Fig. 1.15: Difference between angular motion and spin

ANGULAR MOTION

Basic Terminologies Used in Context of Motion

- **Displacement:**
  - It defines the amount of motion of a body.
  - It is denoted as "s".
  - It is measured in meters and centimeters.
- **Velocity:**
  - It is defined as rate of change of displacement.
  - It is denoted by "v".
  - It is measured in m/sec and cm/sec.
- **Acceleration:**
  - Acceleration is defined as rate of change of velocity.
  - It is denoted as "a".
  - It is measured in m/sec² and cm/sec².

NEWTON'S LAW OF MOTION

Newton's law of motion is the three physical laws describing the relationship between a body and the forces acting on it, and its motion in response to those forces.

The three laws of motion were compiled by Newton in his Mathematical Principles of Natural Philosophy and were first published in 1687.

The three laws described by Newton are as follows:

Newton's First Law

- It is also called as *"law of inertia/law of equilibrium"*.
- It states that *"Every object continues to remain in a state of rest or uniform motion unless and until it is acted upon by an unbalanced force"*.
- It can be restated as *"When an object is in equilibrium, sum of all the forces acting on it is zero"*.

And to maintain this state of equilibrium at least two forces are required.

Determination of equilibrium of a body

- Consider a patient lying on a table in equilibrium. Gravity acts on the patient in downward direction and the force exerted by the upper surface of the table is in upward direction.
- Let the magnitude of these forces be, upward force F_1 and downward force F_2, respectively.
- As the forces are in same plane, same line but in opposite direction, it forms a colinear force system.
- According to force convention, forces acting on the right and in upward direction are considered as positive and the one acting downward and in left are considered as negative.
- Resultant force is zero $(F_2 - F_1 = 0)$.
- Hence, the patient is said to be in equilibrium.

Newton's Second Law

- It is also called as law of acceleration.
- It states that *"Forces acting on a body produces acceleration which is inversely proportional to mass and directly proportional to force"*.

$$a \propto F$$
$$a \propto \frac{1}{m}$$
$$a \propto \frac{F}{m}$$
$$a = K\frac{F}{m} \quad K = 1$$
$$F = ma$$

Clinical, e.g.,

Consider two patients A and B of weight 50 and 30 kg respectively, sitting on a wheel chair.

When equal amount of force is exerted, more acceleration is produced in patient B, than in patient A.

Also as force increases, acceleration also increases.

Newton's Third Law of Motion

- It states that *"For every action, there is equal and opposite reaction."*
- In other words, when one body applies a force on another, the second body in turn applies a force which is equal in magnitude but in opposite direction of the first body.

Mechanical, e.g.,
- When both the palms are placed against each other, one palm applies acting force while the other applies the reacting force.
- In tug of war, acting and reacting force are applied on the rope.

Anatomical, e.g.,
- When a paraplegic patient is made to lie on a table, the body weight of the patient exerts an acting force in downward direction while the upper surface of the table provides a reacting force.
- In standing position body weight passes in downward direction forming the acting force while gravity provides the reacting force.

TORQUE (MOMENT OF FORCE OR MOMENT)

Torque is a force which causes rotation of a body or turning of a lever around a fixed axis.

In human body, it is seen when a bone rotates around a joint.

It is also called as rotatory effect of force.

Mathematically, it is defined as product of force and the perpendicular distance from the axis of rotation to the line of action of force. It is denoted by "τ"

∴ τ = F × perpendicular distance

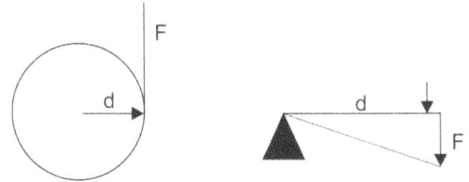

Units:
- **MKS system:** It is measured in Newton.
- **CGS system:** It is measured in Dyne.
- **FPS system:** It is measured in Pounds (lb).

Moment Arm

It is the perpendicular distance from the axis of rotation of a joint to the line of action of force.
∴ From the above mentioned equation,
    τ = Force × Moment arm

Movement According to Joint Position

In human body, joint acts as a fulcrum or axis of rotation and the force is supplied by weight of the body part or by muscle work.

Consider abduction movement of the shoulder joint from the neutral position.

Here, the shoulder joint acts as a fulcrum or axis of rotation.

Weight of upper extremity is the force acting ⅓rd at distance from the shoulder joint.

τ depends upon the momentum and is directly proportional to momentum.

Mechanical, e.g., Opening and closing of door

Anatomical, e.g., Knee extension by the quadriceps, where knee joint is the fulcrum, body weight is the COG of the leg **(Fig. 1.18)**.

If the weight of forearm and hand is 10 lb acting at a distance of 10 inch from the joint axis, Then,

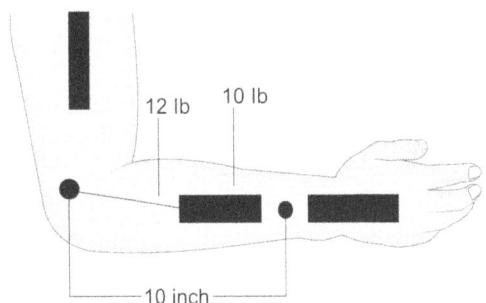

τ produced by biceps brachii muscles
    T_B = 120 lb × 1 inch = 120 lb inch (negative)
τ produced by weight of forearm and hand
    T_G = 10 lb × 10 inch = 100 lb inch (positive)

In anticlockwise direction is negative while in clockwise direction is positive.

Net τ

$τ_R$ = −120 lb inch + 100 lb inch = −20 lb inch

$τ_R$ = 20 lb inch in anticlockwise direction.

It indicates that elbow joint is in the direction of flexion.

If $τ_R$ = 0, the lever system will be in a state of equilibrium (there is no movement at elbow joint).

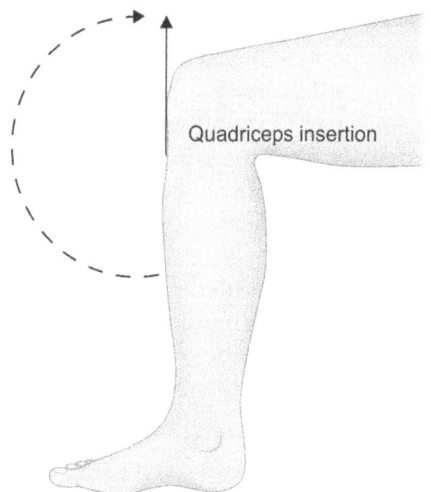

Fig. 1.18: Torque force by the quadriceps

PRACTICAL APPLICATION OF TORQUE

- This effect is seen in balance board or equilibrium board.
- It is a rectangular or a circular board resting on a curved surface.
- It is usually used for strengthening the muscles of lower extremity or for re-education of balance.
- Balance board is based on the principle of moment.
- When a person stands on the balance board, there is equal distribution of weight by both legs. Also the distance is equal from the axis of rotation or fulcrum.

$$F_1 \times d_1 = F_2 \times d_2$$

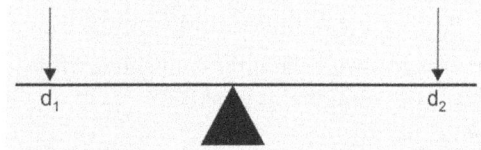

When a muscle is inserted far from the joint axis, it has more rotational effect on the bone than the muscle inserted close to the joint axis.

FRICTION

- Friction is the force that opposes motion between two surfaces.
- It is measured as coefficient of friction.
- It is denoted by "μ"

Coefficient of friction is the ratio between force of limiting friction and the normal reaction between them.

$$\mu = \frac{F}{R}$$

F = Force of limiting friction
R = Normal reaction

Frictional force depends upon the nature of the contact surfaces and the normal reaction.

Rough surfaces provide more coefficient of friction while smooth surfaces provide less coefficient of friction.

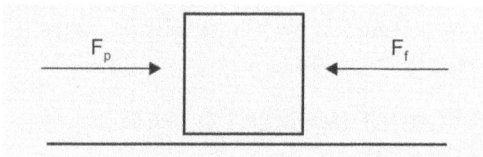

As friction is produced when one body slides over another, it is a shear force.

Units: Newton, Dyne.

It satisfies all the properties of force, such as magnitude, direction, line of action, and point of application.

Properties

- Magnitude
- **Direction:** It is always opposite to the movement of the body.
- Line of action of frictional force: It is always parallel to the contact surface.

Classification

Basically, friction is classified into two types:
1. Static or limiting friction
2. Dynamic or kinetic friction

Dynamic friction is further classified into:
- Sliding friction
- Rolling friction

Static friction: Produced at a point when body tends to move.

Dynamic friction: Produced when a body moves or is in motion.

Sliding friction: It is obtained when a body slides on another.

Rolling friction: It is obtained when one body rolls on another. For example, when a tyre rolls on another.
- Static force > Dynamic force
- Sliding force > Rolling force

For example, it is easier to pull a cylinder by rolling than sliding because rolling friction is lesser than sliding friction.

Application of Friction

- As rough surface have more friction than smooth surface, there is less chances of falling on rough surface.
- Rubber tyre has many grooves that increases friction.
- In axillary crutch, rubber tip is attached to the distal end that increases the friction.
- Oil or powder is applied during massage reduces friction between skin and hand.
- Oil is used in machines to reduce friction.
- In human body, the articulating surfaces of the joints are covered by articular cartilage and lubricative synovial fluid that reduces friction.

GRAVITY

Gravity is a force which attracts all body toward the center.

The weight of the body is the force produced by the gravity and it depends upon the quantity of matter, such as mass.

∴ $W = mg$
Where, m = mass of body
G = acceleration due to gravity

Newton's Law of Gravity

It states that every particle in universe attracts every other particle and the force is directly proportional to the total mass and inversely proportional to the square of distance between them.

$$F \propto m_1 m_2$$

$$F \propto \frac{1}{d^2}$$

$$F \propto \frac{m_1 \cdot m_2}{d^2}$$

$$F = \frac{G \cdot m_1 \cdot m_2}{d^2}$$

Where,
$G = 6.67 \times 10^{-11}$ N m²/kg²
Gravitational constant = G
Anatomical, e.g., when shoulder is in abduction from neutral position.
- Movement occurs against gravity; here muscular force is greater than gravitational force.
- Shoulder wall remains in abduction as long as if, muscular force = gravitational force.
- When shoulder is brought back to neutral, movement occurs with the help of gravity and muscles relax.

Line of Gravity (LOG)

It is an imaginary vertical line that passes through COG of the body **(Fig. 1.19)**.

In normal anatomical position, from lateral view (side) it passes:
- Skull
- Through external ear
- Midpoint of cervical vertebra
- In front of thoracic vertebra
- Midpoint of lumbar vertebra
- Anterior to the 2nd sacral vertebra
- Through midpoint of hip joint axis
- Anterior to the knee joint axis
- Anterior to the ankle joint axis
- Then touches the ground at the level of midtarsal joint.

Base of Support (BOS)

It is an area covered by a body.
- **Mechanical example:**
  - When a book is placed on a table, the lower surface of the book is the BOS.
  - When a table is placed on the ground, the BOS is outer border of the four legs of the table.

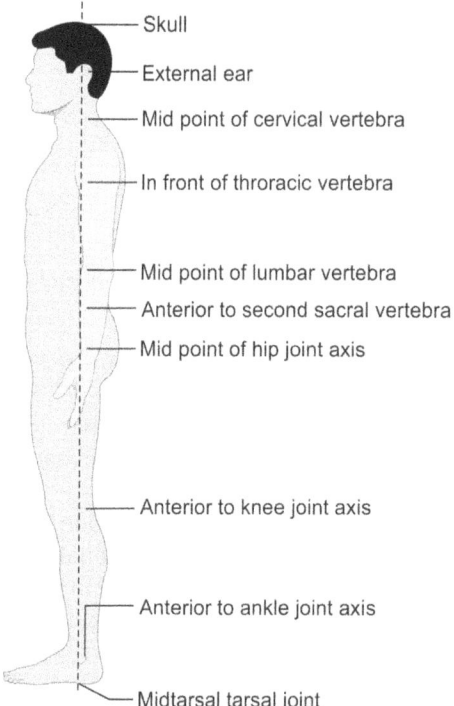

Fig. 1.19: Line of gravity of human body

- **Anatomical example:**
  - When a person is standing, the BOS is outer border of both legs. It can be increased by spreading of legs laterally or anteriorly.
  - When person is supine position, the BOS is posterior part of body.
- LOG and BOG, the stability factors of the body

Center of Gravity

- It is a point where all body masses are assumed to be concentrated.
- COG is a point where all body mass and weight are balanced in all direction.
- It is a point where three planes intersect each other (sagittal, frontal and transverse plane).

COG of Geometrical Objects

- COG of uniform cylindrical rod; lies on the MP of its axis.

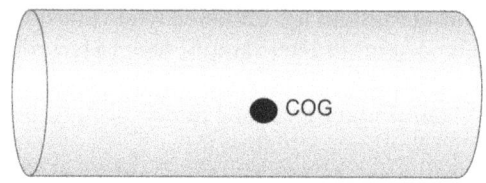

- COG of a triangle; lies at the intersection of median

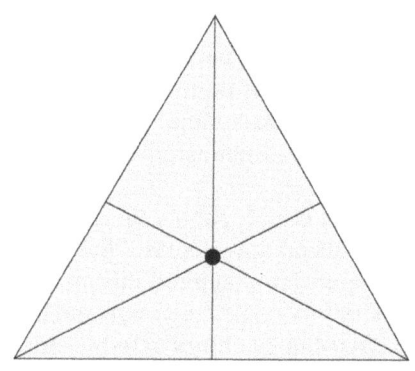

- COG of parallelogram, rectangle, rhombus and square; lies at the intersection of diagonals.

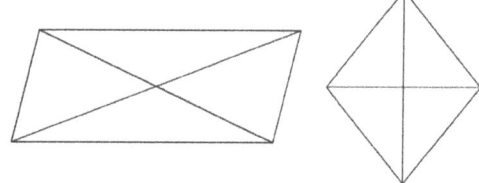

- COG of solid circular cone; lies on its axis at a 1/4th distance from plane base.

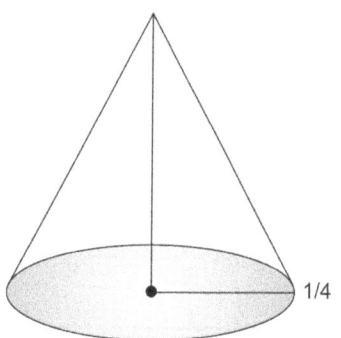

- COG of hollow cone lies on its axis at 1/3rd of distance from the plane base.

Segment	COG
Head	At the level of sphenoid sinus
Head and neck	Just below the occipital bone
Head, neck and trunk	Anterior to the 11th thoracic vertebra
Arm	5 mm proximal to the insertion point of the deltoid muscle
Forearm	11 mm proximal to the insertion point of pronator teres muscle
Hand	Lies on the axis of 3rd metacarpal that is corresponding to the transverse proximal common crease
Upper limb	Just above the elbow joint
Thigh	29 mm below the apex of femoral triangle on the adductor grevis muscle
Leg	35 mm below the popliteus muscle
Foot	In between 2nd and 3rd cuneiform bone
Lower limb	Just above the knee joint

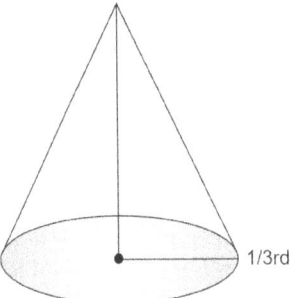

- COG of solid hemisphere lies on its central radius at a distance 3/8th from plane base.

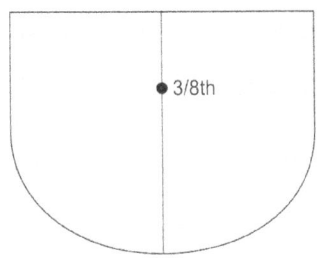

- **COG of hollow hemisphere:** Lies on its central radius at the midpoint.

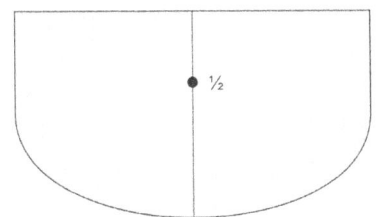

Segmental Weight of Human Body

Segment	% of weight of the segment to the whole body weight	
Head	6.9%	
Head and neck	7.9%	} 59%
Head, neck and trunk	59%	
Arm	2.7%	
Forearm	1.6%	} UL = 4.9%
Hand	0.6%	
Thigh	9.7%	
Leg	4.5%	} LL = 15.6%
Foot	1.4%	

- Segmental COG
- Human body consists of number of segments and each segment has its own COG.

COG of Human Body

When all the segments are combined together and entire body is considered as a single object, in normal anatomical position COG lies slightly anterior to the 2nd sacral vertebra. It is a not a constant point. It changes according to the change in posture.

For example, forward bending of trunk, COG moves anteriorly and falls outside the body.

Relocation of COG

- When there is plaster cast in the right leg and person is walking by the support of crutch, the COG moves down and right.
- When a person is carrying suitcase in right hand, the COG moves up and to the right.
- When both hands are parallel, COG moves up.
- When both hands are vertical, COG moves up.
- During forward bending of trunk, COG moves anteriorly.
- When person is bending toward left side, COG moves toward left side.
- When person standing on right leg COG moves toward weight-bearing side (right side)

- **COG of any segment:** 45% of length from proximal end and 55% of length from distal end.

EQUILIBRIUM

Equilibrium occurs when forces acting on object are perfectly balanced and object remains at rest.

Condition of the Equilibrium
- Summation of all forces is equal to 0, i.e., $\varepsilon f = 0$
- No tendency to move in any direction.
- Summation of all torque = 0, $\varepsilon\tau = 0$
- No tendency to rotate in any direction.

Types of Equilibrium
- Stable equilibrium
- Unstable equilibrium
- Neutral equilibrium

Stable Equilibrium
If a body returns to its original position after being displaced by external forces, this state of equilibrium is called stable equilibrium.

Conditions
- If the position of COG is lower, the object is more stable. The LOG moves to the center of BOS.
- If the position of COG is high, the LOG moves toward the periphery of BOS and the object is less stable.

For example, when a solid cone is placed on a base

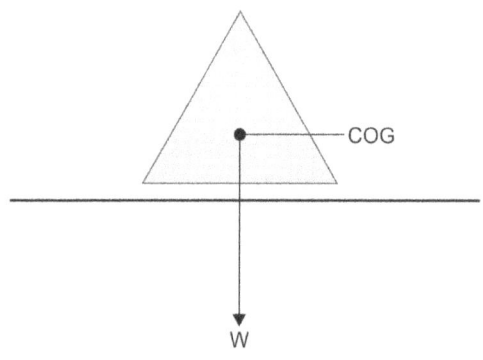

Here, COG is low and the LOG passes within the BOS.

For example, person is in bilateral stance.

Unstable Equilibrium
If the body gets displaced from its original position, with the COG remaining at the same level when subjected to external forces, the state of equilibrium is called as unstable equilibrium.

Conditions
- COG is high and LOG falls outside BOS. For example, when a cone is placed at its apex.
- Toe standing

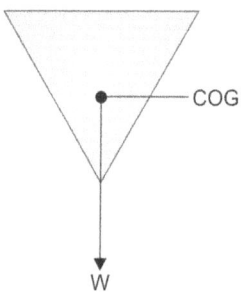

Neutral Equilibrium
If the body does not get displaced from its original position and if the COG remains at the same level when subjected to external forces, this state of equilibrium is called neutral equilibrium. For example, when a ball moves on a plane surface.

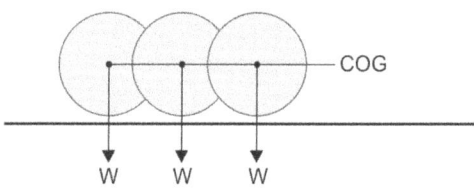

Stability of body: Depends on:
- Size of BOS
- Height of COG
- Position of LOG

Size of base of support: Stability is directly proportional to base of support. In normal anatomical position, maximum stability is attained. When the legs are separated or moved laterally, the base of support increases. As the feet come close together, the base of support decreases and the body becomes less stable. In single leg standing or toe standing, the body is least stable as the base of support is minimum.

Height of COG: The lower the COG, more stable is the body. In comparison to various positions, such as supine lying, standing and sitting, the supine lying position is most stable.

Position of LOG: The distance between the LOG and center of base of support is inversely proportional to stability.

WORK, ENERGY, AND POWER

Work

- Work is said to be done when the point of application of force applied is in same or opposite direction.
- It is measured as product of force and magnitude of its direction.

Consider the work done by the force as positive and work done against it as negative.

Then mathematically,

Work done = F × S
Where S = Magnitude of direction of force
F = Force
WD = Work done

For example,
- When a bucket is drawn into a well, the bucket and the force acting on it are in the same direction. Hence, the work done by the force is positive.
- When the bucket is fetched out of well, the weight of the bucket is in downward direction while the bucket moves in upward direction. Hence, the work is done against the force and is taken as negative.

Anatomical, e.g., when shoulder is abducted, the work is done against gravity and is negative.

When abducted shoulder is brought back to the neutral position, work is done by the force and it is positive.

Measurement of Work

In MKS system, the unit of work is Joule. It measures the work being done when a force of 1 Newton acts through a distance of 1 meter.

1 Joule = 1 Newton × 1 Meter.

In CGS system, it is measured in ERG. It measures the work being done when a force of 1 Dyne acts through a distance of 1 centimeter.

1 Erg= 1 Dyne × 1 centimeter.

In FPS System, it is measured in Calorie.

ENERGY

Energy is defined as capacity to do work.

Principle of Conservation of Energy: It states that "Energy can neither be created nor destroyed, rather it can be transformed from one form to another."

Types of Energy

Mainly, there are two forms of energy, i.e., potential energy and kinetic energy.

Potential Energy

- Energy produced by a body due to its rest is called potential energy.
- It is also called as stored energy.

Potential energy = mgh

Where, m = mass of body
g = acceleration due to gravity
h = height of body

- For example, when a rubber band is stretched and waiting to be released.
  – Anatomical, e.g., sitting posture.

Kinetic Energy

- Energy produced by a body due to its motion, is called as kinetic energy.

Kinetic energy = ½mv^2

Where, m = mass of body
v = velocity of body

For example, when a rubber band is zinged from the fingers.
- Anatomical, e.g., running, walking.

POWER

Power is defined as rate at which work is done.

$$P = \frac{W}{t}$$

Where, P = Power
W = Work
t = Time

Units:
- In MKS System, Power is measured in Watt.
- 1 watt is equal to one joule per second.
- In CGS System, it is equal to one erg per second.

SPRINGS

A spring consists of a number of uniform coils of wire which are used either in tension or compression.

When subjected to tension, the length of the spring increases and vice versa.

Therapeutic Use

It is used either to resist or to assist the force of muscular contraction or to produce passive movements at joints.

In physiotherapy, it is used in suspension therapy, hand grip exercises, and also in multiple gym equipment.

Properties of Spring

- **Extensibility:** Elongation is directly proportional to the applied force. When force is applied to one end of a spring with its other end fixed, the spring elongates in a direction along its long axis.
- **Recoiling of spring:** After the removal of force, the spring returns to its original position. During extension of the spring, potential energy is converted into kinetic energy while the reverse occurs during recoiling.
- **Weight of spring:** The standard springs are available in various weights, e.g., 10, 20, 30 lb (pounds). Internally, the spring consists of a cotton tape which becomes tight when the spring reaches its maximum length thereby, preventing the over stretching of the spring. The weight of the spring depends on the material used, diameter, and thickness of coil.
- **Oscillatory movement produced by spring:** When forces are applied vertically to one end of the spring, and released oscillatory movements are produced. The amplitude of oscillation gradually decreases as the spring comes back to its resting position.

Springs in Series (Figs. 1.20A and B)

It is obtained when springs of equal weight are connected end-to-end.

For example,

Suppose a spring of 5 cm is elongated with 5 kg of weight separately.

Here the force acting is unidirectional.

∴ The total elongation is 5 cm + 5 cm = 10 cm and the resistance offered by the spring is 10 pounds (resistance offered by the spring in series = weight of any one spring).

Springs in Parallel (Figs. 1.21A and B)

It is obtained when springs of equal weight are connected side-to-side.

Here, weight is divided by the spring and 2.5 kg of force is acting on each spring and the elongation is 2.5 cm.

∴ The total elongation offered by the spring in parallel is 2.5 cm and the resistance applied is equal to the sum of weight of the spring, i.e., 10 lb + 10 lb = 20 lb.

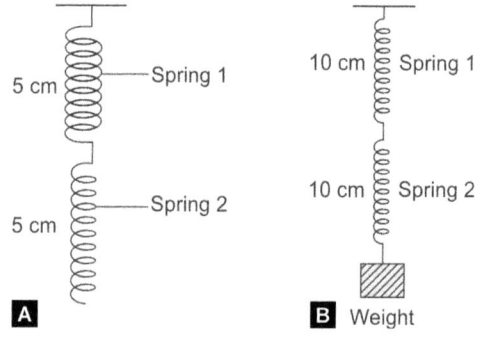

Figs. 1.20 A and B: Springs in series

Chapter 1 | Basic Physics with Biomechanical Perspective

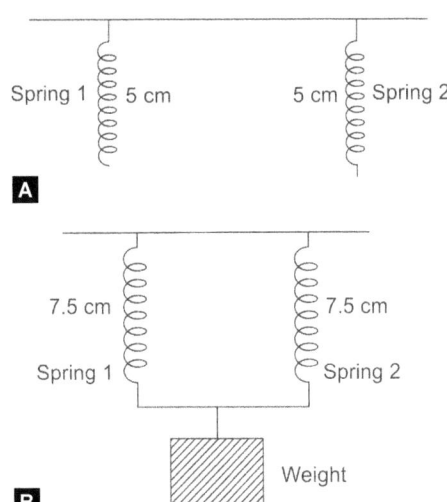

Figs. 1.21A and B: Spring in parallel

LEVERS

A lever is a rigid body which rotates around a fixed axis.

Here, the axis of rotation is called fulcrum and the two forces acting along the length of the lever at particular distance are effort and weight/resistance/load.

In simple terms, it is a simple machine used to transmit force, alter direction and magnitude of force, or to speed up movement.
- Effort tends to produce movement while weight or resistance resists the movement.
- Effort arm is the perpendicular distance from fulcrum to effort.
- Resistance arm is the perpendicular distance from the fulcrum to the resistance applied.

Classification

A lever is classified according to the relative position of fulcrum, effort, and resistance.

There are three types of lever:
1. First order lever
2. Second order lever
3. Third order lever

First Order Lever

In this type, fulcrum lies between effort and resistance. It may be either situated in center or toward effort or resistance.

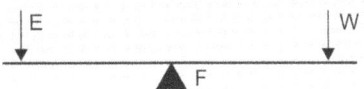

Conditions
- When fulcrum is at center, effort arm is equal to resistance arm.

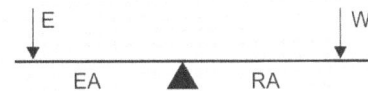

- When fulcrum is nearer to the effort arm, then effort arm is less than resistance arm.

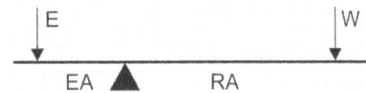

- When fulcrum is nearer to the resistance arm, the effort arm is greater than resistance arm.

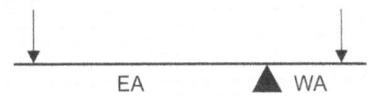

Second Order Lever

In this, resistance lies between fulcrum and effort.

∴ Effort arm is always greater than resistance arm.

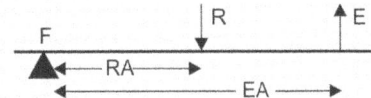

Third Order Lever

In this type, effort lies between fulcrum and resistance.

∴ Resistance arm is always greater than effort arm.

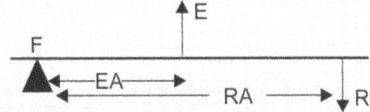

Mechanical Advantage

It is defined as the ratio of resistance to the effort.

OR

It is defined as the ratio of effort arm to the resistance arm.

$$MA = \frac{W}{E} = \frac{EA}{WA}$$

When the value is greater than one, the lever has mechanical advantage and when the value is lesser than one, the lever has mechanical disadvantage.

Mechanical advantage for first order lever: Mechanical advantage for first order lever may be lesser, greater, or equal to one.

Conditions:
- When fulcrum is at the center, EA = RA and MA = 1
- When fulcrum is near to the effort, EA < RA and MA < 1
- When fulcrum is near to the resistance, EA > RA and MA > 1

Mechanical advantage for second order lever:
- As EA > RA
- Mechanical advantage for second order lever is greater than one.
- It is also called as lever of advantage.

Mechanical advantage for third order lever:
- As EA < RA
- Mechanical advantage is lesser than one.
- It is also called as lever of disadvantage.

Mechanical Levers

Example:
- **For first order lever:** See saw, scissors, common balance, cutting player.
- **For second order lever:** Nut cracker, shoulder wheel, closing a door.
- **For third order lever:** Lifting a ladder which rests against a wall, forceps.

Principle of Lever

- If the product of effort and effort arm is equal to the product of resistance and resistance arm, the lever is said to be in equilibrium or mechanical advantage = 1.
- If effort arm is greater than resistance arm then the lever is called as lever of advantage and the mechanical advantage is greater than 1.
- If effort arm is less than resistance arm then the lever is called as lever of disadvantage and the mechanical disadvantage is lesser than 1.

Analysis of Lever

- Find out the fulcrum
- Locate the effort and resistance
- Find out the effort arm and the resistance arm
- Justify the type of lever

LEVERS IN HUMAN BODY

In human body, lever is represented by bone, fulcrum (f) is represented by joint, effort (e) is the contraction of muscle force applied at insertion point, and weight (w) may be either COG of the moving part or the weight placed on the bony segment.

First Order Lever (Figs. 1.22A and B)

- This is the lever of stability and equilibrium with/without mechanical advantage.
- Nodding movement of the head
- Lever—skull
- Fulcrum—atlanto-occipital joint
- Weight—COG of the head
- Effort—insertion point of posterior neck muscles

Second Order Lever (Fig. 1.23)

- This is the lever of power with mechanical advantage.
- Plantarflexion of ankle
- Lever-foot
- Fulcrum-ankle joint
- Weight—COG of the foot
- Effort-insertion point of plantar flexors, i.e., gastrocnemius and soleus.

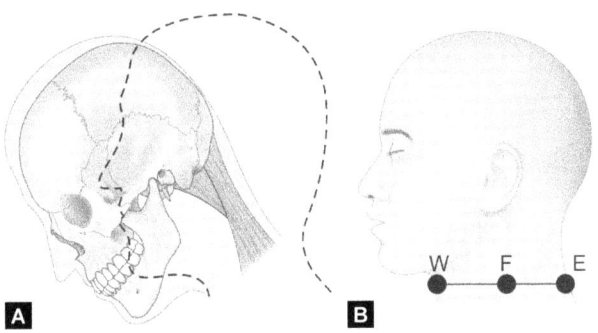

Figs. 1.22A and B: Atlantoaxial joint example of first order lever

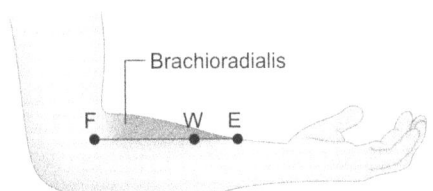

Fig. 1.23: Example of second order lever elbow flexion by brachioradialis
- Lever—forearm
- Fulcrum—elbow joint
- Weight—COG of forearm
- Effort—insertion point of brachioradialis

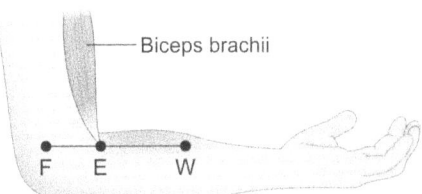

Fig. 1.24: Third order lever

Third Order Lever (Fig. 1.24)

This is the lever of inconvenience with mechanical disadvantage. But this is the most common lever system found in the human body
- Flexion of elbow by biceps brachii
- Lever-forearm and hand
- Fulcrum-elbow joint
- Weight—COG of forearm and hand
- Effort—insertion point of biceps brachii at radial tuberosity.

ELASTICITY

When a body is subjected under load, it may undergo change in shape or size. After removal of force, the body regains its original position. This property is known as elasticity.

Elasticity is expressed in stress or strain.

Stress

It is a force within the body. It is measured as force per cross sectional area.

Where,
$S = F/A$
$F = $ force
$A = $ cross-sectional area, and
$S = $ stress

Anatomical example:

Units of stress:
- In MKS system, the unit of stress is Newton/m².
- In CGS system, the unit of stress is Dyne/m².

Strain

It is defined as ratio of change in shape or size of a body to the original shape and size of a body.
- **There are three types of strain:**
  1. **Linear strain:** Change in length per unit length.
  2. **Shear strain:** Change in area per unit area.
  3. **Volume strain:** Change in volume per unit volume.
  - Strain has no dimensions and units.
  - Strain depends on the applied force, cross sectional area, structure, and design of material.
  - Stress and strain increase with increase in force while it decreases with increase in cross-sectional area.

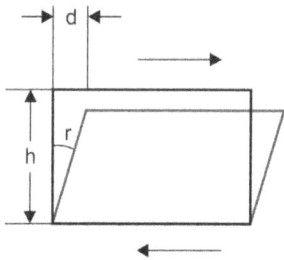

- Unit normal strain = % (dimensionless quantity) or mm/m shear strain = rad
- Tensile strain is positive while compressive strain is negative.
- Factors affecting the extent of deformation:
  - Mechanical properties
  - Size of the body
  - Shape of the body
  - Temperature
  - Humidity
  - Magnitude, direction, and duration of applied forces.

Application of Stress-Strain Curve

Stress-Strain Curve (Fig. 1.25)

- **Elastic region:** When the magnitude of the stress is small, the elastic force can be represented by the relation for an ideal spring (Hooke's law), i.e., the elastic force exerted by the viscoelastic material is proportional to the amount of deformation

$$F = kx$$

where F = elastic force
k = spring stiffness which is a constant
x = amount of deformation

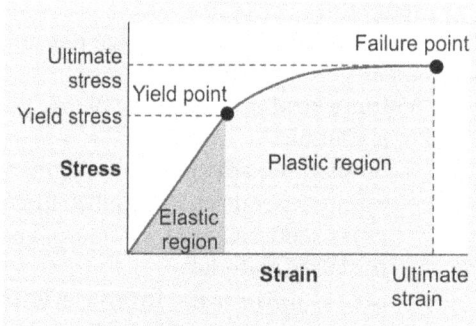

Fig. 1.25: Stress strain curve

- Plastic region
- Yield point
- Failure point

Strength

- Maximum stress that a body can be loaded (ultimate stress).
- Maximum strain that a body can be deformed (ultimate strain).
- Maximum energy stored.

Stiffness

- **Modulus of elasticity (Young's modulus):** For both tensile and compression stress
  - The ratio of the stress to strain in the elastic region of the stress-strain curve
  $$E = \sigma/\varepsilon$$
  - Named after Thomas Young (1773-1829, English scientist)
  - *SI unit:* Pascal
  - *USCS:* psi
- **Hooke's law:** Only for tensile stress
  - For an elastic material, the strain is a linear function of the stress applied
  - Named after Robert Hooke (1653-1703, English scientist)
- **Modulus of rigidity (shear modulus of elasticity)**
  $$G = \tau/\gamma$$
  where $\gamma = d/h$
- **SI unit:** Pascal
- **USCS:** psi

Poisson's Ratio

- When a material is under a tensile stress, the tensile strain and the lateral contraction is proportional.
$$\nu = \varepsilon_{lateral}/\varepsilon_{longitudinal}$$
  - *Assumptions:*
    - The material is homogeneous
    - The material is isotropic
  - *Named after Simeon Denis Poisson (1781-1840)*
- **Unit:** Dimensionless
- $0 \leq \nu \leq \tfrac{1}{2}$
- Relationship between the modulus of elasticity and that of rigidity
$$G = E/2(1 + \nu)$$

- **Brittle vs. ductile materials:**
  - *Brittle material:* The material whose failure occurs at a very low strain, e.g., ceramic or glass.
  - *Ductile material:* The material that is able to resist a very high strain before failure, e.g., aluminum alloys.
- **Creep phenomenon:** Progressive deformation of a material with time as the amount of load remains constant **(Fig. 1.26)**.
- **Load relaxation phenomenon:** Progressive decrease in load with time as the deformation of the structure remains constant **(Fig. 1.27)**.
- **Hysteresis:**
  - Energy stored in a viscoelastic material when a load is given and then relaxed **(Fig. 1.28)**.
  - *Aged heel pad:* Poor ability to absorb the shock **(Fig. 1.29)**.
  - Elastic vs. plastic materials
- **Elasticity:** The ability of a body to resume its original size and shape on removal of the applied loads **(Fig. 1.30A)**.

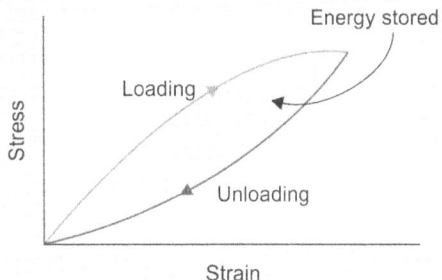

Fig. 1.28: Hysteresis

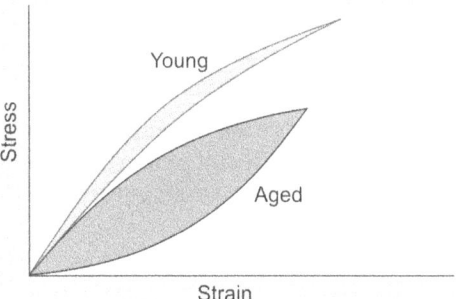

Fig. 1.29: Hysteresis of heel pad

Note: The elastic material is not necessary to have a linear relationship on the stress-strain curve.
- **Plasticity:** When a tissue is stretched to the plastic region and then released, the tissue will assume a new resting length that is longer than the initial length because of plastic changes in its structure **(Fig. 1.30B)**.
- **Clinical application:** Flexibility exercise or joint mobilization.
- **Allowable stress:**
  - When a structural member or mechanical element is designed, the stress must be restricted in a material to a level that will be safe. This is the allowable stress.
  - *Factor of safety (FS):* The ratio of a theoretical maximum load that can be carried by the member until it fails in a particular manner divided by an allowable load

$$FS = F_{fail}/F_{allow}$$

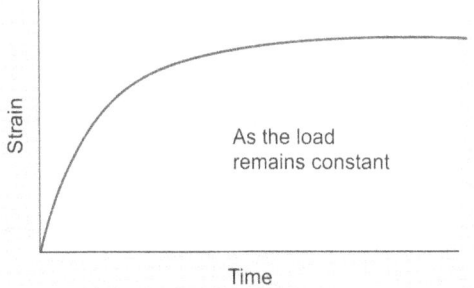

Fig. 1.26: Creep phenomenon

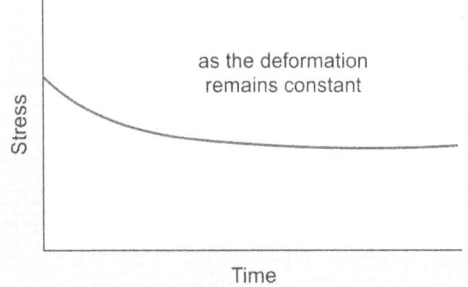

Fig. 1.27: Load relaxation phenomenon

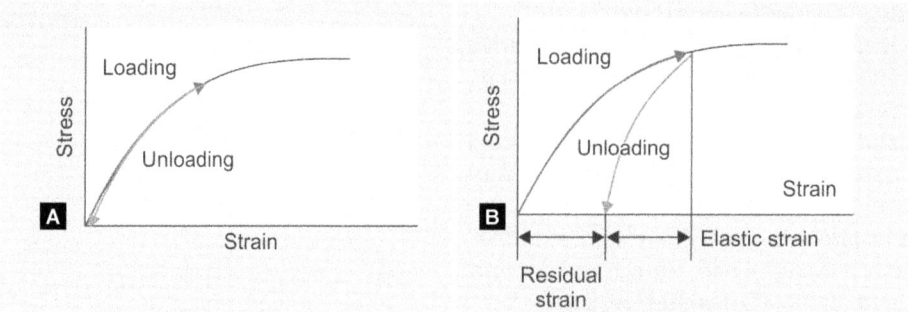

Figs. 1.30A and B: (A) Elastic behavior; (B) Plastic behavior

- The factor of safety is chosen to be greater than 1 to 10 in order to avoid the potential for failure.

When a body is under strain, the deformation produced is directly proportional to the load and the body thus, undergoes the following phases:
- Elastic region
- Plastic region
- Strain hardening
- Necking region
- Rupture/failure point

- **Elastic region:**
  - When a body is subjected to load, it undergoes deformation.
  - It regains its original position after removal of the load.
  - However, when the elastic limit is reached, the body does not regain its original position.
- **Hooks law:** It states that stress is directly proportional to strain within its elastic limit.
$$\therefore \frac{\text{Stress}}{\text{Strain}} = Y = E$$
Where Y = constant = modulus of elasticity.
- **Yield point:** Yield point is achieved when a body stretches for a period without addition of any further load.
- **Plastic region:** Here the deformation produced is permanent and the body attains a new shape.
- **Strain hardening:** During the later stages of plastic phase, molecular changes occur within the body providing resistance to the deformation.
- **Necking region:**
  - This effect is seen when the body is subjected to linear tensile stress.
  - As the body stretches, the cross sectional area of the body decreases reducing the ability of the body against stress.
  - Thus, rupture or point of failure occurs.
- **Rupture or failure point:** This occurs when the tissue breaks. In human body, muscles, ligaments, tendons and other soft tissues are torn whenever injury occurs and this causes weakening of the soft tissues.
- **Result of time on strain:**
  - If a constant pressure is applied to a body, there may be change in shape and size of the body.
  - It can be attributed to the elastic and viscous property of the body.

Viscous property is a slow reaction to stress. It occurs when a constant force is applied for a longer duration of time.
  - After removal of force, the object does not return to its original position.
  - Human body is a combination of elastic and viscous properties which is termed as viscoelasticity and the resulting deformation produced is called as creep.
- **Creep:**
  - It is defined as gradual deformation produced within a body when a force is applied for longer duration of time.
  - In human body, skin produces higher degree of elasticity.
  - In old age, wrinkling occurs due to loss of elasticity of skin.

Springs, sorbo rubber, rubber elastic, and crepe bandage which are commonly used in physiotherapy department show elastic properties.
- **Sorbo rubber:** It is compressible as well as extensible and provides grip for hand movements.
- **Rubber elastic:** It is used either to increase or resist the movements of small joints of hand.
- **Crepe bandage:**
  - Used to control and reduce swelling of the limb.
  - When applied to a limb, muscle contraction occurs increasing the circumference of the limb.
  - When the muscle relaxes, the crepe bandage recoils removing the weight placed on the limb.

In human body, tendons, ligaments, and muscles show elastic properties.

PULLEYS

Definition: A pulley changes the direction of the force, making it easier to lift things.

Anatomic Pulleys

Frequently, the fibers of a muscle or a muscle tendon wrap around a bone or are deflected by a bony prominence. When the direction of pull of a muscle is altered, the bone or bony prominence causing the deflection forms an anatomic pulley. Pulleys (if they are frictionless) change the direction without changing the magnitude of the applied force. As we will see, the change in action line produced by an anatomic pulley (even without affecting force) will have implications for the ability of the muscle to produce torque.

Function of Anatomical Pulley

The function of any pulley is to redirect a force to make a task easier. The "task" in human movement is to rotate a body segment. Anatomic pulleys (in the majority of instances) make this task easier by deflecting the action line of the muscle away from the joint axis, thus increasing the moment arm (MA) of the muscle force. By increasing the MA for a muscle force, a force of the same magnitude (with no extra energy expenditure) produces greater torque.

Types

There are three types of pulleys:
1. **Fixed pulley** is the only pulley that when used individually, uses more effort than the load to lift the load from the ground.
   - The fixed pulley when attached to an unmovable object, e.g., a ceiling or wall, acts as a first class lever with the fulcrum being located at the axis but with a minor change, the bar becomes a rope.
   - The advantage of the fixed pulley is that you do not have to pull or push the pulley up and down.
   - The disadvantage is that you have to apply more effort than the load.
2. **Movable pulley** is a pulley that moves with the load.
   - The movable pulley allows the effort to be less than the weight of the load. The movable pulley also acts as a second class lever. The load is between the fulcrum and the effort.
   - The main advantage of a movable pulley is that you use less effort to pull the load.
   - The main disadvantage of a movable pulley is that you have to pull or push the pulley up or down.
3. **Combined pulley:**
   - Makes life easier as the effort needed to lift the load is less than half the weight of the load.
   - The main advantage of this pulley is that the amount of effort is less than half of the load.
   - The main disadvantage is that it travels a very long distance.

THE PATELLA AS AN ANATOMIC PULLEY

The classic example of an anatomic pulley is that formed by the patella. The quadriceps muscle belly lies parallel to the femur. The tendon of the muscle passes over the knee joint and attaches to the leg (tibia) via the patellar tendon at the tibial tubercle. For knee joint extension, the joint axis is considered to be located through the femoral condyles. The MA for the quadriceps muscle force (QLf) lies in space between the vector and the joint axis. Without the patella, the line of pull of the quadriceps muscle on the leg-foot segment would follow the patellar tendon at the tibial tubercle and would lie parallel to the leg-foot segment. However, the patella lies between the quadriceps tendon and the femur, changing the angle that the patellar tendon makes with the leg (tibia) and changing the line of pull of the quadriceps muscle away from the knee joint axis. The effect of changing the line of pull of the quadriceps muscle on the tibia (QLf) is to increase the MA.

CHAPTER 2

Joint Structure and Function

Chapter Outline

- Classification of joints
- Joint design
- Joint motion—range of motion
  - Osteokinematics
  - Arthrokinematics
  - Concave convex rule
- Joint stability
- Joint function

INTRODUCTION

The articulation of two or more bones whether there is movement or not is referred to as joint. It is also called as arthrosis.

CLASSIFICATION OF JOINTS (FIG. 2.1)

- Joints in the human body can be categorized into simple and complex.
- Simple joints have stability as the primary function whereas complex joints have mobility as its primary function.
- Most joints serve both functions, mobility and stability, and must also provide dynamic stability.
- The joints are surrounded by joint capsules, ligaments, and tendons. These are components of synovial joints, whose primary function is mobility. The ends of synovial joints are covered by hyaline cartilage and enclosed in a synovial sheath and fibrous layer that together constitute the joint capsules. Menisci, disc, and labra synovial joints help to increase stability, provide shock absorption, and facilitate motion. A lubricant, synovial fluid is secreted in synovial joints that help to reduce friction between the bony segments.

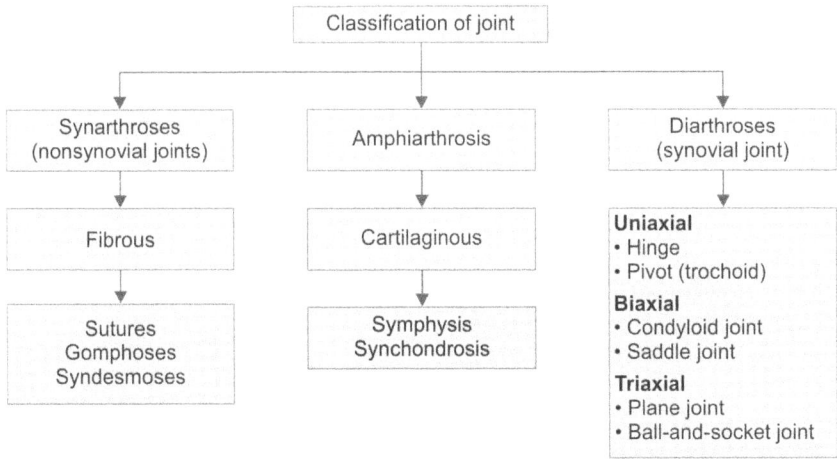

Fig. 2.1: Classification of joints.

- Two traditional method of joint classification, namely—synarthroses (nonsynovial joints) and diarthroses (synovial joints):

Synarthroses

Synarthroses are grouped further based on the type of connective tissue that unites the bony segments. They are divided into:
- **Fibrous joints:** Here the fibrous tissue directly connects bone-to-bone. Three different types of fibrous joints found in human body are sutures, gomphoses, and syndesmoses.
    - *Suture joint:* Two bony components are united by a collagenous sutural ligament or membrane. This type of joint is found in the skull. Early in life, it allows small amount of motion. Fusion of the two opposing bones in suture joints occurs later in life and leads to formation of bony union called synostosis.
        - Example of suture joints: Coronal suture is the suture that joints the parietal and frontal bones of the skull. At birth, the suture allows minimal motion for ease of passage through the birth canal and also allows for the growth of the brain. In adulthood, the sutures fuse and no motion takes place.
    - *Gomphosis joint* is the joint between a tooth and either the mandible or maxilla.
    - *Syndesmoses:* The bony components are joined by interosseous ligaments, a fibrous cord or an aponeurotic membrane. It allows only a small amount of motion.
        - Example: The shaft of tibia is joined directly with shaft of fibula by an interosseous membrane.
- **Cartilaginous joints**
    - *Amphiarthrosis*: Cartilaginous joints are connected by either fibrocartilage and or hyaline cartilage, thus creating bone-cartilage-bone interface.

    The two types of cartilaginous joints are:
    1. **Symphysis (secondary cartilaginous joints):** Here the bony components are covered with hyaline cartilage and directly joined by fibrocartilage in the form of discs or pads. Examples are intervertebral joints between the bodies of vertebrae, joints between the manubrium, and sterna body and symphysis pubis in the pelvis.
    Example: Symphysis pubis is the union of two pubic bones that are joined by fibrocartilage. These joints serve as weight-bearing joint and are responsible for withstanding and transmitting forces. Very little motion is permissible.
    2. **Synchondrosis (primary cartilaginous joint):** Here the bony segments are connected by hyaline cartilage. The function of this joint is to permit bone growth, in addition to providing stability. These joints are found in the skull.

Diarthroses (Synovial Joint) (Fig. 2.2)

Joint Design/Material Made Up in the Joint

The synovial joint consists of:
- Capsule
- Synovial membrane

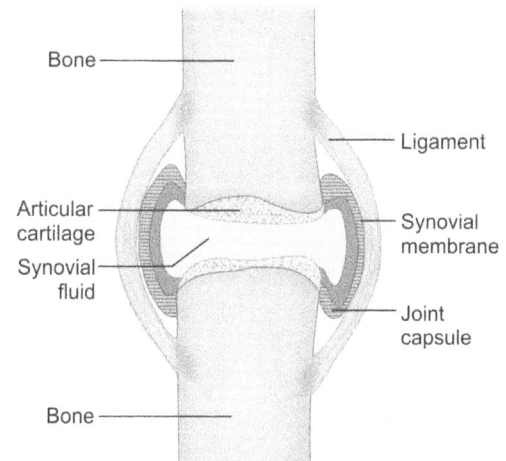

Fig. 2.2: A typical synovial joint.

- Synovial fluid
- Articular cartilage
- Accessory structures (discs, plates, menisci, labrum, fat pad, etc.).

Articular disc, menisci, and synovial fluid help to prevent excessive compression of opposing bony segments by spreading applied forces over larger area. Articular discs and menisci increase joint congruity.

Joint capsule is composed of two layers: An outer layer called stratum fibrosum and inner layer called stratum synovium. The inner layers of stratum synovium are the lining tissue of the capsule. It consists of two layers: The intima and the subsynovial tissue. Joint cavity is enclosed by the capsule. Synovial tissue lines the inner surface of the capsule. Synovial fluid forms a film over the joint surfaces. Hyaline cartilage covers the surfaces of enclosed contiguous bones.

Functions of the capsule:
- Provide stability to the joint
- Allow movement in a certain pattern specific to each joint and prevent extreme range of motion (ROM)
- Acts as a protective layer to the joint
- Provides space for the attachment of ligaments and tendons.

Joint receptors are found in the joint capsule and are sensitive to stretching or compression of the capsule, as well as to any increase in internal pressure due to increased production of synovial fluid (joint swelling).

Synovial fluid: It helps to keep the joint surfaces lubricated and thus reduces friction. This fluid provides nourishment for the hyaline cartilage covering the articular surfaces. The composition of synovial fluid is similar to blood plasma except it contains hyaluronate (hyaluronic acid) and a glycoprotein called lubricin. Lubricin is responsible for cartilage-on-cartilage lubrication and also dissipate energy.

Normal synovial fluid appears clear, pale yellow and is a viscous fluid that is present in synovial joints. The synovial fluid resists shear loads. The viscosity of the fluid varies inversely with the joint velocity or rate of shear. Viscosity is also sensitive to change in temperature. Higher temperature decreases viscosity whereas low temperatures increase the viscosity.

Articular cartilage: It is the protective layer of tissue that lies on the articulating ends.

Functions of articular cartilage:
- It minimizes friction between the joints.
- It spreads the load evenly on the surface of the joint.
- It acts as a protective layer to prevent joint degeneration.
- It facilitates smooth movement between the joint surfaces.

Joint lubrication: Human joints are lubricated by two or more types of lubrication, the two basic types are boundary lubrication and fluid-film lubrication. Boundary lubrication occurs when each load bearing surface is coated with thin layer of large molecules that forms a gel that keeps the opposing surfaces from touching each other. These layers contain lubricin. Fluid-film lubrication involves a thin fluid film that provides separation of the joint surfaces.

Diarthrodial subclassification
The three main traditional categories are:
1. Uniaxial
2. Biaxial
3. Triaxial

Uniaxial involves visible motion of bony components in one plane around a single axis. The axis of motion is usually located near or in the center of the joint or in one of its bony components. It has one degree of freedom. Hinge joint is a joint that resembles a door hinge.
- **Example of hinge joint (Fig. 2.3):** Interphalangeal joints of the fingers. These hinge joints are formed between the distal end of one phalanx and proximal end of another phalanx. Flexion extension motion occurs in sagittal plane and around coronal axis.
- **Another example:** Humeroulnar joint.

Pivot (trochoid) joint is constructed so that one component is shaped like a ring and the

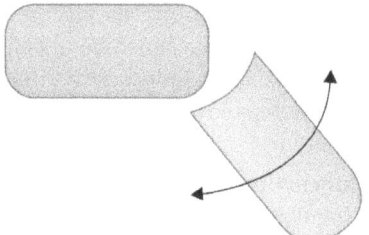

Fig. 2.3: Hinge joint.

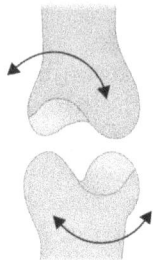

Fig. 2.5: Saddle joint.

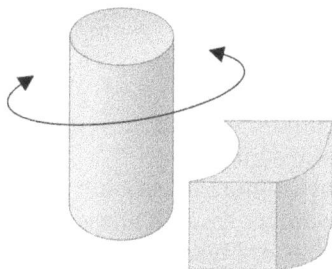

Fig. 2.4: Pivot joint.

other component is shaped so that it rotates within the ring.
- **Example of pivot joint (Fig. 2.4):** Atlantoaxial joint is formed by the atlas and transverse ligament. The odontoid process (dens) of the axis, which is enclosed in the ring, rotates within the osteoligamentous ring. Motion occurs in the transverse plane around longitudinal (vertical) axis.
- **Another example:** Humeroradial joint.

Biaxial joints rejoint in which the bony components are free to move in two planes and around two axes. These joints have two degrees of freedom. Two types of biaxial joints are condyloid joint and saddle joint.
1. Condyloid joints are shaped so that concave surface of one bony component slides over the convex surface of another component in two directions.
2. Saddle joint **(Fig. 2.5)** is a joint in which each joint surface is convex in one plane and concave in the other. These surfaces fit together like a rider on a saddle.

Example: Metacarpophalangeal joint is formed by the convex distal end of the metacarpal bone and concave proximal end of the proximal phalanx. Flexion and extension occur in sagittal plane around coronal axis. Adduction and abduction occur in frontal plane around anteroposterior (A-P) axis.

Another example is carpometacarpal joint of the thumb. It is formed by the distal end of the trapezius and proximal end of the first metacarpal. The motions available are flexion/extension and abduction/adduction.

Triaxial or multiaxial diarthrodial joints are joints where the bony components are free to move in three planes and around three axes. Motion at these joints may occur in oblique planes. Triaxial joints are divided into two categories, namely—plane joints and ball-and-socket joints.
- Plane joints permit gliding between two or more bones.
  - **Example of plane joint (Fig. 2.6):** Carpal joints. Plane joints are found between adjacent surfaces of carpal bones. The adjacent surfaces glide on one another or rotate with regard to one another in any plane.
  - **Another example:** Facet joint of the spine.

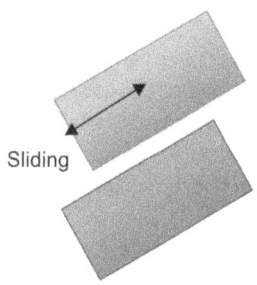

Fig. 2.6: Plane synovial joint

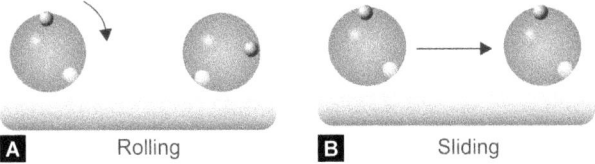

Figs. 2.7A and B: (A) Rolling; (B) Sliding

- Ball-and-socket joints are formed by a ball-like convex surface being fitted into a concave socket. Motions permitted are flexion/extension, abduction/adduction, rotation, and combination of these movements.
  - **Examples of ball-and-socket joint:** Hip joint. It is formed by the convex head of femur and concave socket called acetabulum. Flexion and extension motions occur in sagittal plane around coronal axis. Abduction/adduction occurs in frontal plane around anteroposterior axis. Rotation of femur occurs in the transverse plane around longitudinal axis.

JOINT MOTION

Range of motion: Normal ROM is also called as anatomic or physiologic ROM that refers to the amount of motion available to a joint within the anatomic limits of the joint structure. The extent of anatomic ROM is determined by the shape of the joint surfaces, joint capsule, ligaments, muscle bulk and musculotendinous and bony structures.

The humeroulnar joint at the elbow is limited in extension by bony contact of the ulna on the olecranon fossa of the humerus. The sensation that the therapist experiences while performing passive physiologic movements at each joint is referred to as the end-feel.

A ROM is considered pathological when motion at a joint either exceeds the normal limits (hypermobile) or fails to reach normal anatomic limits of motion (hypomobile).

Osteokinematics refers to rotator movement of the bones in space during physiological joint motion. Movements are typically described by the plane in which they occur, the axis about which they occur and the direction of movement.

Note: Movements are always described as if they are occurring in the anatomical position.

Arthrokinematics/accessory motion: Physiologic joint motion involves rotation of bony segments (osteokinematics) as well as motion of the joint surfaces in relation to one another.

The term roll, slide, and spin are used.

Roll (**Fig. 2.7A**) refers to rolling of one joint surface on another, example of tire rolling on the road. In knee joint, when the subject is squatting, the femoral condyles roll over the fixed tibial surface. The direction of roll is described by the direction of movement of the bone. Thus, the femur rolls backward during squatting.

Sliding (**Fig. 2.7B**) is a pure translatory motion that refers to gliding of one component over another, as when a braked wheel skids. In the hand, proximal phalanx slides over the fixed end of metacarpal during flexion and extension.

Spin is a pure rotatory motion. At the elbow joint, the head of radius spins on the capitulum of the humerus during supination and pronation of the forearm.

The type of arthrokinematic motion that occurs at a particular joint depends on the shape of the articulating surfaces.

CONCAVE CONVEX RULE

When a concave articulating surface is moving on a fixed convex surface. Rolling is considered to occur in the same direction as the moving bony segment. Glide occurs in the same direction as moving segment (**Fig. 2.8**).

When a convex surface moves on a fixed concave surface, the bone rolls in one direction

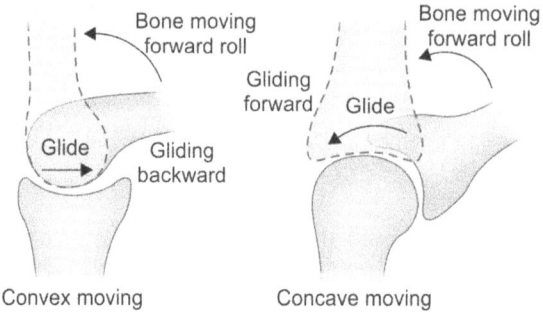

Fig. 2.8: Concave convex rule.

and glides in the opposite direction in order to maintain optimum contact.

JOINT STABILITY

- Orientation of the articulating surfaces
- Type of the joint
- Labrum, disc
- Negative intra-articular pressure
- Joint capsule
- Ligaments
- Fascia

⎫ Static stabilizers

- **Muscles:** Dynamic stabilizers

Close-packed Position

Close pack position is the position assumed by the joint in which the articulating surfaces are in congruency. The capsule and ligaments are taut and the joint is in most stable position. **Example:** For the glenohumeral joint, the close-packed position is abduction of 90° and full external rotation.

Loose-packed Position

Loose pack position is the position assumed by the joint in which the articulating surfaces are in least congruency. The capsule and ligaments are stretched and the joint is in most stable position.

Close pack position	Loose pack position
Maximum congruency	Minimum congruency
Stable position	Least stable position

Contd...

Contd...

Close pack position	Loose pack position
Ligaments, capsule are taut	Ligament, capsule are stretched
Joint surfaces are the nearest	Joint surfaces are the farthest
Assumed during heavy work or load lifting in which stable joint is required	Assumed during injury or rest when maximum joint space is required for healing
Also called as position of work	Also called as position of rest
In the event of an accident in this position chances of fracture is more	In the event of an accident in this position, chances of soft tissue (ligament, capsule) injury is more

Degrees of Freedom

It is the number of planes or axes the joint moves about. There are a total of 3 angular degrees of freedom and 3 translatory degrees of freedom. For practical purposes only the angulatory degrees of freedom are discussed in any joint.

- **1° of freedom:** If the joint moves in only one plane, it is said to be having 1° of freedom. Example humeroulnar joint moves in only sagittal plane (flexion-extension) thus it has only 1° of freedom.
- **2° of freedom:** If the joint moves in 2 planes, it is said to be having 2° of freedom. Example, knee joint moves in 2 planes; sagittal plane (flexion-extension) and transverse plane (medial rotation-lateral rotation) thus it has 2° of freedom.

- **3° of freedom:** If the joint moves in all the 3 planes, it is said to be having 3° of freedom. Example, hip joint moves in all the 3 planes; sagittal plane (flexion-extension), frontal plane (abduction-adduction), and transverse plane (medial rotation-lateral rotation) thus it has 3° of freedom.

Close Pack Position

Joint(s)	Position
Facet (spine)	Extension
Temporomandibular	Clenched teeth
Glenohumeral	Abduction and lateral rotation
Acromioclavicular	Arm abducted to 30°
Sternoclavicular	Maximum shoulder elevation
Ulnohumeral	Extension
Radiohumeral	Elbow flexed 90°, forearm supinated 5°
Proximal radioulnar	5° supination
Distal radioulnar	5° supination
Radiocarpal (wrist)	Extension with ulnar deviation
Metacarpophalangeal (fingers)	Full flexion
Metacarpophalangeal	Full opposition (thumb)
Interphalangeal	Full extension
Hip	Full extension and medial rotation
Knee	Full extension and lateral rotation of tibia
Talocrural (ankle)	Maximum dorsiflexion
Subtalar	Supination
Midtarsal	Supination
Tarsometatarsal	Supination
Metatarsophalangeal	Full extension
Interphalangeal	Full extension

Loose Pack Position

Joint(s)	Position
Facet (spine)	Midway between flexion and extension

Contd...

Contd...

Joint(s)	Position
Temporomandibular	Mouth slightly open (free way space)
Glenohumeral	55° abduction, 30° horizontal adduction
Acromioclavicular	Arm resting by side in normal physiological position
Sternoclavicular	Arm resting by side in normal physiological position
Ulnohumeral (elbow)	70° flexion, 10° supination
Radiohumeral	Full extension and full supination
Proximal radioulnar	70° flexion, 35° supination
Distal radioulnar	10° supination
Radiocarpal (wrist)	Neutral with slight ulnar deviation
Carpometacarpal	Midway between abduction/adduction and flexion/extension
Metacarpophalangeal	Slight flexion
Interphalangeal	Slight flexion
Hip	30° flexion, 30° abduction and slight lateral rotation
Knee	25° flexion
Talocrural (ankle)	10° plantar flexion, midway between maximum inversion and eversion
Subtalar	Midway between extremes of range of movement
Midtarsal	Midway between extremes of range of movement
Tarsometatarsal	Midway between extremes of range of movement
Metatarsophalangeal	Neutral
Interphalangeal	Slight flexion

Joint Function

The primary function of any joint is to provide mobility. Depending on the type of the joint the joint may either be mobile, less mobile or nonmobile. Nonmobile joints main function is to provide stability, e.g., sutures of a skull. Less mobile joints provide both, a bit of stability and a bit of mobility, e.g., symphysis pubis. The mobile joints are the main joints of motion, and are mostly synovial joints. The joint motions are already previously discussed; of osteokinematics, arthrokinematics, degrees of freedom, etc.

Further the joint functions can be discussed in terms of open kinetic chain (OKC) and closed kinetic chain (CKC).

OKC versus CKC

Kinetic chain is nothing but a chain of series of joints joining together to perform a functional movement and the joints are interdependent.
- **Open kinetic chain (OKC):** It is the chain of the joints in which the distal segment is free and the proximal segment is fixed, e.g., walking.
- **Close kinetic chain (CKC):** It is the chain of the joints in which the proximal segment is free and the distal segment is fixed, e.g., push-ups.

Closed kinetic chain exercises to allow for multijoint activities that simulate everyday as well as athletic movements. Performing a squat can aid in functional activity.

Kinetic link model is a biomechanical model that is helpful in analyzing sport activities. Human body is linked wherein the segments are interdependent and works in a proximal to distal fashion. Model highlights the contribution of entire body rather than focusing on individual segments. Muscle activation is believed to occur in a proximal-to-distal sequence in order to elicit efficient normal motion. This proximal-to-distal sequencing should be kept in mind when attempting to restore function via a rehabilitation protocol.
- The joints which are in series in the human body are not independent but are interlinked to each other. This forms a chain like system called as kinetic chain where one bony segment affects the other.
- The extremity can either be in OKC or CKC depending on which end of the kinetic chain is free. If the distal end is free and proximal end is fixed, it is called as OKC and vice versa for CKC. OKC allows movement of the distal joint without causing movement to the adjacent joints. Core stabilization and proximal stabilization is important for eliciting motion in distal segments. Examples of upper extremity in open chain are shoulder shrug and biceps curls. Example of lower extremity in OKC is a person walking. Performing exercises in open kinetic chains helps to focus on individual muscle groups and on a particular joint.
- An extremity is said to be in a CKC when the distal segment is fixed and the proximal segment is moving. Movement of one segment would produce substantial movement of adjacent segments. While performing activities in closed kinematic chain, example, push-ups, dip, squat or dead lift, leads to multiple joint activity and involves use of numerous muscle groups simultaneously.
- When incorporating conditioning exercises, open versus closed kinetic chain exercises should be taken into consideration.

■ EFFECT OF DISEASE ON THE JOINTS

Impact of disease, injury or aging could have an impact on complex joints more than on simple joints.

Rheumatoid arthritis could affect the normal function of the synovial membrane. The normal function of synovial membrane is to produce synovial fluid. Thus, the production and composition of synovial fluid will be altered. Alterations in synovial fluid could affect joint lubrications.

In another type of arthritis, osteoarthritis which may be genetic or mechanical in origin, the cartilage is primarily involved. Here, the cartilage is unable to withstand normal stress. Under stress the cartilage erodes and splitting of cartilage is evident. Thus, increasing friction between joint surfaces and thus increasing the erosion process.

EFFECTS OF INJURY ON THE JOINTS

When joints or ligaments are subjected to injury. Example, tearing of a ligament will result in lack of stability at that joint. Further damage and disruption of function will take place resulting in instability at that joint. The once stabilized joint will now show increased mobility.

EFFECTS OF IMMOBILIZATION ON THE JOINTS (STRESS DEPRIVATION)

A limb can be immobilized either by an external cast, bedrest, weightless or denervation or it can be self-imposed as a reaction to pain and inflammation.

When a joint is injured, it will show signs of inflammation, such as pain and swelling. The joint assumes a loose packed position to accommodate the increased volume of fluid within the joint space. It is referred to as the position of comfort as there is reduction in pain in this position. Each joint has a position of minimum pressure and maximum volume. Example, knee and hip joints, the position of comfort is between 30 and 45° of flexion; for ankle it is 15° of plantar flexion. If the joint is immobilized in the comfort position, the joint capsules will shorten and contractures will develop in surrounding soft tissues; thus, limiting ROM at the joint.

Effect on ligaments and tendon: Ligaments adapt to decrease load by decreasing collagen content and reducing cross-linking among collagen molecules. Tissues are thus weakening. The musculotendinous junction of tendons loses its interdigiting structure when not loaded, which makes it weaker. Ligaments and tendons show a 50% decrease in tensile strength and stiffness after 8 weeks of immobilization.

Gradual reloading is necessary to restore tendon and ligament strength.

Effects on articular surfaces and bone: Biochemical and morphological changes include proliferation of fibrofatty connective tissue within the joint space, adhesions between folds of the synovium, atrophy of cartilage, regional osteoporosis, weakened ligaments at the insertion point as a result of osteoclastic resorption of bone and Sharpey's fibers, decrease in PG content and increase in water content.

Thinning and softening of articular cartilage occur. There will be loss of ROM at the joint.

Adverse effects of immobilization have led to the development of many strategies to help minimize the effects of immobilization, (1) use of continuous passive motion (CPM) devices after joint surgery, (2) reduction in duration of casting, (3) development of dynamic splinting devices to allow joint motion, (4) use of graded loading after immobilization, (5) extension of recovery period to months rather than days or weeks.

EFFECTS OF EXERCISE

Low frequency compressive loading will increase cartilage formation while higher frequencies will enhance bone synthesis. Higher magnitude or sustained loading will induce fibrocartilage formation whereas tensile loads will induce tissue formation resembling that found in tendons and ligaments.

- **Bone response to exercise:** Bone deposition is increased with weight bearing exercises. Very low magnitude high-frequency vibration has been shown to increase trabecular bone formation by 34%.
- **Cartilage response to exercise:** Exercise increases the PG synthesis.
- **Tendon response to exercise:** Tendons respond to increase tensile loads by increasing their collagen concentration, collagen cross-linking, tensile strength, and stiffness. Chronic increased loading causes tendon hypertrophy and increased cross-linking.

- **Ligament response to exercise:** Effects of exercise on normal ligament are less clear.

Overuse

When joints and their surrounding structures are subjected to repetitive loading, they are highly susceptible to injury. It may result in injury as they do not have enough time to recover before they are subjected to another loading cycle, even though the load magnitude maybe within normal loading range. An injury resulting from this type of repetitive strain loading may be called as overuse injury or syndrome, repetitive motion disorder, or repetitive strain injury.

CHAPTER 3

Connective Tissue Structure and Function

Chapter Outline

- Classification
- Ligaments
- Tendons
- Bursae
- Cartilage
- Bone
- General properties of connective tissue

INTRODUCTION

Connective tissue includes bone, bursa, capsule, cartilage, discs, fat pads, labrum, menisci, plates, ligaments, and tendons.

Connective tissue is characterized by widely dispersed cells (cellular component) and large volume of extracellular matrix.

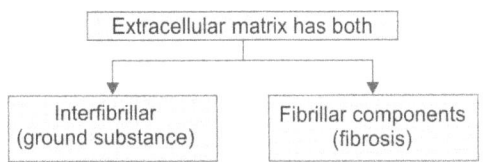

Cells: Fibroblast is the basic cell of most connective tissue, it produces extracellular matrix.

Depending on its mechanical (compressive forces) and physiological environment, fibroblast produces different types of connective tissue and receives new name namely fibroblast specialize to become chondroblast (cartilage), tenoblast (tendon), and osteoblast (bone). These cells are called fibrocytes, chondrocytes, and osteocytes when they mature and become less metabolically active.

Extracellular matrix:
- Is the part of connective tissue outside the cells.
- Contains protein and water and is organized into a fibrillar component and a surrounding matrix.

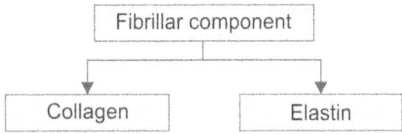

Two proteins, i.e., collagen (most abundant protein) and elastin.

1. **Collagen:** It is present in abundance. Collagen has tensile strength and is responsible for functional integrity of connective tissue structures and their resistance to tensile strength.
   - Fibril-forming collagens (Type 1, 2, 3, 5, 11)
     - **Type 1 collagen:** 90% of total collagen in the body. Found in tendon, ligaments, menisci, fibrocartilage, joint capsules, synovium, bones, labra, and skin, and is responsible for tensile strength of tissues.
     - **Type 2:** Cartilage and intervertebral discs
     - **Type 3:** Skin, joint capsules, muscles and tendon sheath, and healing tissues.
2. Elastin is found in skin, the tracheobronchial tree, and walls of arteries (aorta).

Interfibrillar component:
Interfibrillar component contains water and proteins, primarily glycoproteins and

proteoglycans (PGs). Ground substance is a mixture of PGs and water. Carbohydrate portion of PGs consists of long chains of repeating disaccharide units called glycosaminoglycans (GAGs).

Components of collagenous tissues:
- **Cell:** Fibroblast or chondrocyte
- **Extracellular matrix:**
  - *Fiber:*
    - Collagen fiber: For strength
    - Elastin fiber: For flexibility
  - Ground substance

COLLAGEN

Structure
- The most abundant protein in the body
- To resist tensile stress
- **Tropocollagen:** Three procollagen polypeptide chains (α chains) coiled about each other into a right-handed triple helixes **(Fig. 3.1)**.

Types
Type I: Found in bone, tendon, ligament, and skin.
Type II: Found in articular cartilage, nasal septum, and sternal cartilage.

SPECIFIC CONNECTIVE TISSUE STRUCTURES

Ligaments
Connect one bone to another, usually at or near a joint. Ligaments blend with joint capsules and appear as thickenings in the capsule. It consists of cells 10-20%—fibroblast, 80-90%—extracellular matrix, 0.2%—PGs, and dermatan sulfate GAG. Fibrillar component of extracellular matrix-type 1 collagen. Ligament resists tensile forces (collagen fibers). The arrangement of collagen fibers and the collagen/elastin fiber ratio in various ligaments determines the relative abilities of these structures to provide stability and allow mobility for a particular joint.

Properties
- The physiologic response of ligaments to intermittent tension (application and release of tensile force) is an increase in the thickness and strength.
- Immobilized ligaments become weaker rapidly and take over 12 months to recover their mechanical properties.
- Ligaments more variable than tendons as they are designed to withstand both compressive and shear forces as well as tensile forces.

Tendons
Connect muscle to bone and transmit forces developed by the muscles to their bony attachments, e.g., Biceps tendon. Tendons contain Type 1 collagen (95% more)—for tensile strength. Collagen fibrils of tendon form larger subunits, primary bundles known as fibers. Its diameter increases with age and increases tensile loads.

Group of fibers, enclosed by a loose connective tissue sheath called the endotendon, forms a secondary bundle called a fascicle. Several fascicles form a larger group (tertiary bundles) that is enclosed in the endotendon. Sheath that encloses the entire tendon—epitenon. Paratenon is a double-layered sheath that is loosely attached to outer surface of epitenon. Epitenon and paratenon together are sometimes called peritenon. Paratenon protects tendon from friction, allows it to slide past adjacent structures, and provides a source of replacement cells if tendon is injured **(Fig. 3.2)**.

Tendons have two types of bone attachment: Fibrocartilaginous (enthesis) and fibrous. Tendon insertion is subjected to both compressive and tensile forces. The fibrous enthesis subdivided into two categories: Periosteal and bony. In the former, tendon fibers attach to the periosteum which thus indirectly attaches tendon to bone. In the latter,

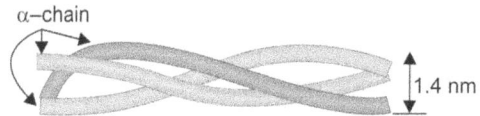

Fig. 3.1: Structure of tropocollagen

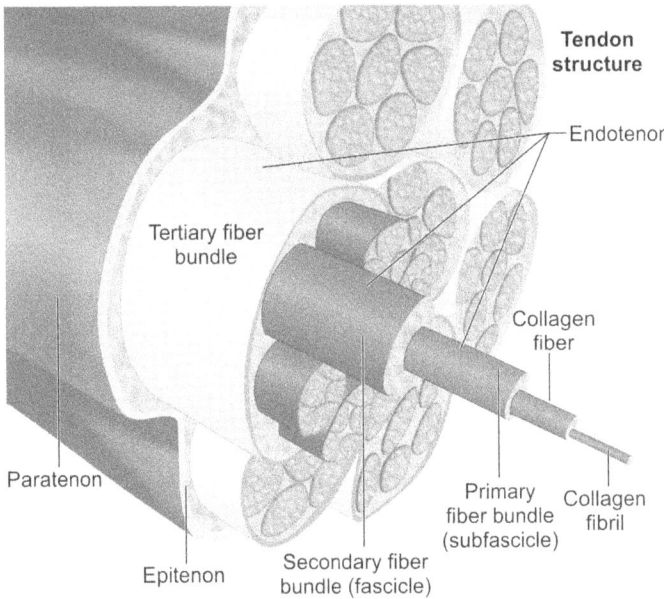

Fig. 3.2: Structure of tendon

tendon attaches directly to bone. Attachment of tendon to muscle at the myotendinous junction (MTJ) comprises interdigitation between collagen fibers and muscle cells.

Properties

- Tendon exhibits creep when subjected to either constant or uninterrupted cyclic tensile loading, e.g., stress applied to a tendon through muscle contraction.
- Cross-sectional area, composition of tendon, and length of tendon determine the amount of force that a tendon can resist and the amount of elongation that it can undergo.
- Tendons adapt readily to changes in the magnitude and direction of loading.

Bursae

Bursae are located where moving structures are in tight approximation that is between tendon and bone, bone and skin, muscle and bone, or ligament and bone. Bursae located between skin and bone, such as those found between patella and the skin and between olecranon process of ulna and skin are called subcutaneous bursae. Subtendinous bursae lie between tendon and bone. Submuscular bursae lie between muscle and bone.

Cartilage

Components: Low cellular density
- **Chondrocyte:** <10%
- **Extracellular matrix:**
  - Collagen fibers
  - *Ground substance:* Proteoglycans
  - *Water (65–80%):* Interstitial fluid movement is important in mechanical property and joint lubrication.

Divided into following types: Fibrocartilage (white), elastic (yellow), and (articular) hyaline cartilage. It contains mainly type 2 collagen and large amounts of aggregating PGs.
- White fibrocartilage forms the bonding cement in joint that permit little motion and is present in the intervertebral discs. It contains type 1 collagen.
- Yellow elastic fibrocartilage found in ears and epiglottis and has higher ratio of elastin to collagen fibers.
- Hyaline articular cartilage (**Fig. 3.3**) forms a thin covering on the ends of bones in

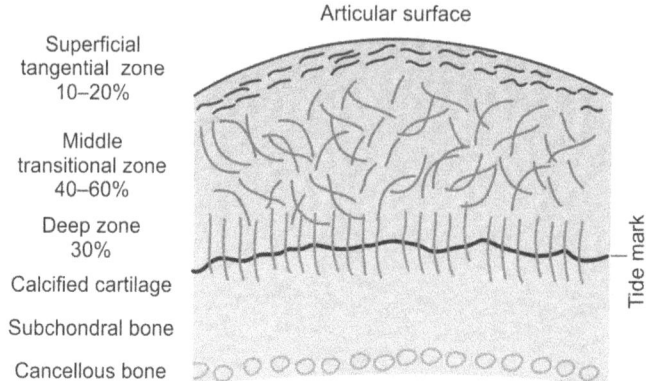

Fig. 3.3: Collagen arrangement of the articular cartilage

majority of joints. It provides smooth, resilent, low-friction surface for the articulation of one bone with another. They are capable of bearing and distributing weight.

When a cartilage is subjected to injury, it has limited and imperfect mechanisms for repair. Cells of articular cartilage are chondrocytes and chondroblasts. The ability of cartilage to resist compressive force depends large volume of aggregating PGs and an intact collagen network.

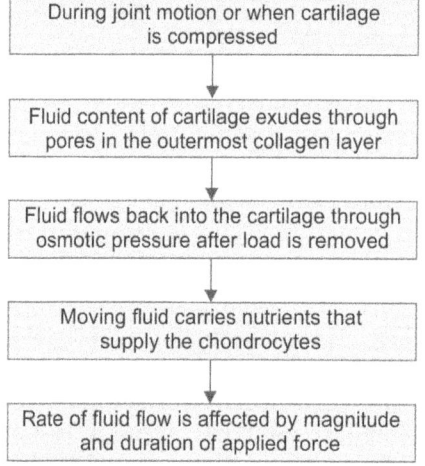

Because hyaline cartilage is devoid of blood vessels and nerves in adults, its nourishment is derived solely from the back and forth flow of fluid. Thus free flow of fluid is essential for survival of articular cartilage. Diminished flow occurs with decreased loading. Hyaline cartilage thus undergoes degenerative changes after prolonged loading or unloading.

Functions of articular cartilage:
- Spread load over a wide area
- Allow movement of two articulating bones with minimal friction and wear
- Deformed under loading, exuding synovial fluid.

Collagen fibers in articular cartilage:
- **Biological unit:** Tropocollagen
- **Mechanical properties:** Tensile stiffness and strength
- **Distribution of collagen in articular cartilage:**
  - *Superficial tangential zone:* Parallel to the articular surface
  - *Middle zone:* Randomly distributed
  - *Deep zone:* Perpendicular to cartilage-calcified cartilage interface (tidemark).

Proteoglycans in articular cartilage:
(Figs. 3.4 and 3.5)
- **Basic unit:** GAGs
- Mutually repelled between neighboring GAGs
- **Proteoglycan:**
  - Hyaluronic acid
  - Link protein
  - *GAG chains:* 200–400 nm in length
    - Protein core
    - Chondroitin sulfate chains (CS): Decrease with aging
    - Keratan sulfate chains (KS): Increase with development and aging

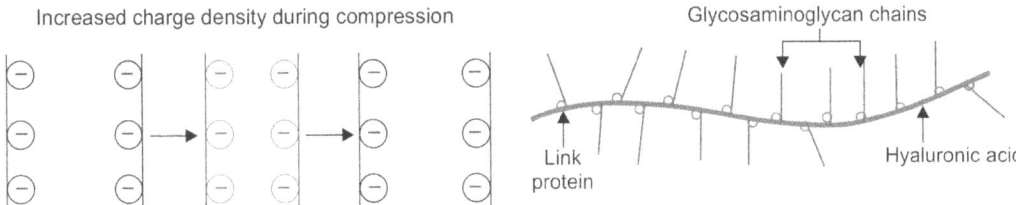

Fig. 3.4: Repulsive force on GAG of articular cartilage

Fig. 3.5: Structure of proteoglycan

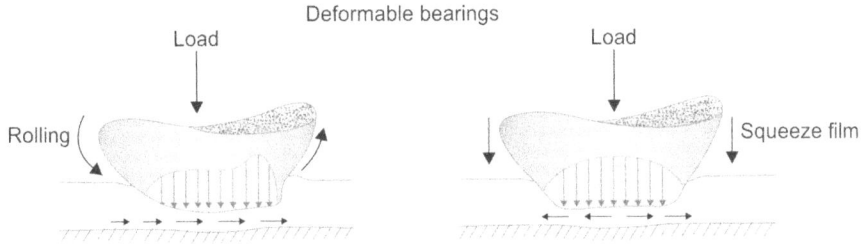

Fig. 3.6: Thick fluid film and low pressure

- CS/KS ratio: 10:1 at birth and 2:1 in adult.

Mechanical Properties of the Articular Cartilage

- **Biphasic creep response:**
  - *Exudation of fluid:* Up to 50% of the fluid can be squeezed out **(Fig. 3.6)**
  - Creep phenomenon of the collagen fiber
- **Biphasic load relaxation phenomenon:**
  - Stress increased as fluid exudation
  - Stress decreased as fluid redistribution

Lubrication Mechanism

Boundary lubrication:
- The chemical adsorption of a monolayer of lubricant molecules onto the articular surfaces
- Depends on the chemical property of lubricants.

Fluid film lubrication:
- A much thicker film of lubricant causing a relatively large separation of the two bearing surface.
- Elastohydrodynamic fluid films of both the sliding and the squeeze type probably play an important role in lubricating the joint.
- With high load and low speeds of relative motion, the fluid film will decrease in thickness as the fluid is squeezed out from between the surfaces.
- Under very high-loading conditions, the fluid film may be eliminated, allowing surface-to-surface contact.

Failure of the Cartilage

- Mechanical loading and unloading prevent cartilage degeneration.
- Limited ability to remodel itself if articular cartilage is damaged.

Types of failure:
- **Interfacial wear:** Wear resulting from the direct interaction of bearing surfaces.
  - Adhesion or abrasion wear only takes place in an impaired or degenerated joint.
  - Traumatic arthritis
- **Fatigue wear:** Wear resulting from bearing deformation under repetitive loads
- Failure of collagen-PG matrix + loss of PG, e.g., chondromalacia patella
- Damage from a high impact **(Fig. 3.7)**
- **Loads leading to wear:**
  - *Acute injury:* Active loading or impact loading
  - *Chronic injury:* Interfacial or fatigue loads.

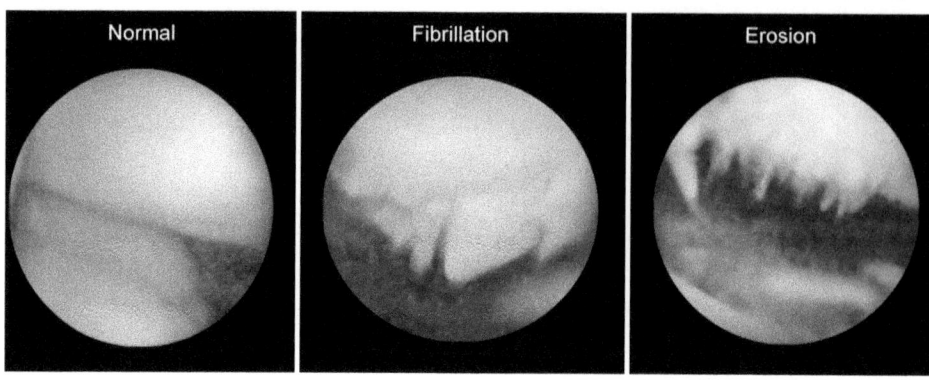

Fig. 3.7: Wear of articular cartilage viewed by arthroscopy

Bone

- **Cortical bone**
  - Compact bone, cortex
  - 5–30% of porosity
- **Cancellous bone**
  - Spongy bone
  - 30–90% of porosity

It is the hardest of all connective tissues. Osteoblasts are primary bone-forming cells that are responsible for synthesis and for its deposition and mineralization. Osteoblasts also secrete procollagen (precursor of type 1 collagen) into the surrounding matrix. When osteoblasts cease their bone-making activity they are called osteocytes. Osteoclasts are responsible for bone resorption.

Architecture of bone: The innermost layer is called cancellous (also trabecular or spongy) bone and outer layer is called compact or cortical bone. Cancellous bone, calcified tissue forms thin plates called trabeculae that are laid down in response to stresses placed on the bone. Trabeculae are capable of distributing the load optimally. Cancellous bone is covered by a thin layer of dense compact bone called cortical bone, which is laid down in concentric layers. The fibrous layer covering all bones is the periosteum. Periosteum is well-vascularized and contains many capillaries that provide nourishment for the bones. It contains an osteogenic layer that contains cells that are precursor to osteoblasts and osteoclasts and thus act as reservoir for cells needed for growth and repair. Damage to periosteum as a result of trauma or surgery will decrease the healing capacity of bone. At microscopic level, both cortical and cancellous bone may contain two distinct types of bone architecture: Woven and lamellar bone.

Osteoporosis: An imbalance between bone synthesis and resorption, in which osteoclasts break down or absorb bone at a faster rate than the osteoblasts can remodel or rebuild the bone, results in osteoporosis. Bones will have decrease mineral density.

- **Mechanical functions:**
  - To protect internal organs
  - To provide rigid kinematic links
  - To provide attachments sites for muscles
  - To facilitate muscle action and bone movement
- **Physiological functions:**
  - To produce blood cells (hematopoiesis)
  - To maintain calcium metabolism (mineral homeostasis)

Properties
- Cortical bone is stiffer than cancellous bone (trabecular) bone.
  Cortical bone can withstand greater stress but less strain than cancellous bone.
- Rate, frequency, duration, magnitude, and type of loading—affect bone
- Repeated loading, either high repetition coupled with low load or low repetition with high load—cause permanent stress and leads to bone failure.
- Bone losses stiffness and strength with repetitive loading as a result of creep strain

- Creep strain occurs when a tissue is loaded repetitively during the time the material is undergoing creep.

Bone Modeling and Remodeling

- **Bone modeling:** The process by which bone mass increased to alter the size, shape, and structure of the bone.
- **Bone remodeling:** The process by which bone mass adapts, by change its size, shape, and structure, to the mechanical demands placed upon it.

Anisotropic Behavior of the Bone (Figs. 3.8A and B)

- **Anisotropy:** The property of a material which exhibits different mechanical properties when loaded in different direction.
- Stiffness with respect to tension is maximal for axial loads and minimal for perpendicular loads.

Factor Affecting Bone Strength

- For ultimate stress of cortical bone: Compression > tension > shear
- Contraction of muscle alters the stress distribution in the bone.
- Contraction of the gluteus medius muscle produces great compressive stress on the superior cortex of the neck of the femur, neutralizing the tensile stress, and thereby allowing the femoral neck sustain more load.
- **When loads are applied at higher rate within the physiological limit, the bone:**
  - Becomes stiffer
  - Sustains a higher load to failure
  - Stores more energy before failure
- **When a bone fractures, the stored energy is released:**
  - Single bone crack for a low-energy fracture
  - Comminuted fracture of bone for a higher-energy fracture
  - Severe destruction of bone before failure
- **Possible causes of bone failure:**
  - Excessive acting forces
  - Unfavorable acting moments
  - Small bone dimension
  - Excessive repetition of load application

GENERAL PROPERTIES OF CONNECTIVE TISSUE

Mechanical Behavior

Force and elongation—

Load refers to an external force or forces applied to a structure. When force acts on an object, it will produce a deformation. A tensile load will produce elongation.

The load-deformation curve is the result of plotting the applied load (external force) against the deformation and provides information regarding the strength properties of a particular material or structure. It provides information about elasticity, plasticity, ultimate strength, and stiffness of the material as well as amount of energy that the material can store before failure.

Region of the curve between point A and B is the elastic region. In this region deformation of the material will not be permanent, and

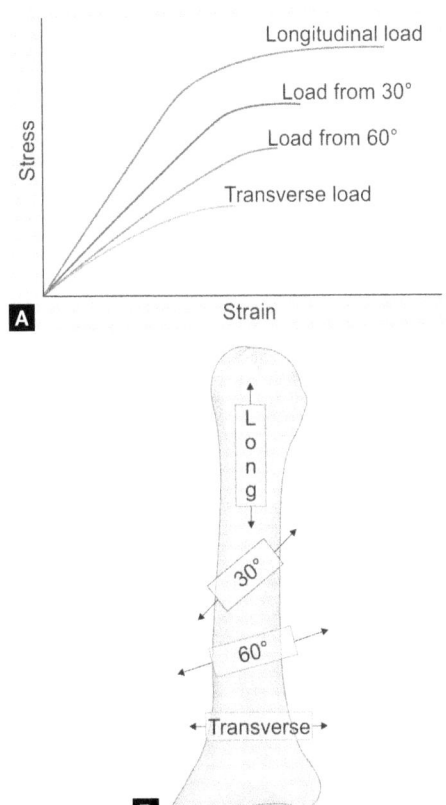

Figs. 3.8A and B: Anisotropic behavior of the bone

structure will return to its original dimensions immediately after removal of the load.

Point B, the yield point signifies end of elastic region. After this point, the material will no longer immediately return to its original state when the load is removed, although it may recover in time.

The region from B to C is the plastic region. In this region, deformation of the material will be permanent when the load is removed, although the structure is still intact

If loading continues into the plastic range, the material will continue to deform until it reaches the ultimate failure point, C. The load being applied when this point is reached is the failure load (**Fig. 3.9**).

The force values in the load-deformation curve depend on both size of the structure and its composition. A larger structure (cross-sectional area) will be able to withstand more forces and a longer structure will elongate further when a force is applied. The load-deformation curve is said to reflect the structural properties of the structure being treated.

Young's Modulus

The modulus of elasticity defines the mechanical behavior of the material and is a measure of the material's stiffness (resistance offered by the material to external load). A value of stiffness is found by dividing the load by the deformation for any two successive sets of points in the elastic range of the curve. Inverse of resistance is called compliance.

Load deformation and stress strain curve:

- **The first region of the curve from 0 to A is the toe region:** Very little force is required to deform the tissues—proteoglycans (PGs) and glycosaminoglycans (GAGs) allow interfibrillar sliding
  - Minimal amount of force produces a large amount of deformation (elongation)
  - Stress is low and strain is 1–2% range
  - Equated to the area in which an evaluator clinically tests the integrity of a ligament by the application of a tensile force or the slack in a tendon that must be taken up by the muscle before the tendon begins to move bone.
- **Second region of curve A to B is elastic region**—in this phase tissue is subjected to stress leading to tissue strain thus there is linear relationship between stress and strain.
  - Collagen fibrils are being elongated and resisting the applied force.

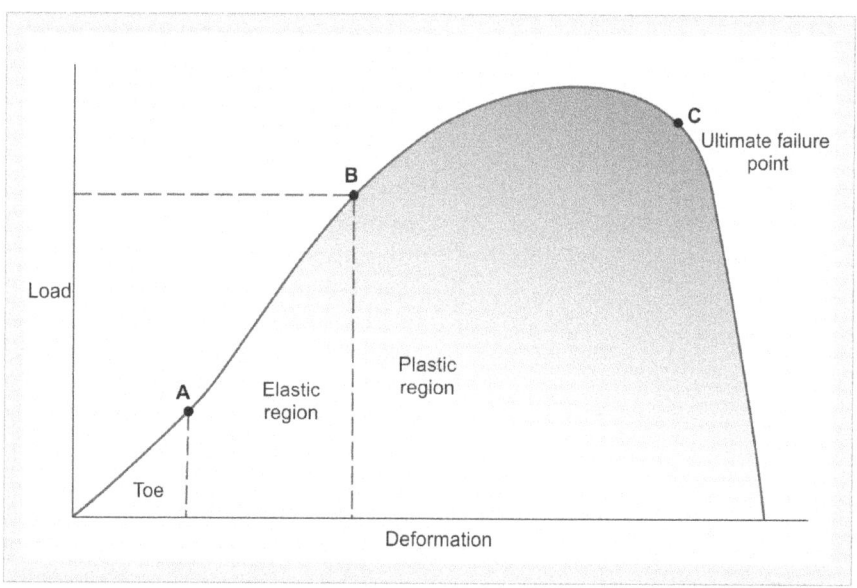

Fig. 3.9: Load deformation curve

- Thus, linear relationship of stress strain curve reflects the type of collagen, the fibril size and cross-linking among collagen molecules.
- When load is removed, ligament or tendon returns to its prestressed dimensions (is time-dependent).
- **Third region:** B to C (plastic region) progressive failure of collagen fibers begins and ligaments or tendon is no longer capable of returning to its original length—recovery will require considerable time.
- As plastic range is exceeded and force continues to be applied.
Remaining collagen fibrils rapidly experience increased stress and fail, creating overt failure or macrofailure of tissue
  - Tendon/ligaments—tearing and disruption of connective tissue fibers; this is called a rupture.
  - If failure occurs through a tearing off of the bony attachment of the ligament or tendon—called as avulsion.
  - When failure occurs in bone tissue—fracture
  - Low loading rates—create avulsion/fracture
  - Fast loading rates—creates midsubstance tears

Viscoelasticity

- Elasticity refers to materials ability to return to its original state after deformation (change in dimensions, i.e., length or shape) after removal of the deforming load
- Elastic qualities in connective tissue primarily depend on collagen and elastin content and organization
- When material is stretched work is done and energy increases, e.g., during walking.
- A lengthening (eccentric) muscle contraction stretches the attached tendon.
- This elastic energy is returned during the subsequent shortening (concentric) contraction of the muscle-tendon unit.
- Elasticity implies that length changes or deformations are directly proportional to the applied forces or loads.

Strain-rate Sensitivity

- Most tissues behave differently if loaded rapidly in comparison to slowly.
- If connective tissues have a load applied rapidly, a larger peak force can be applied to the tissue than if the load was applied slowly.
- Subsequent force relaxation will be larger than if the load is applied slowly.
- Creep will take longer to occur under conditions of rapid loading.

Hysteresis

- When force and length of tissues are measured, as force is applied (loaded) and removed (unloaded), the resulting load-deformation curves do not follow the same path.
- The energy gained as a result of lengthening work is not recovered 100% during the exchange from energy to shortening work
- Some energy is lost usually as heat.

Age-related Changes

- **Before adolescent:** Ligament strength < bone strength
- **Maturation:**
  - Increase in number and quality of cross-links
  - Increase in diameter of collagen fibril
  - Increase in tensile strength and stiffness
- **Aging:**
  - Decrease in number of collagen fibers
  - *Collagen fibril concentration in the collagen fibers:* Controversial
  - Decrease in tensile strength and stiffness.

Pregnancy and the Postpartum Period

- Increase in laxity of the tendons and ligaments in pubic area
- Decrease in tensile strength of tendons and ligaments during later stages of pregnancy and the postpartum period
- Decrease in stiffness during the early stage of postpartum period.

CHAPTER 4

Muscle Structure and Function

Chapter Outline

- Types of muscles
- Basic behavior of skeletal muscle
- Mechanical model of a muscle
- Structure and function of skeletal muscle
- Generation of cross-bridge interaction
- Characteristics of slow twitch and fast twitch muscle fibers
- Types of muscle contraction
- Motor unit
- Muscle function
- Passive and active insufficiency
- Classification of muscle
- Delayed onset muscle soreness
- Effects of immobilization, injury, and aging

INTRODUCTION

Skeletal muscles have primarily two role, namely—mobility that is movement of a bony lever around joint axis and stability meaning resisting extraneous movement of joint surfaces.

TYPES OF MUSCLES

- **Smooth muscles/involuntary muscles:** Smooth muscles are not directly under our conscious control. The walls of blood vessels are covered with smooth muscles thus allowing them to constrict or dilate in order to regulate blood flow. Also seen in walls of most internal organs allowing them to contract and relax.
- **Cardiac muscles:** Found only in the heart and not under conscious control. It is controlled by fine tuning of nervous and endocrine system.
- **Skeletal muscles:** Voluntary muscle can control by conscious. It attaches to and moves the skeleton.

Basic Behaviors of the Skeletal Muscle

- **Extensibility:** The ability of the muscle to elongate itself or to increase in length.
- **Elasticity:** The ability to return to its original length after its being elongated.
- **Irritability:** The ability of a muscle to respond to a stimulus.
- **Ability to develop tension:** The ability to reduce in length.
- Increase in tension does not imply decrease in muscle length.

Mechanical Model of a Muscle (Fig. 4.1)

- **Contractile component:** Muscle fiber
- **Series elastic component (SEC):** Tendon
- **Parallel elastic component (PEC):** Muscle membrane

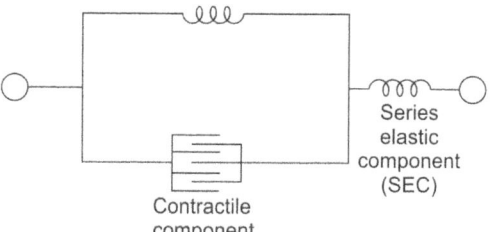

Fig. 4.1: Mechanical model of a muscle.

Elements of Muscle Structure

- Skeletal muscle is composed of contractile (muscle tissue) and noncontractile (connective tissue).
- Muscle tissue has the ability to develop tension in response to chemical, electrical, or mechanical stimuli.
- Connective tissue develops tension in response to passive loading.

STRUCTURE AND FUNCTION OF SKELETAL MUSCLE (FIG. 4.2)

- **Epimysium** is the connective tissue that covers the entire muscle.
- Small bundles of fiber wrapped in a connective tissue sheath. These bundles are called fascicles. Connective tissue surrounding each fascicule is called **perimysium.**
- Sheath of connective tissue covering each muscle fiber (single muscle cell) is called **endomysium.**
- Basic functional unit of myofibril is called **sarcomere.**
- The length of the longest muscle fibers is about 12 cm (4.7 in).
- **Sarcolemma:**
  - Muscle fiber is surrounded by a plasma membrane called sarcolemma.
  - Terminal part of muscle fiber involves the fusion of sarcolemma with the tendon that finally inserts into the bone
  - Tendons comprises fibrous connective tissue that transmits force from muscle fibers to bone.
- **Sarcoplasm:**
  - It is the cytoplasm of muscle fiber.
  - It forms a gelatine-like substance that fills the gaps between myofibrils.
  - It comprises glycogen, fats, minerals, proteins, and organelles.
- **Transverse tubules (T-tubules):**
  - Extensions of sarcolemma that pass laterally through the muscle fiber
  - Main function of transverse tubules is to transmit nerve impulses from sarcolemma to myofibrils.
  - Provides pathways from outside the muscle fiber to its interior, enabling the substance to enter and waste products to leave.
- **Sarcoplasmic reticulum (L-tubules):** Within the muscle fibers, sarcoplasmic reticulum form longitudinal network. It is the primary site where calcium ions are stored that is essential for muscle contraction.
- **Myofibril:** Contractile element of skeletal muscle
  - Skeletal muscle is called striated muscle because of alterations of dark region

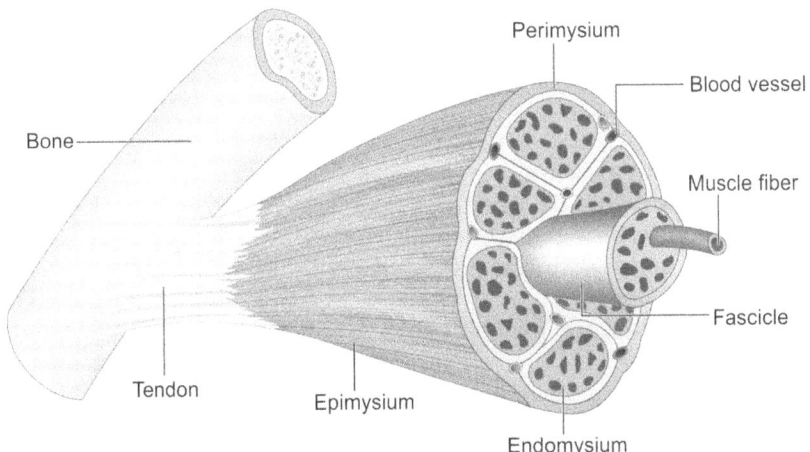

Fig. 4.2: Structure of skeletal muscle

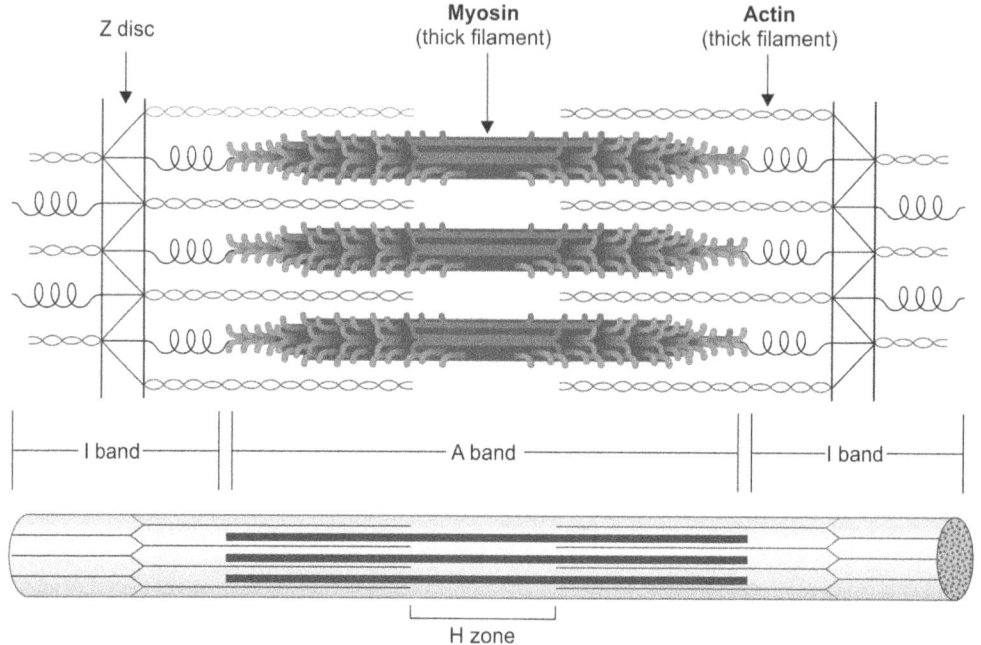

Fig. 4.3: Sarcomere

(known as A band) and light region (known as I band) that can be seen under a microscope **(Fig. 4.3)**.
- Light I band is interrupted by a dark stripe known as Z-disc.
- Sarcomere is the distance between two Z-lines.
- Sarcomere consists of:
  - I band: Thin filament
  - A band: Thick filament
  - H zone: Central portion of A band that appears only when the sarcomere is in a resting state.
- **Myosin filament (Fig. 4.4):**
  - Each myosin molecule is twisted together with protein strands
  - Myosin head—protrude out from myosin filament to form cross-bridges during muscle action with active sites on the actin filament
  - *Titin* stabilizes the myosin filaments in the longitudinal axis.
  - *Nebulin* is anchoring protein for actin, coextends with actin and myosin. It plays a role in mediating actin and myosin interactions.

- **Actin filament:**
  - Each actin filament contains active sites to which myosin head can bind
  - It is composed of three different protein molecules:
    1. Actin
    2. Tropomyosin coves active sites of actin at rest.
    3. Troponin pulls tropomyosin to allow myosin head to attach to active sites of actin.
  - *Tropomyosin and troponin* work together along with calcium ions to maintain relaxation and contraction of muscle.
  - End of each actin filament is attached to a Z-disc.
- **Muscle fiber action:**
  - Neuromuscular junction **(Fig. 4.5)** is the synapse/gap between motor nerve and muscle fiber. It transmits information between nervous system and muscular system.
  - *Motor unit:* Motor nerve and all the muscle fibers it innervates.

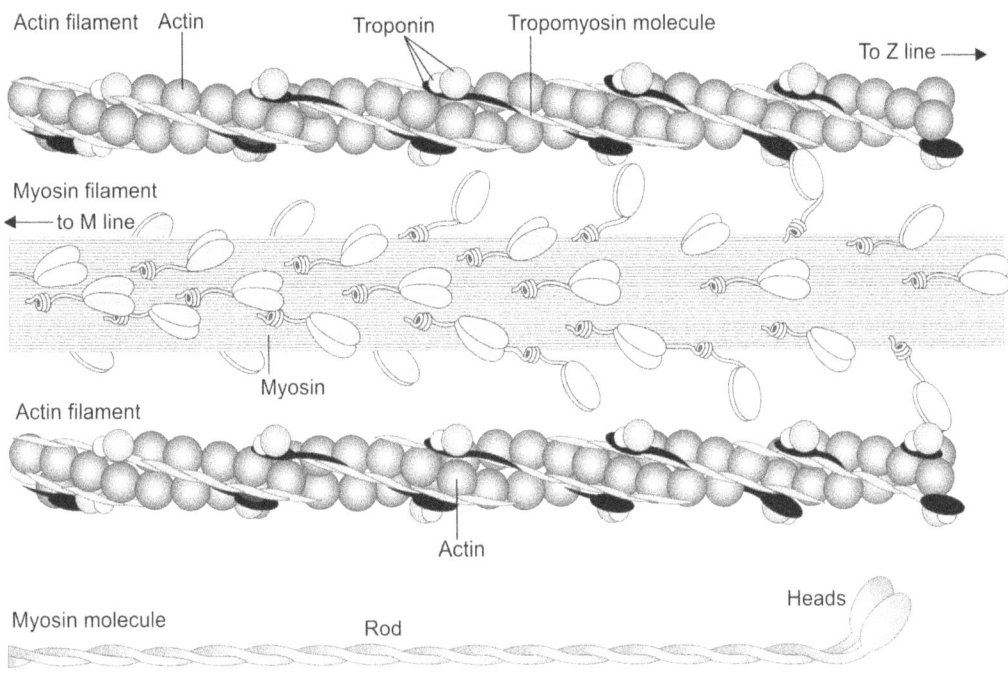

Fig. 4.4: Actin and myosin filaments.

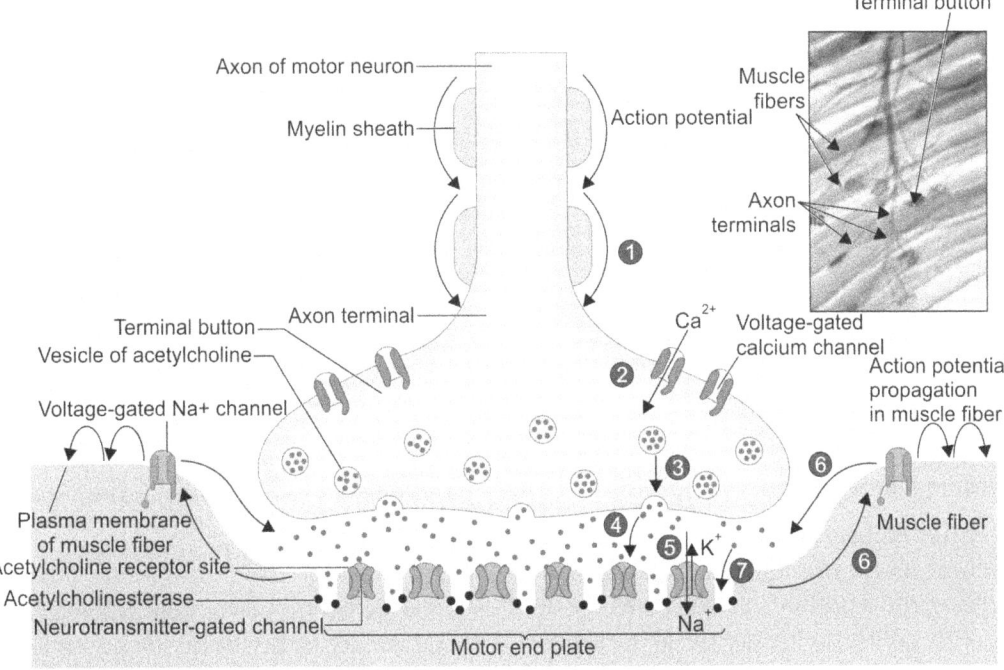

Fig. 4.5: Neuromuscular junction

GENERATION OF CROSS-BRIDGE INTERACTION

```
Neural impulse that arrives at the axon terminals
                    ↓
Nerve ending secrete a neurotransmitter substance
called acetylcholine (ACh) which binds with
receptor on sarcolemma
                    ↓
When enough ACh binds to the receptors an
electrical charge will be transmitted
throughout the length of the muscle fiber
                    ↓
Ion gates open in the muscle cell membrane
                    ↓
Allows sodium to enter—this is called as
depolarization
                    ↓
Thus resulting in firing or generating an
action potential
                    ↓
The electrical impulse travels through
the T and L tubules
                    ↓
Electrical charge cause sarcoplasmic
reticulum to release large amounts of calcium ions
                    ↓
In resting state, tropomyosin molecules cover the
active sites of actin filaments
                    ↓
Thus calcium released binds to troponin
on actin filaments
                    ↓
Troponin lifts the tropomyosin molecules off the
active sites on active filament
                    ↓
Thus allowing the myosin heads to attach to the
active sites on the actin filaments
                    ↓
Resulting in cross-bridge formation
```

Sliding Filament Theory (Fig. 4.7)

- After myosin head tilts, it breaks away from active sites of actin, rotates back to its original position, and attaches to a new active site further along the actin filament.
- Repeated attachments and power strokes causes the filaments to slide past one another

- This process continues until the ends of myosin filaments reach the Z-discs.
- This is termed as sliding filament theory.

```
When the myosin bridges are activated
                    ↓
They bind strongly with actin filaments
                    ↓
This causes the myosin head to tilt
(called power stroke)
toward the arm of the cross-bridge
                    ↓
This drags the actin and myosin
filaments in opposite direction
                    ↓
Leading to muscle contraction
```

Energy for Muscle Action

- Myosin head contains a binding site for adenosine triphosphate (ATP).
- The ATP splits into ADP (adenosine diphosphate) and Pi (inorganic phosphorous) and energy.
- The energy released from this breakdown of ATP is used to bind the myosin head to the actin filaments.
- Thus, ATP is the chemical source of energy for muscle action.

End of Muscle Action

- Muscle action ends when calcium ions are pumped back into the sarcoplasmic reticulum for storage.
- This leads to relaxation and creation of weak binding site between the myosin heads and active sites, also requires energy supplied by ATP.

SKELETAL MUSCLE AND EXERCISE

Slow twitch and fast twitch muscle fibers **(Table 4.1)**:

- Slow twitch (ST) takes approximately 110 ms to reach peak tension when stimulated
- Fast twitch (FT) reaches peak tension in about 50 ms and can create more force than slow twitch fibers.

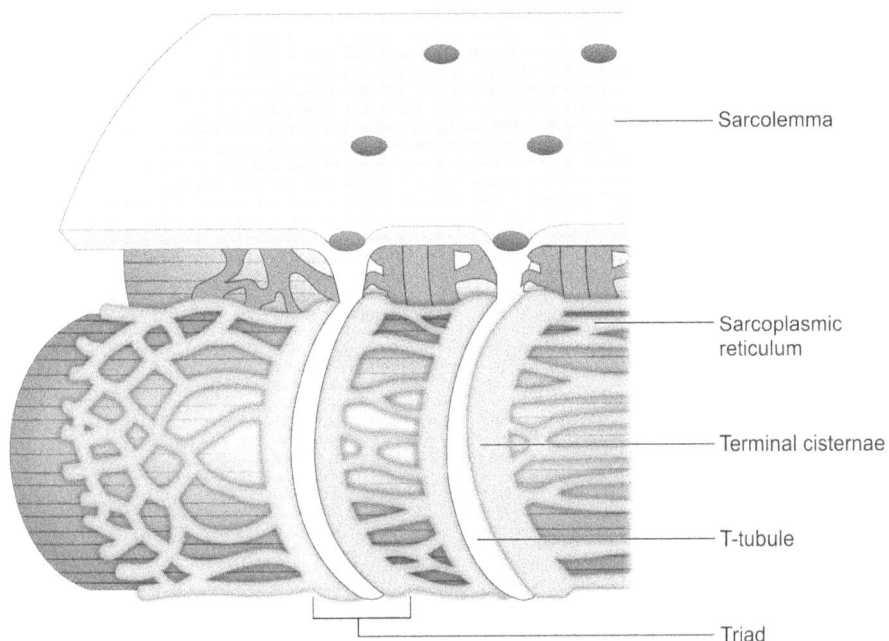

Fig. 4.6: Internal structure of skeletal muscle

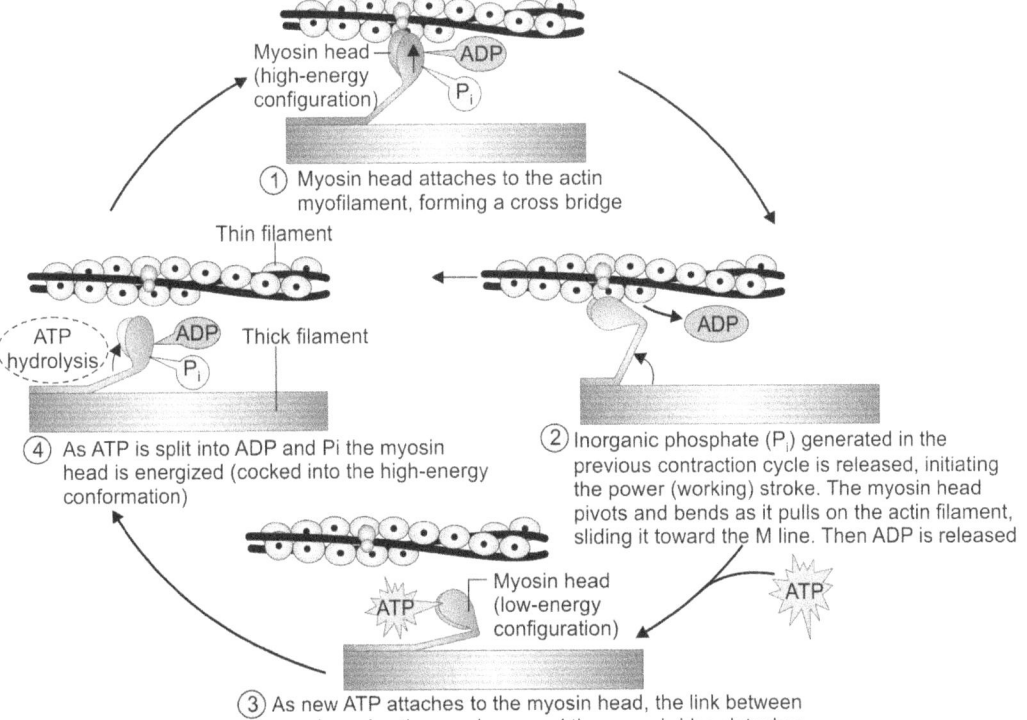

Fig. 4.7: Sliding filament theory

▲ **Table 4.1:** Classification of muscle fiber types.

Characteristics	Slow twitch (ST)	Fast twitch a (FTa)	Fast twitch b (FTb)
	Type I	Type IIa	Type IIb
	Slow oxidative	Fast oxidative glycolytic	Fast glycolytic
Oxidative capacity	High	Moderately high	Low
Glycolytic capacity	Low	High	Highest
Contractile speed	Slow	Fast	Fast
Resistance to fatigue	High	Moderate	Low
Motor unit strength	Low	High	High
Fiber per motor neuron	10–180	300–800	300–800
Motor neuron size	Small	Large	Large
Nerve conduction velocity	Slow	Fast	Fast
Contraction speed (ms)	110	50	50
Type of myosin ATPase	Slow	Fast	Fast
Sarcoplasmic reticulum development	Low	High	High
Motor unit force	Low	High	High
Aerobic capacity	High	Moderate	Low
Anaerobic capacity	Low	High	High

Figure 4.6 shows internal structure of skeletal muscle.

Types of fast twitch fibers are:
- Fast twitch type a (FTa)—most frequently recruited
- Fast twitch type b (FTb)
- Fast twitch type c (FTc)—least used
- Therefore, most muscles are composed of roughly 50% slow twitch, 25% FTa, 25% FTb, and 1 to 3% FTc.

Characteristics of slow twitch and fast twitch fibers:
- **ATPase:**
  - ST fibers have a slow form of myosin ATPase.
  - FT fibers have a fast form of myosin ATPase.
  - Myosin ATPase is the enzyme that splits ATP to release to drive contraction or allow relaxation.
  - As a result FT fibers have energy for contraction more quickly than do ST fibers.
- **Sarcoplasmic reticulum:**
  - FT fibers comprise highly developed sarcoplasmic reticulum than do ST fibers.
  - FT fibers can distribute calcium ions more into the cell. Resulting in faster speed of action of FT fibers.
  - Speed of action in FT fibers is 5 to 6 times faster than ST fibers
  - Thus, the predominance of FT fibers in leg muscles of sprinters is higher than ST fibers.
- **Motor unit:**
  - Motor neuron in an ST motor unit has small cell body and innervates a cluster of 10 to 180 muscle fibers.
  - Motor neuron of FT motor unit has a larger cell body and more axons and innervates from 300 to 800 muscle fibers.
  - Thus, peak power of FT fibers is higher than ST fibers.
  - Also FT motor fibers reach peak tension faster and generate for force than ST fibers.

Types of muscle action/muscle contraction:
- **Concentric action (Figs. 4.8A to C):**
  - Shortening of the muscle
  - The actin filaments are pulled closer together. Because joint movement is

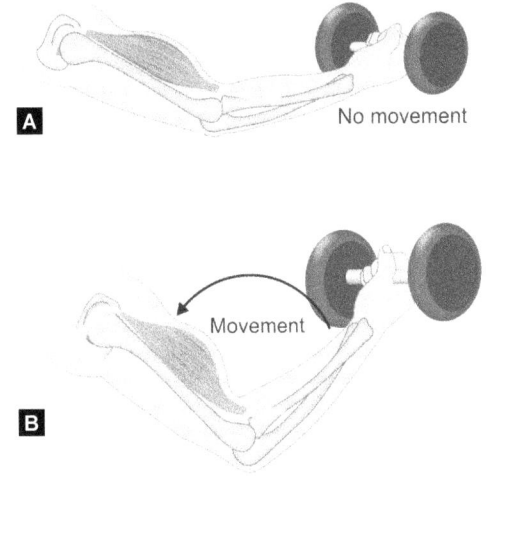

Figs. 4.8A to C: Types of muscles contraction. (A) Isometric contraction (muscle contracts but not shorten); (B) Concentric contraction; (C) Eccentric concentration

- Occurs when muscle actively resists motion created by an external force (such as gravity). That is external force more than internal force.
- Tension is generated by the muscle as cross-bridges are reformed.
- Work done is called negative work because work is done on the muscle rather than by the muscle.
- Speed of lengthening increases
- Tension increases
- **Isotonic contraction:** Refers to equal or constant tension.
- **Muscle action under controlled conditions:**
  - *Isokinetic exercise:* Constant velocity; resistance produced by isokinetic device is directly proportional to torque produced by a muscle at all points in the range of motion, e.g., isokinetic device such as Biodex.
  - *Isoinertial exercise:* Muscle acts against a constant load or resistance and measured torque is determined while the constant load is accelerating or decelerating.

If torque produced by muscle equals the resistance—muscle contracts isometrically.

If torque produced by muscle is greater than the resistance—muscle shortens (concentric) **(Fig. 4.9)**.

If torque produced by muscle is less than the resistance—muscle eccentrically contracts.

produced, concentric actions are said to be dynamic actions.
- Internal force more than external force
- Positive work is done because joints move through a range of motion.
- Speed of shortening decreases
- Tension increases
- **Static isometric muscle action:**
  - Muscles act without moving.
  - Its length remains static (unchanged).
  - Its joint angle does not change.
  - In static action, the external and internal forces are equal.
- **Eccentric action:**
  - Dynamic action, i.e., lengthening of muscle
  - Thin (actin) filaments are pulled farther away from thick (myosin) filaments and cross-bridges are broken and reformed as the muscle lengthens.

Motor Unit (Fig. 4.10)

It consists of alpha motor neurons and all the muscle fibers it innervates.
- Muscles that control fine movements or make small adjustments are the small sized motor units that have small cell bodies and small diameter axons. They are primarily type I fibers.
- Muscles that produce large increments in force and large movements are large-size motor units that have large cell bodies and large diameter axons. These are primarily type II fibers.

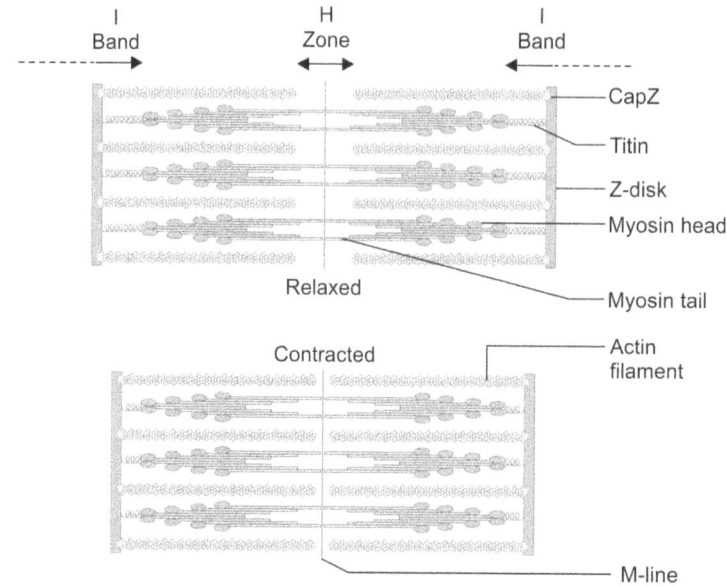

Fig. 4.9: Concentric contraction

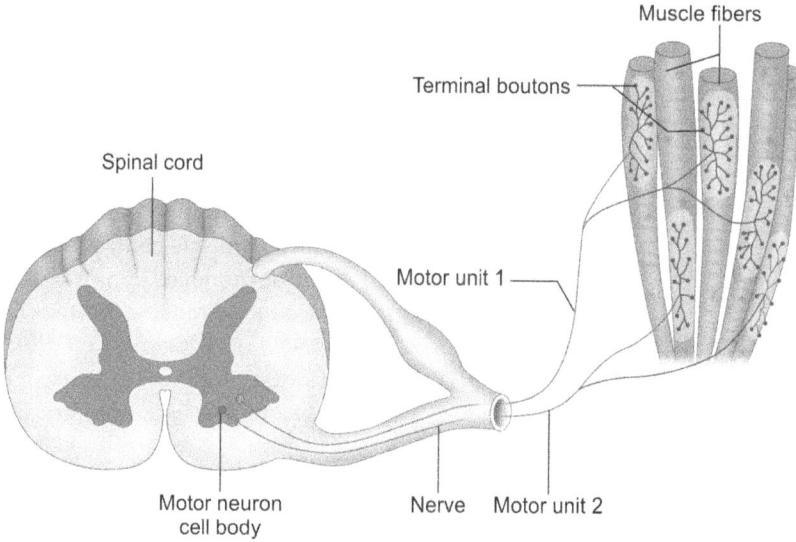

Fig. 4.10: Motor unit

Recruitment of Motor Units

Isometric muscle contraction:
- During an isometric muscle contraction, the motor units with small cell bodies and few motor fibers are recruited first.
- As force increases the large motor units are recruited.
- This recruitment strategy is energy conserving. Recruitment strategy may be based on previous experience, nature of the task and type of muscle contraction.

Muscle Architecture: Size, Arrangement and Length

Two important architectural characteristics that affect muscle function are fiber length and physiologic cross-sectional area (PCSA).

Fiber length (or number of sarcomeres): Long fibers are able to move the bony lever to which it is attached through a greater distance than is a muscle with short fibers. Muscle fiber length and moment arm (MA) affects the muscle length-shortening relationship. Amount of force is directly proportional to number of sarcomeres, e.g., quadriceps have larger physiologic cross-sectional area thus designed for greater force production. Hamstrings have longer fibers thus designed for movements requiring a large range of motion.

Fasciculi may be parallel to long axis or may be at an angle to long axis or may spiral around long axis. Muscles that have parallel fiber arrangement are called strap or fusiform muscle example sternocleidomastoid muscle. Muscles with parallel fiber arrangement will produce greater range of motion of a bony lever than with muscles with a pennate fiber arrangement. Fusiform has longer fiber length than pennate muscles **(Fig. 4.11)**. Muscles that have fiber arrangement oblique to muscles long axis called pennate muscles. A muscle is said to have pennate fiber arrangement if it forms an angle to the longitudinal axis of the muscle example rectus femoris, deltoid, etc. The greater the angle of pennation, smaller amount of force is transmitted to the tendon. The angle of pennation is directly proportional to the tension that develops within the muscle. Thus as the angle of pennation increases, it causes progressive increase in tension within the muscle. The pennate muscles namely are unipennate, bipennate, and multipennate. Example of unipennate muscles is flexor pollicis longus with obliquely set fascicles fan out on only one side of a central muscle tendon. Example of bipennate muscle is gastrocnemius with obliquely set on both sides of central tendon. Examples of multipennate muscles are soleus and subscapularis, oblique fascicles converge on several tendons.

MUSCLE FUNCTION

Passive Tension

It is the tension developed in parallel elastic component of the muscle. It is generated when the muscle is lengthened beyond the slack length of the tissues.

Total amount of tension developed during active muscle contraction is sum of passive tension (noncontractile) + active tension (contractile).

Active Tension

It refers to tension developed by the contractile elements of the muscle. It is initiated by cross-bridge formation and movement of thick and thin filaments.

Amount of active tension depends on neural factors and mechanical properties.

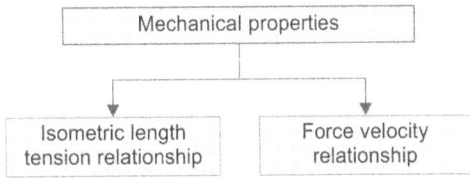

Neural factors include frequency, number, and size of motor units that are firing.
- Isometric length tension relationship at optimal sarcomere length of muscle fibers contributes to maximal isometric tension.
  - Maximal isometric tension is developed when the muscle fiber is at optimal sarcomere length as actin and myosin filaments are positioned such that maximum number of cross-bridges within the sarcomere can be formed.

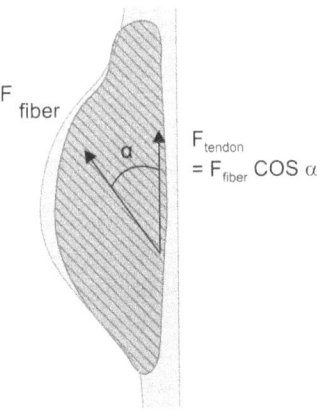

Fig. 4.11: Pennate muscle

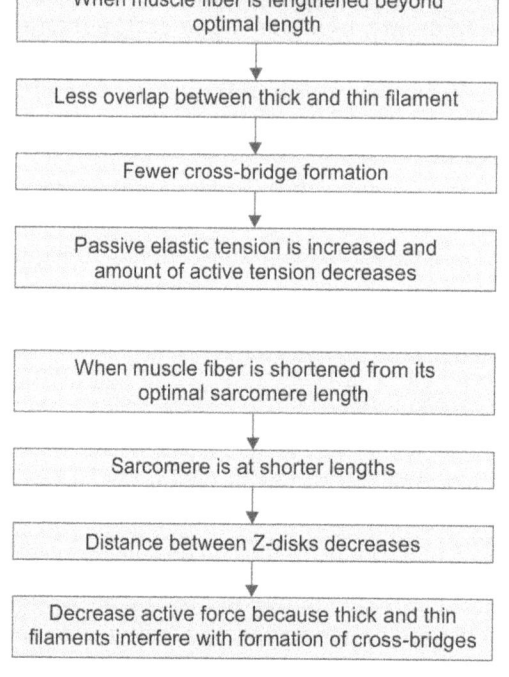

- **Force velocity relationship:**
  - Speed of shortening that is rate at which actin and myosin slide to form and reform cross-bridges
  - It is the relationship between velocity of muscle contraction and force production.

Note:
- Concentric contraction—shortening speed decreases, tension in muscle increases.
- Isometric contraction—speed of shortening is zero and tension is greater than concentric contraction
- Eccentric contraction—speed of lengthening increases and tension increases.

Types of muscle contraction	Speed	Tension
Concentric	Speed of shortening decreases	Increases
Isometric	Speed of shortening is zero	Tension > concentric
Eccentric	Speed of lengthening increases	Tension increases

CLASSIFICATION OF MUSCLE

Based on Muscle Role

Prime mover (agonist): Role is to produce a desired motion at a joint, e.g., flexion of elbow—biceps brachii are prime movers.
- Muscles that are directly opposite to desired motion (extensors), i.e., triceps is called **antagonists**.
- If agonist and antagonist contract simultaneously then co-contraction occurs.
  Muscle that helps agonist to perform a desired action are called **synergists,** e.g., if flexion of wrist is desired.
  - Flexor carpi radialis and flexor carpi ulnaris are agonists or prime movers.
  - Finger flexors are synergists that may directly help wrist flexion
  - Wrist extensors are antagonists.

Application of the length tension relationship:
- It occurs only in the muscles that cross more than one joint (two-joint or multijoint muscles).
- A decrease in the torque produced by the muscle when full range of motion is attempted simultaneously at all joint crossed by multijoint muscle. Thus, decrease in torque is called active insufficiency.

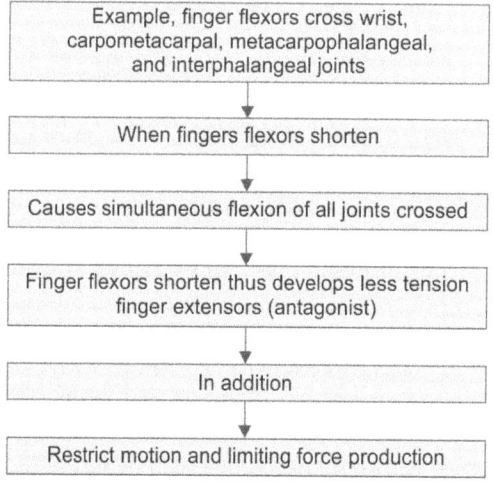

Chapter 4 | Muscle Structure and Function

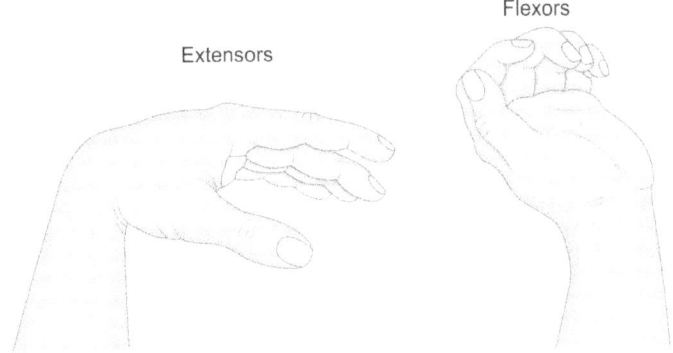

Fig. 4.12: Passive insufficiency

Based on Muscle Architecture
- Knee extensors short fiber length and large physiological cross sectional area.
- Knee flexors have longer fibers and smaller physiological cross sectional area.

Based on Length of Moment Arm
Length of moment arm and fiber length determine torque and range of motion through which muscle move the joint.

Factors Affecting Muscle Function
- **Type of joints and location of muscle attachments:**
    - Structure of the joint determines type of motion and range of motion (flexion and extension)
    - Muscles location determines which motion muscle will perform, for example, anterior aspects flexors and posterior aspect extensors
    - Muscles which distal attachments are close to joint axis are able to produce wide range of motion and muscles which distal attachments are at a distance from joint axis, provide stability.
- **Number of joints crossed by the muscle:**
    - Single joint muscles are recruited during activities that involve concentric and isometric contractions.
    - Multijoint muscles are recruited to control fine regulation of torque during dynamic movements involving eccentric more than concentric muscle actions.

- **Passive insufficiency (Fig. 4.12):** Mostly seen in muscles that cross two joint or multijoint muscles.

    If person's elbow is placed on the table with forearm in vertical position and hand is allowed to drop forward into wrist flexion
    ↓
    Fingers tend to flex (flexion of fingers)
    ↓
    Due to insufficient length of finger extensors that are being stretched over flexed wrist
    ↓
    This insufficient length is termed as passive insufficiency
    ↓
    If person moves wrist backward into wrist extension
    ↓
    Fingers tend to flex (flexion of fingers)
    ↓
    As a result of insufficient length of finger flexors

- **Sensory receptors:**
    - Two important sensory receptors are Golgi tendon organ and muscle spindle
    - Golgi tendon organ—located at myotendinous junction (sensitive to tension) and activated by either active muscle contraction or by excessive passive stretch of muscle.
    - Muscle spindle consists of 2–10 muscle fibers (intrafusal fibers). That is sensitive to length and velocity of lengthening of muscle fibers (extrafusal fibers).

These send information about state of stretch. Muscle spindle sends message to muscle to contract when tendon of a muscle is tapped with a hammer.
Deep tendon reflex (DTR)/muscle spindle reflex (MSR)/simple stretch reflex

```
┌─────────────────────────────────────────────┐
│ Quick stretch of muscle caused by tapping   │
│ the tendon activates the muscle spindle     │
└─────────────────────────────────────────────┘
                      ↓
┌─────────────────────────────────────────────┐
│ Muscle responds by a brief contraction      │
└─────────────────────────────────────────────┘
```

- Thus, both muscle spindle and Golgi tendon help protect the muscle from injury by monitoring changes in muscle length.

EFFECT OF IMMOBILIZATION, INJURY, AND AGING

Immobilization:
- Depends on the position of shortened or lengthened, percentage of fiber types, and immobilization period
- In shortened position, it produces following structural changes:
  - Decrease number of sarcomeres
  - Increase sarcomere length
  - Increase amount of perimysium
  - Thickening of endomysium
  - Increase amount of collagen
  - Increase ration of connective tissue to muscle fiber tissue
  - Loss of weight and muscle atrophy
- In lengthened position:
  - Increase number of sarcomeres
  - Decrease in length
  - Muscle hypertrophy that may be followed by atrophy

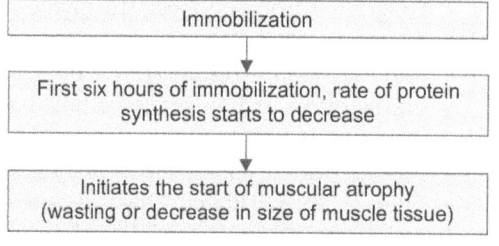

- Lack of muscle use results in muscle atrophy and loss of muscle protein
- Strength decreases during the 1st week of immobilization
- Muscle atrophy is associated with decrease neuromuscular activity of the immobilized muscle.
- Immobilization affects slow twitch muscle fibers.
- Muscle atrophy causes decrease in cross-sectional fiber area and percentage of slow twitch fibers.
- Recovery period is longer than the period of immobilization.

Injury:
- Overuse causes injury to tendons, ligaments, bursae, nerves, cartilages, and muscles.

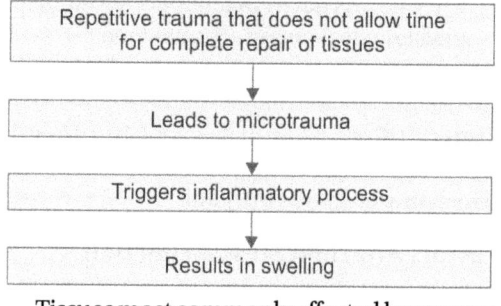

Tissues most commonly affected by overuse injuries are musculotendinous unit.
- **Muscle strain:** Muscle usually fails at the junction between the muscle and tendon.
- **Eccentric exercise-induced muscle injury:** Injury to muscles usually occurs while performing eccentric exercises. Delayed onset muscle soreness (DOMS) reaches a peak of 2-4 days after exercise. Histochemical studies show collagen breakdown.
- **DOMS:** DOMS includes structural damage to muscle cells and inflammatory reactions within the muscles.

Structural Damage

- Muscle soreness felt a day or two after a heavy bout of exercise.
- Because the pain does not occur immediately, it is called as delayed onset muscle soreness.

Chapter 4 | Muscle Structure and Function

- Eccentric training is the primary indicator of delayed onset muscle soreness.
- It is associated with muscle damage due to increase concentration of muscle enzymes in blood after intense exercise.
- Muscle tissue breakdown might occur.
- During eccentric actions or stretching of tightened muscle fibers, the Z discs are pulled apart. Thus responsible for localized pain, tenderness, and swelling that are associated with DOMS.

Inflammatory Reactions

- White blood cells tend to increase.
- Mononucleated cells in muscle are activated.
- Neutrophils invade the injury site and release cytokines which attract and activate additional inflammatory cells.
- Microphages invade the damaged muscle fibers thus removing debris through a process known as phagocytosis.
- Soreness results from inflammatory reactions in the muscle.
  Sequence of events in DOMS:
  - Armstrong's proposed model of the sequence of events that cause DOMS includes:
    - Structural damage
    - Impaired calcium homeostasis leading to necrosis
    - Accumulation of irritants
    - Increased macrophage activity
  DOMS and performance:
  - When an individual experiences DOMS, there is reduction in the force generating capacity of the affected muscle

Eccentric muscle action (downhill running)

↓

High muscle forces damage sarcolemma causing release of cytosolic enzymes and myoglobin

Contd...

Contd...

↓

Damage to the muscle contractile and noncontractile structures

↓

Metabolites (e.g., calcium) accumulate to abnormal levels in the muscle cell to produce more cell damage and reduced force capacity

- Loss in strength is due to:
  - The physical disruption of muscle
  - Failure within the excitation-contraction coupling process
  - Loss of contractile protein
- Muscle glycogen resynthesis is also impaired when a muscle is damaged.

Reducing the negative effects of DOMS:
- Muscle soreness can be prevented or minimized by:
  - Reducing the eccentric component of training
  - Beginning training with low intensity exercises and gradually increasing it
  - Beginning with a high exhaustive bout of eccentric action exercise, which will cause much soreness initially but will decrease future pain
- *Aging:* Fiber number and fiber type changes—skeletal muscle strength decreases. Decrease in number and size of Type II fibers and increase in Type I fibers. Decrease in number of motor units.

Connective tissue damage: Increase amount of connective tissue within endomysium and perimysium

↓

Results in decrease range of motion and increase muscle stiffness

- Aging results in decrease muscle strength, loss in muscle power thus risk of falls increases.

SECTION 2

Joint Segments in Detail

SECTION OUTLINE

- Temporomandibular Joint
- Shoulder Joint
- Elbow Complex
- Wrist and Hand Complex
- Hip Joint
- Knee Joint
- Ankle and Foot Complex
- Vertebral Column

CHAPTER 5

Temporomandibular Joint

Chapter Outline
- Stabilization
- Ligaments
- Osteokinematics
- Arthrokinematics
- Kinetics
- Pathomechanics

INTRODUCTION

- Most continuously used joint—talking, eating, and swallowing
- Temporomandibular joint (TMJ) is unique—horseshoe-shaped mandible articulates with the temporal bone at each end giving it two completely separate but solidly connected joints.
- Each TMJ formed by the articulation of the **condyle of the mandible** with the **articular eminence** of the **temporal bone** and an interposed **articular disc (Figs. 5.1 and 5.2)**.

OSTEOLOGY

Individual bones:
- Mandible
- Maxillae
- Temporal
- Zygomatic
- Sphenoid
- Hyoid

Are all related to the structure and function of the TMJ.

Mandible **(Fig. 5.3)**
- The largest of the facial bones
- **Very mobile:** Suspended from cranium by muscles, ligaments, and capsule of TMJ
- Muscles of mastication attach directly or indirectly to it

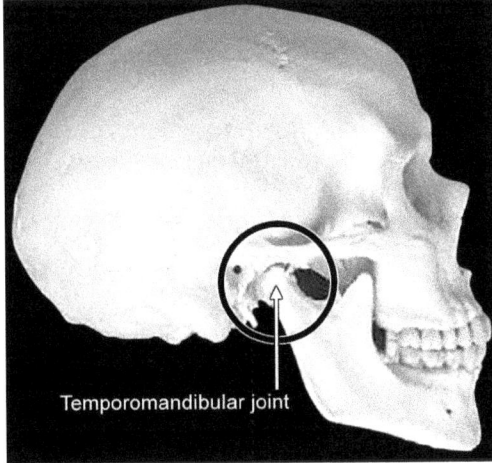

Fig. 5.1: Temporomandibular joint—articulation between mandibular condyle and articular eminence of temporal bone

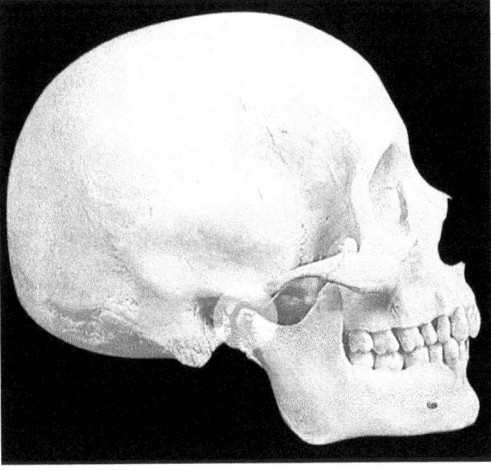

Fig. 5.2: Mandibular condyle sits in mandibular fossa

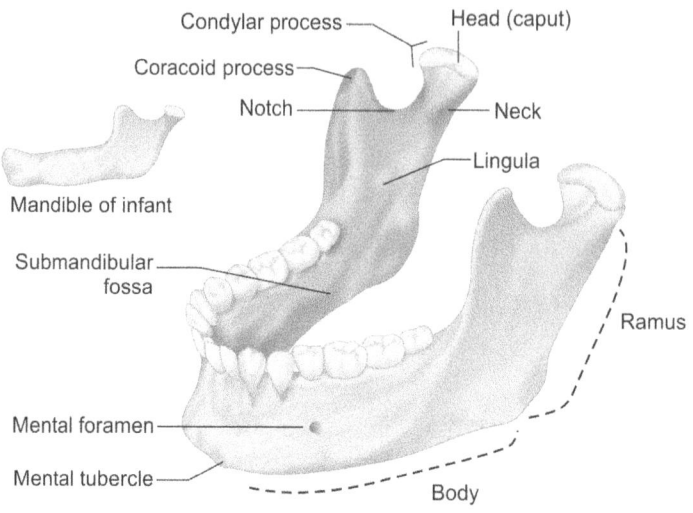

Fig. 5.3: Parts of mandible

Maxillae (**Fig. 5.4**)
- Right and left fuse to form a single maxilla or upper jaw
- Fixed within the skull

Temporal bone (**Fig. 5.5B**)
- Mandibular fossa
- Articular eminence
- Postglenoid tubercle
- Styloid process
- Zygomatic process
- Zygomatic bone

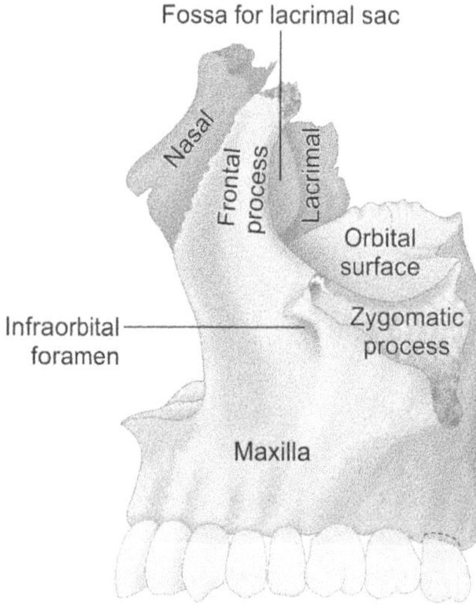

- Constitute the major part of the cheeks and the lateral orbits of the eyes
- Temporal process of zygomatic bone contributes to anterior zygomatic arch
- A large part of masseter muscle attaches to it

Sphenoid bone (**Fig. 5.5A**)
- Does not contribute to the structure of the TMJ but provides proximal attachments for the medial and lateral pterygoid muscles
- **Parts**
  - Greater wing
  - Medial pterygoid plate
  - Lateral pterygoid plate

Hyoid bone
- U-shaped
- Located at base of throat
- Suspended primarily by its bilateral stylohyoid ligaments.
- Several muscles involved with moving of the tongue, swallowing, and speaking attach to it.

These bones and other bones of skull are shown in **Figure 5.6**.

ARTHROLOGY

Glenohumeral joint is the most mobile joint in the human body, i.e., it moves at a varied degree of angle in all the planes.

Fig. 5.4: Maxilla

Chapter 5 | Temporomandibular Joint

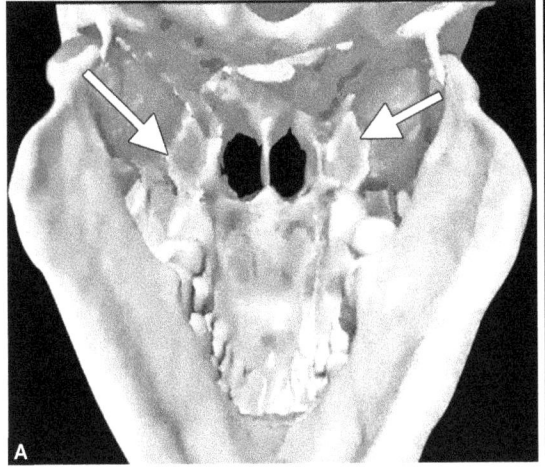
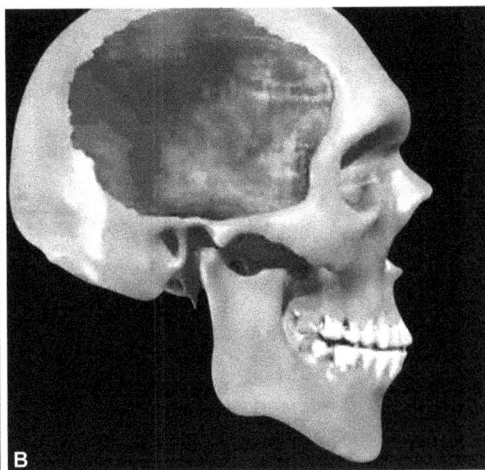

Figs. 5.5A and B: (A) Sphenoid bone; (B) Temporal bone

Type of Joint
Condylar type of synovial joint.

Degrees of freedom:
- Two rotatory degrees of freedom (depression-elevation, lateral deviation)
- One translatory degree of freedom (protrusion-retrusion)

Articulating surface:
- **Proximal articulating surface:** Articular eminence of temporal bone
- **Distal articulating surface:** Mandibular condyle

Close pack position:
Clenched teeth

Loose pack position:
Mouth opening

Neutral position:
Anatomic position

STABILIZATION

The stabilization of the joint can be discussed in two parts:
1. Static stability
2. Dynamic stability
   The factors responsible for the stability of the TMJ are:
- Joint design ⎫
- Articular disc ⎬ Static Stabilizers
- Joint capsule ⎭
- Ligaments
- Muscles—dynamic stabilizers

Joint Design
The articulating structure is in the form of a condyle and socket. This itself serves as a stable structure.

Articular Disc (Fig. 5.7)
- Cushions the potentially large and repetitive muscle forces inherent to mastication
- Separates the joint into two synovial joint cavities
- Biconcave allows the convex surface of the condyle and the convex surface of the articular eminence to remain congruent throughout the motion.
- Anterior and posterior portions are innervated and vascular, middle band is not innervated and avascular.

Functions
- Increased congruence
- Shape of the disc (i.e., thin in the center and wider anteriorly and posteriorly) allows greater flexibility of the disc so it can conform to the articular surfaces as the condyle first rotates and then translates over the articular eminence.
- Self-centering mechanism

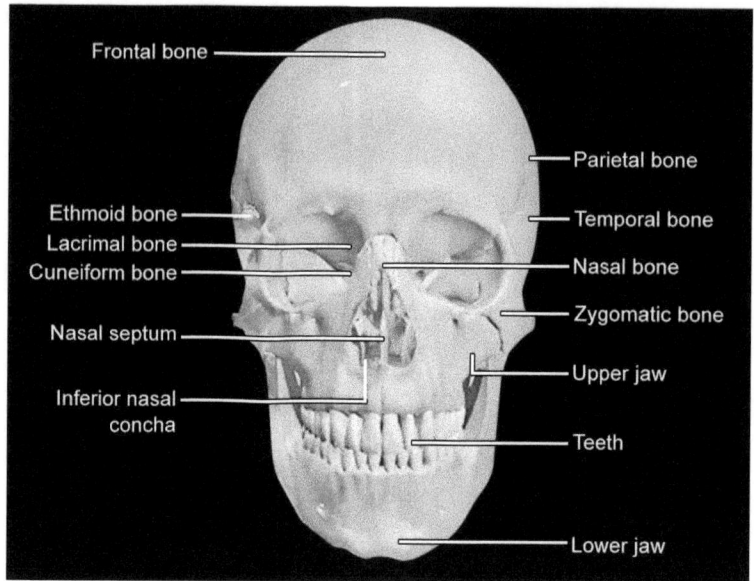

Fig. 5.6: Parts of the skull

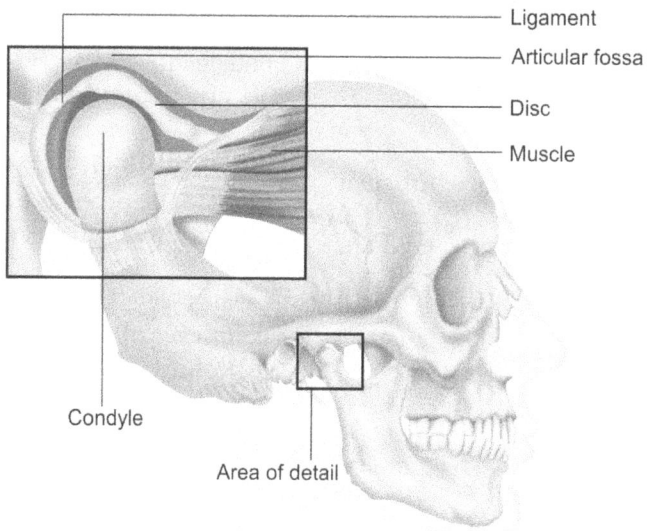

Fig. 5.7: Temporomandibular joint depicting articular disc, muscle

Resting Position

Mouth slightly opens, the lips together, and the teeth not in contact.

Capsular Pattern

Limitation of mouth opening.

CAPSULE AND LIGAMENTS

The temporomandibular joint (TMJ) is the most complex joint in the body. It is disc permits different types of jaw movement and different degrees of mouth opening, including (1) hinge action, and (2) gliding action **(Fig. 5.8)**.

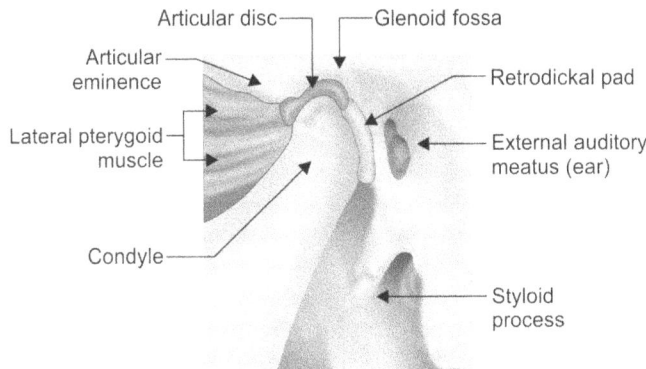

Fig. 5.8: Temporomandibular joint internal view

Capsule (Fig. 5.9)

- **Capsule is attached:**
  - *Superior:* Rim of mandibular fossa, as far ant as articular eminence
  - *Inferior:* Collateral ligaments that form the periphery of the articular disc
  - *Anterior:* Tendon of sup head lateral pterygoid muscle
- Not well-defined
- Short capsular fibers running from temporal bone to disc and from disc to neck of condyle
- Portion of capsule above disc is loose and below it is tight
- Thin and loose in anterior, medial and posterior aspects, firm laterally
- Highly vascular and innervated—good information about position and movement
- Capsule and ligaments

Ligaments (Fig. 5.9)

- Temporomandibular ligament (lateral ligament)
- Stylomandibular ligament
- Sphenomandibular ligament

Temporomandibular Ligament
- Strong
- **2 parts**
  - *Outer oblique:* Limits downward and posterior motion of mandible as well as limits rotation of condyle
  - *Inner:* Resists posterior motion of condyle thus protects retrodiscal pad
- Neither limit forward translation of condyle or disc but do limit lateral translation.

Stylomandibular Ligament
- Band of deep cervical fascia
- Function controversial
  - Limits protrusion of the jaw
  - Draws the disc posteriorly during closing
  - No function.

Sphenomandibular Ligament
- Spine of sphenoid bone to middle surface of ramus of mandible
- **Function controversial:** Suspends the mandible and checks excessive forward translation of mandible

Joint Articulation

- The disc divides the joint into two separate joint spaces; upper and lower
- Each has its own synovial lining
- Synovial fluid provides nutrition.

Upper joint
- Gliding joint
- Formed by articular bone and superior surface of articular disc
- Translatory movement

Lower joint
- Hinge joint
- Formed by anterior surface of condyle of mandible and inferior surface of articular disc
- Condyle and disc are firmly attached at medial and lateral poles of condyle, allow for free rotation of disc on condyle or

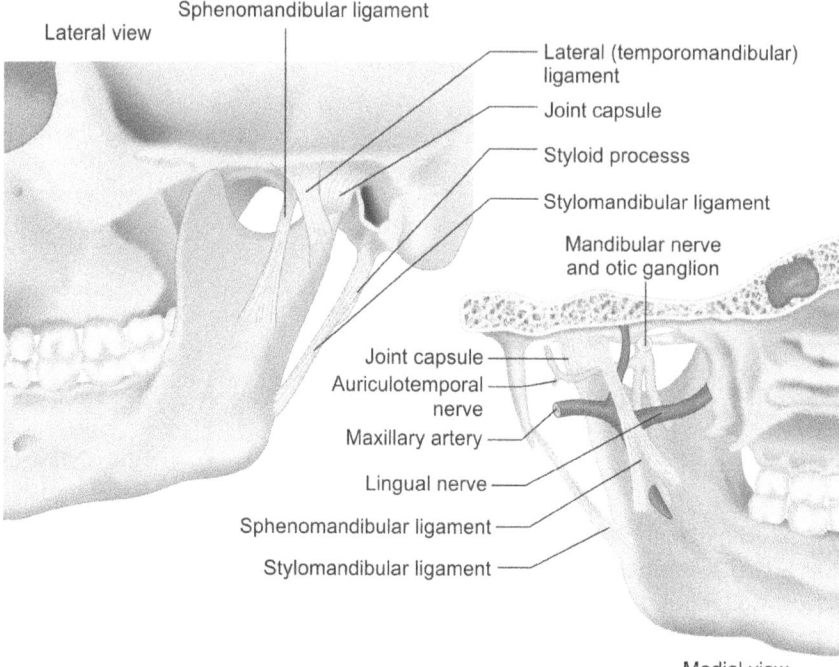

Fig. 5.9: Temporomandibular joint (medial and lateral views)

condyle under disc around axis passing through both poles.
- Firm medial and lateral attachments b/w disc and condyle cause both to translate forward (glide) together as a unit with minimal translation between the two.
- Capsular pattern of TMJ—mouth opening is more limited.
- Resting position of TMJ—mouth slightly open, teeth not in contact but the lips closed.
- Closed-packed position—clenching teeth is in closed packed position.

OSTEOKINEMATICS AND ARTHROKINEMATICS

Mandibular Motions
- Mandibular depression (mouth opening)
- Mandibular elevation (mouth closing) **(Fig. 5.10A)**
- Mandibular protrusion (jutting the chin forward)
- Mandibular retrusion (sliding the teeth backward)
- Lateral deviation (sliding the teeth to either side)

Planes and Axis
- Mandibular depression and elevation happens in sagittal plane
- Mandibular protrusion and retrusion happens in transverse plane
- Lateral deviation occurs in frontal plane.

Mandibular Depression/Jaw Opening (Fig. 5.10B)
- **Max opening:** Yawning and singing
- **In adult:** Opening is average around 50 mm (3 knuckles of PIP joint) mastication: 18 mm–36 mm (2 knuckles of PIP joint)
- The arthrokinematic motions in this joint are both gliding and rolling. Gliding happens in upper compartment while rolling happens in lower compartment.

Rotation and Translation
See **Figures 5.11A and B**.

Mandibular Elevation/Jaw Closing
Jaw closure (mandible elevation) is accomplished through contraction of the mandibular

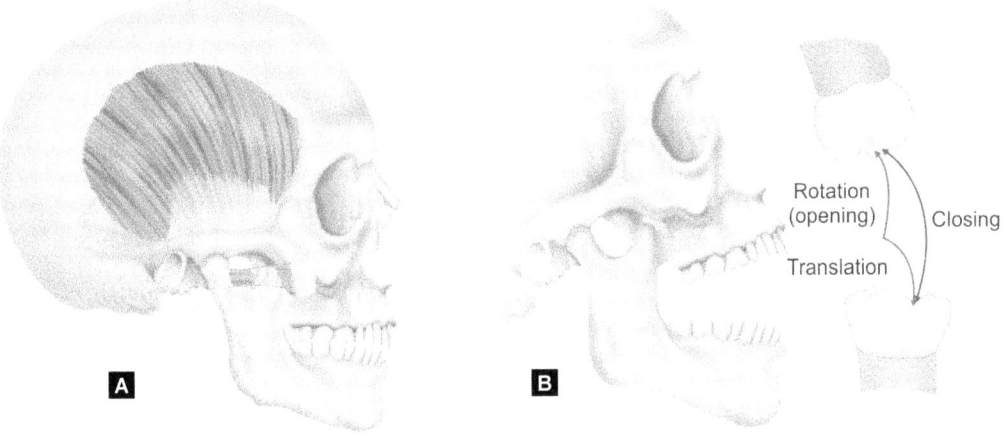

Figs. 5.10A and B: (A) Mandibular elevation; (B) Mandibular depression

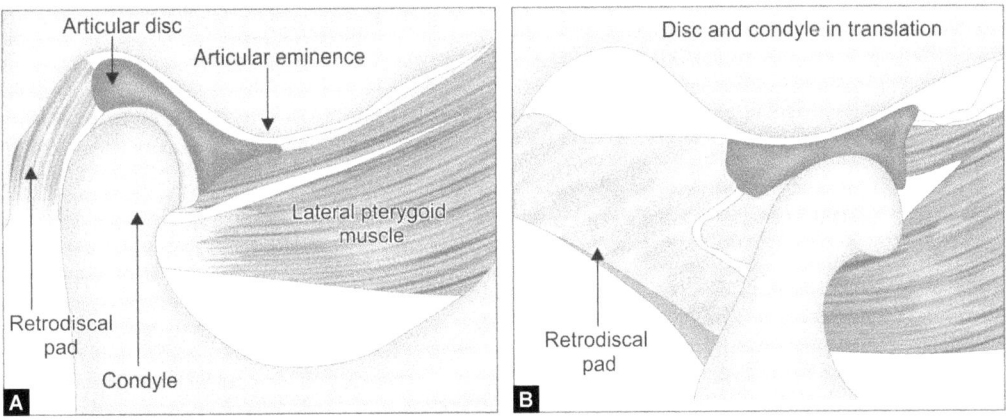

Figs. 5.11A and B: Articular disc during normal jaw opening: (A) At rest; (B) Translation

elevators and retraction of the disc by the elastic fibers of the posterior capsule.

Articular disc during normal jaw opening are shown in **Figure 5.10A**.

Protrusion and Retrusion

- During protrusion, the two heads of the lateral pterygoid contract and cause the discs and condyles to slide anteriorly and inferiorly. This takes place in the upper compartment.
- During mandibular retrusion, these structures slide posteriorly and superiorly while still in the superior cavity. This is accomplished by the temporalis.
- Protrusion
- Retrusion

Lateral Movement

- Lateral movement of the jaw requires that different movements occur concurrently in the TMJs. In adult: Average 11 mm.
- For example, through the contraction of the two heads of the left lateral pterygoid, lateral movement to the left occurs. This necessitates a rotation occurring in the left joint (the mandibular head rotates in relation to the disc in the inferior compartment) and an anterior gliding taking place in the right joint (the disc and mandibular head glide ventrally in the upper compartment).
- Normal chewing

- The lateral pterygoids advance the condyles, thereby opening the mouth with the assistance of the digastric.
- The oblique orientation of the masseters and medial pterygoids create a sling. The nonworking side medial pterygoid contacts simultaneously with the opposite side working masseter.
- It is this oblique orientation of the medial pterygoids and masseters that create the functional "shift" of the mandible, not a *unilateral contraction of a lateral pterygoid*.
- In normal chewing function, the mandible opens, and then, while initiating closing, there is a shift slightly to the side of the bolus, due to the orientation of the masseter and medial pterygoid
- Functional working movement

ARTHROKINEMATICS

The arthrokinematic movement is both gliding and rolling. The gliding follows the concave-convex rule. Rolling does not follow concave-convex rule.

In the TMJ, the moving surface is the mandibular condyle which is convex and nonmoving surface is the fossa which is concave thus gliding happens in the opposite direction to that of the osteokinematic movement.

Rolling happens in the same direction in all the cases.

Movement	Direction of glide	Direction of the roll
Depression	Superior	Inferior
Elevation	Inferior	Superior
Protrusion	Posterior	Anterior
Retrusion	Anterior	Posterior
Lateral deviation	Medial rotation	Lateral rotation

KINETICS

Primary Muscles

- **Temporalis muscle:** it is a flat, fan shaped muscle. Superior fibers attach to the cranium and inferior fibers attach to the coronoid process and medial surface of ramus of mandible. Its main function is elevation of mandible and retrusion.
- **Masseter (Fig. 5.12):** Its superior attachment on zygomatic bone and inferior attachment on external surface of ramus of mandible. Its main action is elevation of mandible and protrusion.
- **Lateral pterygoid:** Superior and inferior segments originates from the infratemporal surface and infratemporal wing of sphenoid bone. It travel in horizontal direction and combine posteriorly to attach to the neck of mandible, articular disc and joint capsule. Superior fibers–stabilize the condyle and disc during mandibular loading. Inferior fibers protrude the mandible and contribute to lateral movements and mandibular depression.
- **Medial pterygoid:** Consists of two heads. The bulk of the muscle arises as a deep head from just above the medial surface of the lateral pterygoid plate. The smaller, superficial head originates from the maxillary tuberosity and the pyramidal process of the palatine bone. Its fibers pass downward, lateral, and posterior, and are inserted, into the medial surface of the ramus and angle of the mandible. Medial pterygoid elevates the mandible and contribute to protrusion.

Secondary Muscles (Fig. 5.13)

- Suprahyoid muscles include digastric, geniohyoid, mylohyoid and stylohyoid

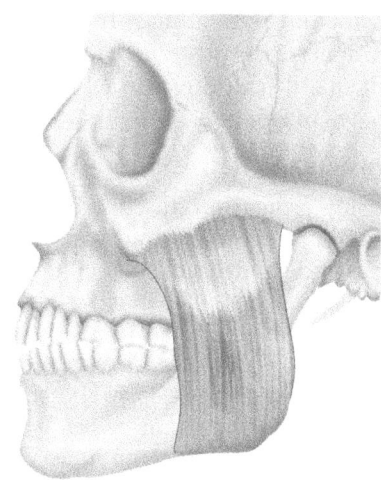

Fig. 5.12: Masseter

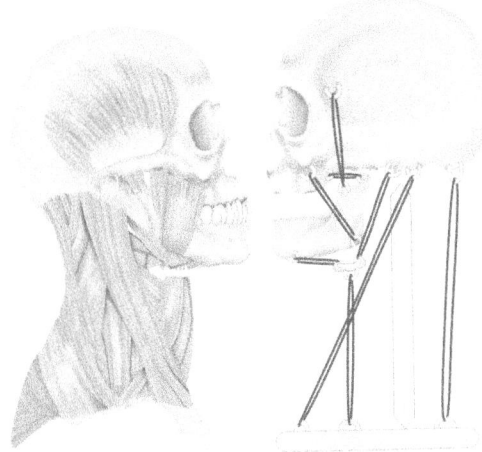

Fig. 5.13: Secondary muscles of mastication

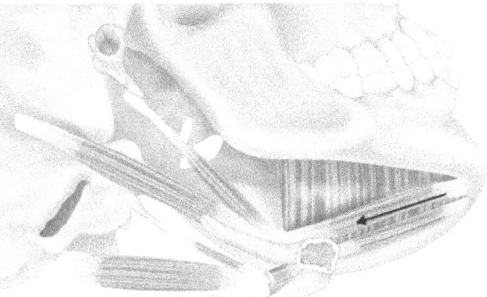

Fig. 5.14: Muscles of TMJ—digastric

infrahyoid muscles include omohyoid, sternothyroid, sternohyoid and thyrohyoid
- Suprahyoid and infrahyoid muscle groups are involved in speech, tongue movements and swallowing.
- Suprahyoid muscle assist with mandibula.

Digastric Muscle (Fig. 5.14)
- The digastric muscle is the muscle most responsible for opening the lower jaw (in combination with the coordinated contraction of the lateral pterygoid muscles).
- Composed of two muscles connected in the middle by a strong tendon. The tendon loops under the hyoid bone which is the only bone in the human body not directly connected to at least one other bone by ligaments.
- Digastric muscle is less bulky and leveraging under a bone not directly connected to the rest of the skeleton makes it quite a weak muscle when *compared with the tremendous upward pressure* that can be exerted on the jaws by the combined force of the temporalis, masseter, and medial pterygoid which oppose it. This accounts for the inability of a patient to open his mouth against spasms of any of the three closing muscles.
- Digastric activity
Actions of the muscles of mastication on the mandible are shown in **Table 5.1**.

PATHOMECHANICS/TMJ DISORDERS

The Classification of Joint Derangements (Figs. 5.15A to C)
- Type IA—popping in the TM joints without pain, very common, said to affect as much as 50% of normal subjects.
- Type IB—popping in the TM joints associated with pain.
- Type II—similar to type IB but patient experiences occasional jaw locking.
  - Closed lock—in this the condyle fails to slide below the meniscus during mouth opening

Table 5.1: Actions of the muscles of mastication on the mandible.

Muscle	Elevation (mouth closing)	Depression (mouth opening)	Lateral excursion	Protrusion	Retrusion
Masseter	Strong	—	Weak (ipsilateral)	Weak	—
Medial pterygoid	Strong	—	Strong (contralateral)	Weak	—
Lateral pterygoid (superior)	Stabilizes	—	Strong (contralateral)	Strong	—
Lateral pterygoid (inferior)	—	Strong	Strong (contralateral)	Strong	—
Temporalis	Strong	—	Weak (ipsilateral)	—	Strong
Suprahyoid group	—	Strong	—	—	Weak

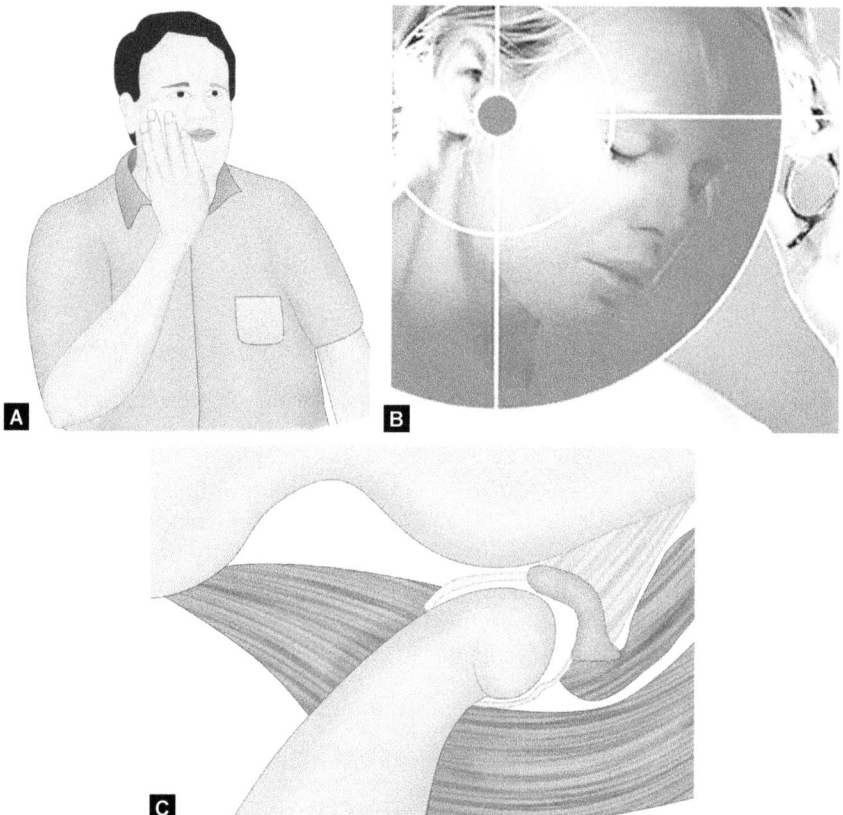

Figs. 5.15A to C: (A and B) Temporomandibular joint dysfuncttion; (C) TMJ subluxation

- Open lock—in this the condyle fails to come back under the meniscus during mouth closing
- Type III—a persistent lock, usually on trying to open. Since the patient cannot open the mouth beyond this point, there is no popping. This condition (unlike all type I and II derangements) requires aggressive therapy with reduction of the lock under anesthesia and physical therapy. If no improvement is seen in three weeks, surgery is generally indicated.

Torn Meniscus
- Decreased shock absorption
- The trick is to press down hard with the thumbs while rotating the body of the mandible up so that the patient's mandible pivots around the thumbs.
- Once a patient dislocates one or both condyles, the ligaments remain stretched out for a long time making further dislocations all too easy.
- A soft diet and a bruxing appliance are probably the best recommendations.

CHAPTER 6

Shoulder Joint

Chapter Outline

- Stabilization
- Ligaments
- Osteokinematics
- Arthrokinematics
- Kinetics
- Scapulohumeral rhythm
- Pathomechanics
- Scapulothoracic joint
- Acromioclavicular joint
- Sternoclavicular joint

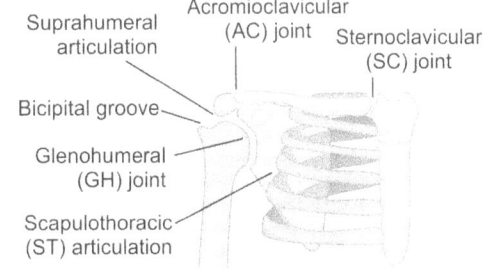

Fig. 6.1: Shoulder complex

INTRODUCTION

The shoulder girdle consists of four joints. They are (Fig. 6.1):
1. Glenohumeral joint (GH joint)
2. Acromioclavicular joint (AC joint)
3. Sternoclavicular joint (SC joint)
4. Scapulothoracic joint (ST joint)

JOINTS AT THE SHOULDER COMPLEX

Glenohumeral Joint

Glenohumeral joint is the most mobile joint in the human body, i.e., it moves at a varied degree of angle in all the planes.

Type of Joint

Synovial joint of ball and socket variety.

Degrees of Freedom

Three degrees of freedom.
- Three rotatory degrees of freedom
- Three translatory degrees of freedom

Articulating Surface (Fig. 6.2)

- **Proximal articulating surface:** Glenoid fossa of the scapula
- **Distal articulating surface:** Head of the humerus

Orientation of the Articulating Surface

- The glenoid fossa is oriented laterally, slightly anterior, and slightly superior.
- The head of the humerus is oriented medially and slightly posterior.

Close Pack Position

90° of shoulder abduction and full external rotation.

Loose Pack Position

30° flexion, 30° abduction, internal rotation.

Capsular Pattern

External rotation > abduction > flexion > internal rotation.

Neutral Position

Anatomic position.

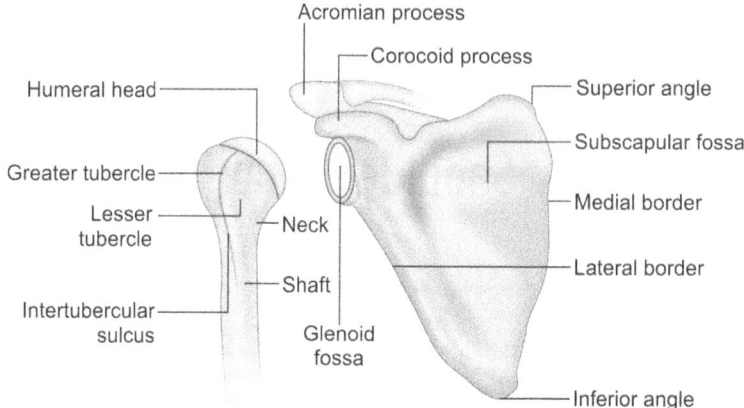

Fig. 6.2: Parts of scapula and upper part of humerus

Resting Position
70° of shoulder abduction and 30° of flexion (horizontal adduction).

STABILIZATION

The stabilization of the joint can be discussed in two parts:
1. Static stability
2. Dynamic stability

The factors responsible for the stability of the shoulder joint are:
- Orientation of the articulating surfaces
- Glenoid labrum
- Negative intra-articular pressure
- Joint capsule
- Ligaments
- **Rotator cuff muscles:** Dynamic stabilizers

} Static stabilizers

Static Stability
- **Orientation of the articulating surface:** As the glenoid fossa faces slightly superiorly (5°) when the arms hang freely. The vertical force produced by the arm is supported by the lower surface of the glenoid fossa.
- **Glenoid labrum (Fig. 6.3):** Glenoid labrum is a ring-like structure presents all along the border of the glenoid fossa. This is like a washer in the pressure cooker. The glenoid labrum increases the depth of the glenoid

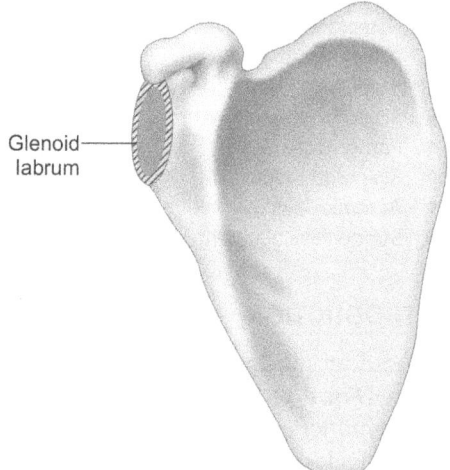

Fig. 6.3: Glenoid labrum

fossa by 50%, thus increasing the stability of the joint.

Functions of the glenoid labrum:
- Distribute transmission of forces equally on the joint
- Creates negative intra-articular pressure as it acts as a vacuum
- The glenoid labrum gives a rubbery grip (example, rubber ferrule of the crutch)
- Serves as an attachment site for the glenohumeral ligament and long head of biceps.

- **Negative intra-articular pressure:** The joint is in the form of ball and socket with the edges of the socket covered by the washer-like structure called glenoid labrum. This

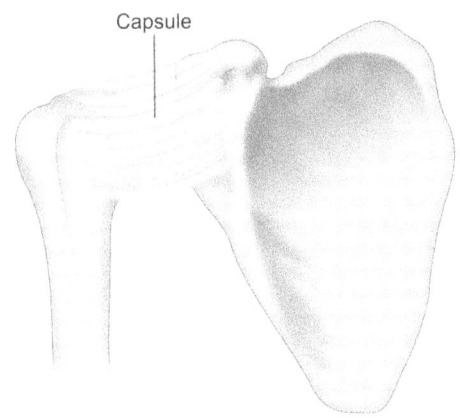

Fig. 6.4: Joint capsule

gives the joint a vacuum insight. This negative intra-articular pressure in the joint contributes to the stability of the joint.

- **Joint capsule (Fig. 6.4):** The glenohumeral joint has a large capsule which is taut superiorly and loose inferiorly and anteriorly. The looseness in the inferior side is in the form of several folds. This is important as the capsule should allow full abduction of the shoulder. The capsule does not provide much stability inferiorly and anteriorly. Thus, there is a requirement of ligaments in the anterior side.

  Functions of the capsule:
  - Mild stability of the shoulder joint, especially, superiorly, and posteriorly
  - Allows the complete abduction of shoulder
  - Acts as a protective layer to the joint
  - Provides space for the attachment of ligaments and tendons

- **Ligaments (Fig. 6.5):** The ligaments of glenohumeral joint are:
  - **Superior glenohumeral ligament:** The superior glenohumeral ligament is attached to the superior part of the glenoid labrum, glenoid fossa, and to the upper part of the neck of humerus. This ligament primarily stabilizes the joint in neutral position, i.e., it has maximum efficiency in 0° abduction. This ligament becomes loose as the shoulder abduction increases.
  - **Middle glenohumeral ligament:** The middle glenohumeral ligament is attached from the anterosuperior side of the glenoid labrum to the anterior neck of the humerus. This ligament runs obliquely. It stabilizes the joint at the angle of 60° abduction. This ligament is absent in 30% of the population.
  - **Inferior glenohumeral ligament complex:** This ligament has three components:
    1. Anterior band
    2. Posterior band

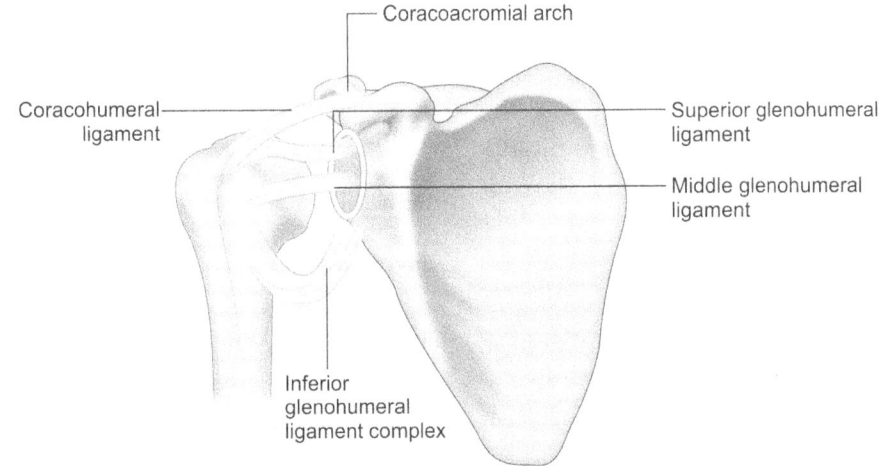

Fig. 6.5: Ligaments

3. Axillary pouch
   - This complex is very essential as it has to allow full range of abduction in the shoulder and also to stabilize the joint.
   - The axillary pouch has several folds which will take up the sack when shoulder is in full abduction. With abduction, this ligament resists inferior humeral head translation.
   - The anterior band is useful in stabilizing when humeral lateral rotation is added to the abduction.
   - The posterior band is useful in stabilizing the joint when medial rotation is added to the shoulder abduction.

Note: The main objective of the three glenohumeral ligaments is to resist anterior translation at various angles of range of motion (ROM).

- **Coracohumeral ligament:** It is attached from the base of the coracoid process, splits into two bands—first band attaches to the supraspinatus and greater tubercle, second band attaches to the subscapularis and lesser tubercle. The long head of biceps passes through these two slips. The coracohumeral ligament is a part of rotator interval capsule. Coracohumeral ligament resists lateral rotation when the arm is in adduction. This ligament also prevents superior translation of humerus.
- **Coracoacromial ligament:**
- *Coracoacromial arch:* The coracoacromial ligament attaching from the inferior part of the acromioclavicular joint and to the coracoid process forms the coracoacromial arch. The coracoacromial arch is an osteoligamentous vault present on the humeral head which protects the joint from any hit or fall by an object. The arch also acts as a physical barrier to prevent superior translation of the joint.

The space between the arch and the joint is called as the subacromial space or

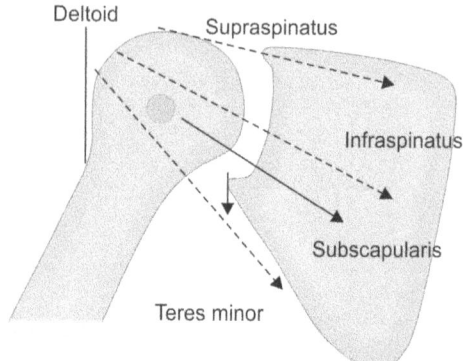

Fig. 6.6: Dynamic stability of rotator cuff

supraspinatus outlet or suprahumeral space. The contents of the subacromial space are subacromial bursa, rotator cuff tendon, and long head of biceps. This space is around 1 cm in healthy population. When the arm is elevated, the space is 0.5 cm.

Dynamic Stability (Fig. 6.6)
Rotator Cuff Muscle
- Supraspinatus
- Infraspinatus
- Teres minor
- Subscapularis

Dynamic stability is brought about by the rotator cuff muscles. When the deltoid and trapezius act to perform flexion, the rotator cuff muscles act as a cuff and hold onto the joint and prevent it from translations. If there were no rotator cuff muscle the gross movements are not possible and shoulder will end up have translator motion with the humeral head coming out of the glenoid fossa. Example abduction without rotator cuff muscles will only results in superior translation of the humeral head.

Special Mention

Rotator interval capsule (Fig. 6.7): The rotator interval capsule is a complex consisting of superior glenohumeral ligament, superior glenohumeral capsule, and coracohumeral ligament. These three are the interconnected structures which fill the space between supraspinatus and subscapularis.

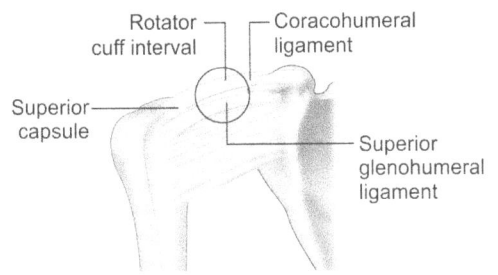

Fig. 6.7: Rotator cuff interval

Bursae of the Shoulder Joint

The most common bursae in the shoulder joint are:
- Subacromial bursa
- **Subdeltoid bursa:**
  - *Subacromial bursa:* It is between the humerus and supraspinatus tendon. It helps in smooth gliding movements.
  - *Subdeltoid bursa:* It is under deltoid muscle and allows free movements between humerus and deltoid muscle.

KINEMATICS

Osteokinematics

The possible movements are:
- Flexion
- Extension
- Abduction
- Adduction
- Medial rotation
- Lateral rotation

Planes and Axis

- Flexion and extension happen in sagittal plane around frontal axis. The axis is not exactly rigid but moves in a curvy manner. This is the instantaneous axis of motion.
- Abduction and adduction happen in frontal plane around AP axis
- Medial and lateral rotations happen in transverse plane around vertical axis.

Range of Motion

Movement	ROM
Flexion (combined GH and ST)	160°
Flexion (only glenohumeral)	90°
Extension	45°–60°
Abduction	160°
Adduction	0°
Medial rotation	80°
Lateral rotation	90°

- **Functional range:** 30°–120°
- **Close kinematic chain motion:** Push-ups, Pull-ups
- **Open kinematic chain motion:** Free hand exercise with dumbbell, hand swing during walking
- **Shoulder flexion restricted by:**
  - Inferior glenohumeral ligament complex
  - Taut posterior capsule
- **Shoulder extension restricted by:**
  - Superior and middle glenohumeral ligament
  - Passive tension created by elbow flexors
  - Passive tension created by collateral ligaments
  - Taut anterior capsule
- **Factors restricting shoulder abduction:**
  - Inferior glenohumeral ligament complex
  - Taut inferior joint capsule
  - Tightness of costoclavicular and interclavicular ligaments and the subclavius muscles at the SC joint
  - Head block
- **Factors restricting abduction:** Trunk block
- **Factors restricting medial rotation:** Posterior joint capsule
- **Factors restricting lateral rotation:**
  - Coracohumeral ligament
  - All 3 glenohumeral ligaments
  - Myofascial tightness

Codman's paradox: Conjunct rotation occurs during sequential motion. Standing with dependent arm position with the palm of the hand facing medially and the thumb facing anteriorly. Shoulder flexion of 180° or shoulder abduction of 180°, the thumb faces posteriorly.

Arthrokinematics (Figs. 6.8A and B)

The arthrokinematic movement is both gliding and rolling. More dominant being the gliding. The gliding follows the concave convex rule. Rolling does not follow concave convex rule.

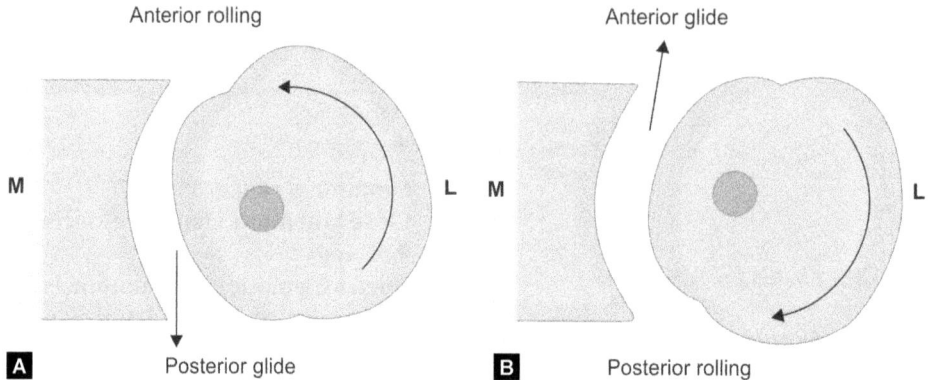

Figs. 6.8A and B: Arthrokinematics of: (A) Shoulder internal rotation; (B) Shoulder external rotation

▲ **Table 6.1:** Rolling happens in the same direction in all the cases.

Movement	Direction of glide	Direction of the roll
Flexion	Posterior	Anterior
Extension	Anterior	Posterior
Abduction	Inferior	Superior
Adduction	Superior	Inferior
Medial rotation	Posterior	Anterior
Lateral rotation	Anterior	Posterior

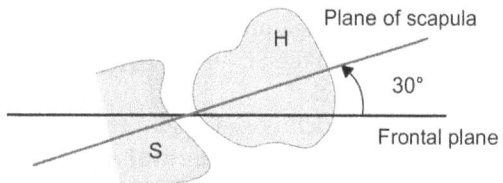

Fig. 6.9: Plane of scapula (superior view)

In the shoulder, the moving surface is head of humerus which is convex and nonmoving surface is glenoid fossa which is concave thus gliding happens in the opposite direction to that of the osteokinematic movement.

Rolling happens in the same direction in all the cases shown in **Table 6.1**.

Plane of Scapula

Plane of scapula also called as scaption plane is the plane where the scapula lies. It is in-between the sagittal plane and frontal plane. It is about 30° to the frontal plane. Functional movements take place in this plane **(Fig. 6.9)**.

KINETICS

See **Tables 6.2** and **6.3**.

Deltoid Muscle

Deltoid is a multipennate muscle. It is a single joint muscle.
It has three parts:
1. Anterior deltoid
2. Posterior deltoid
3. Middle deltoid

Since it is a single joint muscle, it does undergo passive insufficiency. However, active insufficiency can be seen in extreme abduction. The deltoid is mainly a phasic type and can undergo fatigue on sustained activity. However, it can perform short bursts of heavy activity like any other phasic muscle. It is not a postural muscle. This muscle is most effective at the mid-range. The lever of this muscle is of 2nd order.

Table 6.2: Muscles contributing to shoulder motions.

Motion	Prime movers
Shoulder flexion	• Deltoid, anterior fibers • Coracobrachialis • Biceps brachii, long head • Pectoralis major, clavicular head
Shoulder extension	• Latissimus dorsi • Teres major • Triceps brachii, long head • Deltoid, posterior fibers
Shoulder abduction	• Deltoid • Supraspinatus • Biceps brachii, long head
Shoulder adduction	• Pectoralis major • Latissimus dorsi • Teres major • Triceps brachii, long head • Deltoid, posterior fibers
Shoulder external rotation	• Infraspinatus • Teres minor • Deltoid, posterior fibers
Shoulder internal rotation	• Subscapularis • Teres major • Pectoralis major, latissimus dorsi, deltoid, anterior fibers

Table 6.3: Muscles for scapulothoracic (shoulder girdle) motions.

Motion	Prime movers
Scapular elevation	• Upper trapezius • Levator scapulae • Rhomboid major • Rhomboid minor
Scapular protraction	• Serratus anterior • Pectoralis major • Pectoralis minor
Scapular upward rotation	• Trapezius • Serratus anterior
Scapular depression	• Pectoralis minor • Lower trapezius • Latissimus dorsi • Subclavius
Scapular retraction	• Trapezius • Rhomboid major • Rhomboid minor
Scapular downward rotation	• Levator scapula • Rhomboid major • Rhomboid minor

Scapulohumeral Rhythm/ Glenohumeral Rhythm

Scapulohumeral rhythm is the coordinated movement between the joints; glenohumeral joint and scapulothoracic joint to bring about a larger range of motion and lesser instability. This mechanism helps in distributing the work load between the two joint thus no single joint is overloaded.

The scapulohumeral rhythm has a ratio of 2:1 motion between glenohumeral joint and scapulothoracic joint. That means for every 10° of glenohumeral motion there will be 5° of scapulothoracic motion.

Advantages of Scapulohumeral Rhythm

- Larger range of motion
- Shared load between the two joints.
- Less compromise in the joint stability
- Less chance of injury
- Convenient to do activities of daily living
- Increased performance in sporting activities, e.g., throwing, batting, bowling, etc.

The scapulohumeral rhythm can be further explained during shoulder abduction mechanism.

Shoulder Abduction Mechanism (Fig. 6.10)

The shoulder abduction mechanism can be divided into three phases:
- Phase I (0°–60°)
- Phase II (60°–120°)
- Phase III (120°–180°)

Phase I

The abduction is initiated by supraspinatus muscle. Thus, the muscle is also called as **abduction initiator muscle**. During the initial 30° of abduction, the scapula is at an inconvenience to move. Thus, it requires some range of motion to get set and stable. Thus, the first 30° of shoulder abduction is also called as **scapular setting phase (0°–30°)**.

In this phase, the motion predominantly occurs at glenohumeral joint and as the abduction ROM increases the contribution from the scapulothoracic increases.

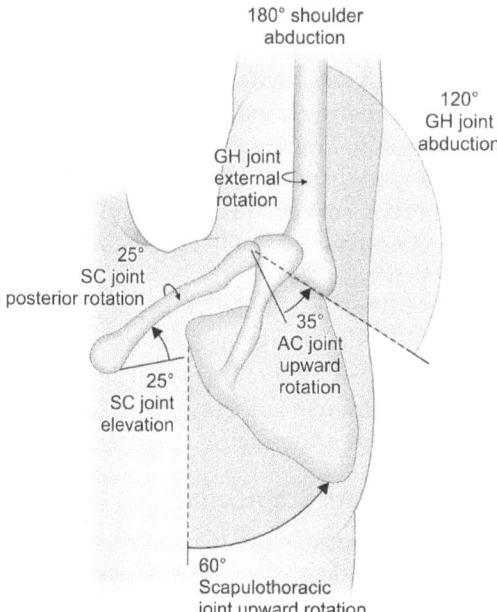

Fig. 6.10: Shoulder abduction mechanism

The muscles responsible for the abduction during this phase are supraspinatus and deltoid.

Phase II

The scapula is stable; the shoulder is at an optimal position to do any kind of activities. In this phase there is synchronized movement between the glenohumeral and scapulothoracic joints. At 60° the greater tubercle of humerus nears the acromion process. To avoid the impact between the two there is an automatic lateral rotation of the humerus thus the tubercle skips the acromion process and the abduction continues further. If the lateral rotation does not take place, there would be no further abduction as can be seen in some pathological cases or simply by demonstrating it manually.

As both the joints contribute in this phase the muscles responsible for the movement are supraspinatus, deltoid, serratus anterior, and upper trapezius. Serratus anterior and upper trapezius make a force couple for the scapulothoracic joint.

Phase III

In this phase, the ROM is more in the scapulothoracic and less in the glenohumeral. The muscles responsible for the movement during this phase are upper trapezius and serratus anterior. The abduction stops at 160°. Beyond 160° is not an actual movement at the shoulder but a body alignment at the spine making it apparently visible that the abduction has achieved 180° of motion.

PATHOMECHANICS

- Impingement syndrome (rotator cuff pathology, supraspinatus tendinitis, bicipital tendinitis, painful arc syndrome, etc.)
- Frozen shoulder (adhesive capsulitis)
- Shoulder dislocation.

Impingement Syndrome/Painful Arc Syndrome

Impingement of the soft tissues (rotator cuff tendon, biceps tendon, subacromial bursa) between the tubercle of head of humerus and coracoacromial arch gives rise to impingement syndrome/painful arc syndrome/rotator cuff tendinitis/supraspinatus tendinitis/biceps tendinitis/subacromial bursitis (**Fig. 6.11**).

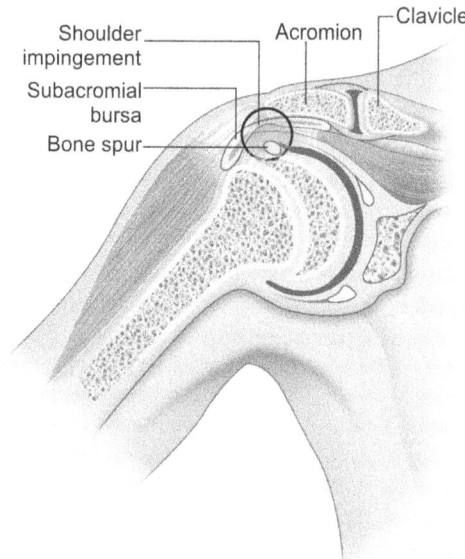

Fig. 6.11: Shoulder impingement syndrome

Shoulder impingement occurs if,
- The subacromial space is insufficient or overcrowded.
- Insufficient inferior glide of the humeral head during arm elevation.
- Insufficient external rotation of the humerus during arm elevation.

Typical painful arc that is pain at abduction between 60 and 120 during which the greater tubercle comes in contact with the coracoacromial arch.

Subacromial Bursitis

It is a condition caused by inflammation of the bursa that separates the superior surface of the supraspinatus tendon (one of the four tendons of the rotator cuff) from the overlying coracoacromial ligament, acromion, coracoid (the acromial arch), and from the deep surface of the deltoid muscle. The subacromial bursa helps the motion of the supraspinatus tendon of the rotator cuff in activities, such as overhead work.

Inflammation is the primary cause of symptoms. Inflammatory bursitis is usually the result of repetitive injury to the bursa. In the subacromial bursa, this generally occurs due to microtrauma to adjacent structures, particularly the supraspinatus tendon.

Frozen Shoulder

- Frozen shoulder is also called as adhesive capsulitis.
- It is characterized by development of dense adhesions and capsular restrictions. Inflammation of the capsule can also be seen.
- This condition results in inability of the person to raise his arm either actively or passively.
- It is commonly seen in age group of 40–60 years
- The restrictions are based on capsular pattern. That is external rotation which is most restricted followed by abduction then flexion and internal rotation. This pattern is just that the capsule is not a uniform cylinder but different thickness at different areas.
- The treatment is gradual stretching of the capsule and pain relieving modalities.

Dislocation of the Shoulder

Most of the shoulder dislocation is anterior (95%) and very less posterior (5%).

This is because of the orientation of the joint surfaces, tight posterior capsule and most of the activities involve forward motion of the joint.

Types of anterior dislocation:
- Subcoracoid
- Subglenoid
- Infraclavicular
- Intrathoracic

Mechanism of injury is usually fall on an outstretched hand or a direct blow. The patient comes with the arm held in abduction and external rotation. Reduction of the dislocation is done by a professional (medical doctor, physiotherapist) performing TEAM technique (Traction External rotation, Adduction, and Medial rotation).

SCAPULOTHORACIC JOINT

The scapulothoracic joint is not a true synovial joint but a functional unit. The scapula just rests on the rib cage joining it with muscular attachments.

Resting Position of Scapula

The scapula rests on the posterior side of the rib cage about 5 cm away from the vertebral spine. It is positioned between 2nd rib and 7th rib. The scapula is internally rotated 35° to 45°, anteriorly tilted 10° to 15°, and upward rotation 5° to 10°.

Functions of the Scapulothoracic Articulation

- The main function being sharing the range of motion with glenohumeral joint to bring about a larger range of motion of the shoulder.
- To provide movement base for the humerus

- To maintain length-tension relationship for the deltoid muscle to function above 90° of arm elevation
- To provide stability of the GH joint working overhead
- To absorb the shock for forces applied to the outstretched arm
- To permit push-up during crutch walking

Movements at the Scapula
(Figs. 6.12 and 6.13)

The movements which are seen at this joint are primarily brought about by the movements at the acromioclavicular joint, glenohumeral joint, and sternoclavicular joint.

The movements in this joint are:
- Upward and downward rotation
- Internal and external rotation
- Anterior and posterior tilt
- Elevation and depression
- Protraction and retraction

Degrees of freedom: Three rotational degrees of freedom and two translatory degrees of freedom.

- Upward and downward rotation, internal and external rotation, anterior and posterior tilt are rotational motions
- Elevation and depression, protraction and retraction are translator motions

Upward and Downward Rotation

- **Upward rotation:** Glenoid fossa facing upward with inferior angle of scapula sliding laterally and anteriorly
- **Downward rotation:** Glenoid fossa facing downward with inferior angle of scapula sliding medially and posteriorly
- This is the principal movement which is required in elevation of the arm. This movement forms a part of the scapulohumeral rhythm.
- **Osteokinematic movement first 30°:** Elevation of the clavicle through the axis at the base of the spine of scapula.
- **Last 30°:** Posterior rotation of the clavicle and scapular rotation around AC joint.
- **Total ROM:** 60°.

Internal and External Rotation

Internal and external rotations are the angular motion. These movements are not apparently visible but are very important movements happening at the scapula. These rotations occur as the ribcage is curvy and the scapula moves along its contour. These rotations occur along with protraction and retraction of scapula (**Fig. 6.14**).
- **Total ROM:** 15°
- Excessive internal rotation can be a result of weak serratus anterior which is attached

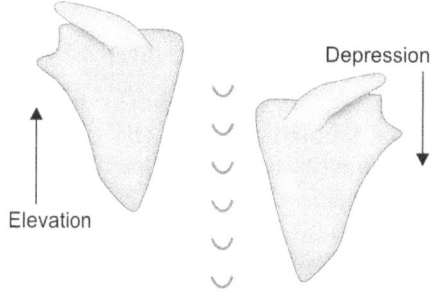

Fig. 6.12: Frontal plane motions of scapula (posterior view)

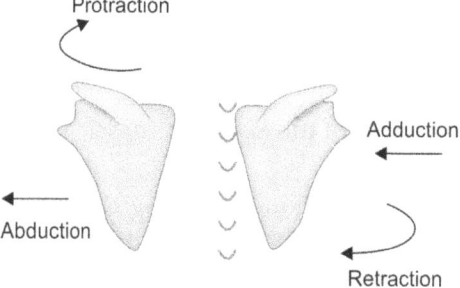

Fig. 6.13: Transverse plane motions (Posterior view)

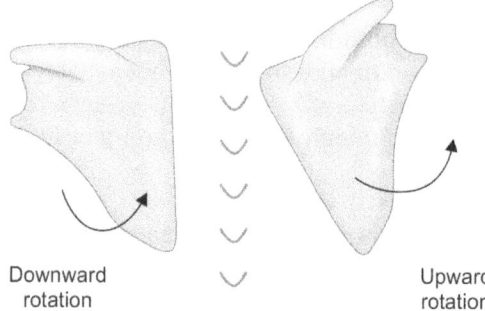

Fig. 6.14: Rotation of shoulder girdle

to the medial border of scapula. In this, the muscle fails to keep the scapula in its position. This is referred to it as winging of scapula.

Anterior and Posterior Tilt
- Anterior and posterior tilts are angular motions at the scapula. It happens in sagittal plane. This movement is not clinically visible. These happen because of the different movement axis of the AC joint and SC joint. Excessive anterior tilting results in tipping of inferior angle of scapula outward.
- **ROM:** 5°

Elevation and Depression
- Elevation and depression are translator motion seen at the scapula. In this, the scapula moves up and down on the ribcage. This motion happens in frontal plane. Upward and downward shrugging of the shoulder result in the elevation and depression. The actual motion occurs at the sternoclavicular joint.
- The movement is limited by the costoclavicular and interclavicular ligaments and the subclavius muscle.
- **Range:** 10–15 cm (translatory motions are not measured in angles).

Protraction and Retraction
- Protraction and retraction are also translatory motions. This also occurs in frontal plane. In this, the scapula moves away from the vertebral column is called as protraction. The scapula moving toward the vertebral column is called as retraction. These movements are also called as abduction and adduction. However, pure abduction and adduction is not possible as the scapula does not move in strict frontal plane but moves along the contours of the rib cage. Thus, sometimes it is considered as angular motion and the range can be calculated in angles.
- **Range:** 25°.

Scapulothoracic Stability
The scalability at the scapulothoracic joint is determined by:
- Scapulothoracic musculature
- Acromioclavicular joint
- Sternoclavicular joint
- Glenohumeral joint

The primary stability is provided by the scapulothoracic musculature. Serratus anterior and rhomboidus keep the scapula conformed to it position. The muscular balance between the upper trapezius, middle trapezius, and lower trapezius helps in dynamic stability. The supraspinatus, infraspinatus, subscapularis, teres minor which are the rotator cuff muscle coordination with the glenohumeral joint to main a rhythmic motion. Teres major also balances out levator scapular which together act as a force couple.

ACROMIOCLAVICULAR JOINT

The acromioclavicular joint attaches the scapula to the clavicle. The main function of the joint is to allow the scapula to move in three dimensions during the movement of the arm so as to increase the motion of the upper extremity.

Articulating Surfaces (Fig. 6.15)
The proximal articulating surface is formed by the lateral end of the clavicle and the distal articulating surface is formed by a small facet on the acromion of the scapula. The articulating surface is incongruent and may vary from being flat, reciprocally concave-convex or reciprocally convex-concave. There is also the difference observed in the angle of inclination formed by the two articulating surfaces.

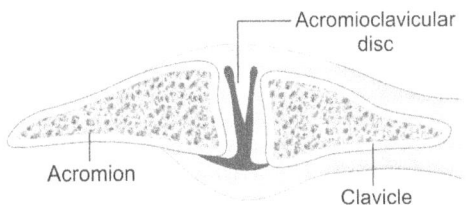

Fig. 6.15: Articular disc in the acromioclavicular joint

Acromioclavicular Joint Disc (Fig. 6.16)

The disc varies in size in different individuals and at different ages. Through the first couple of years of life the disc is fibrocartilaginous and with the use of upper extremity there is a development of joint space which may leave a meniscoid fibrocartilage within the joint.

Acromioclavicular Capsule and Ligaments

The capsule is weak and thus requires the reinforcement of the ligaments to maintain the stability of the joint.

Ligaments (Fig. 6.17)

- **Superior and inferior acromioclavicular ligament:** The fibers of the superior acromioclavicular ligament are reinforced by the aponeurotic fibers of trapezius and deltoid muscle thus giving it a stronger superior joint support than inferior. The main function of the acromioclavicular joint is to act as a primary restraint to posterior translation and posterior axial rotation.
- **Coracoclavicular ligament:** The ligament runs from the coracoid process to the underside of the clavicle near the acromioclavicular joint acting as a primary support to the joint. The ligament has two parts that is the medial portion, the conoid ligament and the lateral portion, the trapezoid ligament. The conoid ligament is fan-shaped vertically oriented, whereas the trapezoid ligament is quadrilateral and horizontally oriented. The two portions are separated from each other by adipose tissue and a large bursa. The ligament restrains the large translatory forces of the AC joint. The conoid portion acts as a primary restraint to translatory motion due to superior directed forces applied to the distal clavicle. The trapezoid portion acts as a restrain to the translatory motion caused by posterior directed forces applied to the distal clavicle. The coracoclavicular ligament as a whole limits the upward rotation of the scapula at the acromioclavicular joint it also prevents the medial displacement of the scapula on the clavicle when immediately directed force is transferred from the humerus to the glenoid fossa.

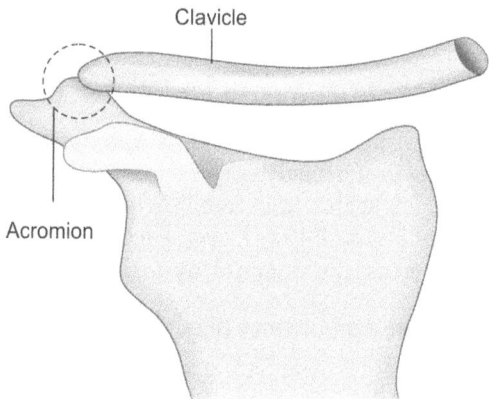

Fig. 6.16: Acromioclavicular joint

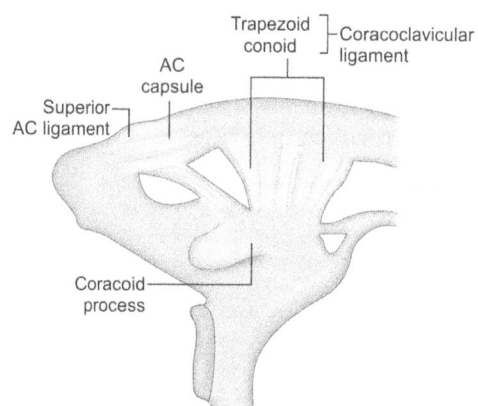

Fig. 6.17: Ligaments of the acromioclavicular joint

Acromioclavicular Motions

The motions usually occur around an axis that is oriented to the plane of the scapula rather than the cardinal planes.
The rotatory motions are:
- Internal/external rotation **(Fig. 6.18)**
- Anterior/posterior tilting or tipping **(Fig. 6.19)**
- Upward/downward rotation **(Fig. 6.20)**.

Internal and external rotation: The motion takes place around an approximately vertical axis through the acromioclavicular joint. During protraction the scapular internally rotates on the AC level to fit on the posterior lateral thorax, whereas during retraction the scapular externally rotates. The combined internal and external rotation range of motion is around 30°.

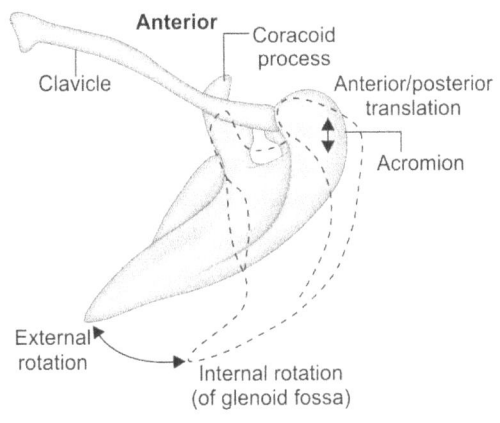

Fig. 6.18: Internal and external rotation of acromioclavicular joint

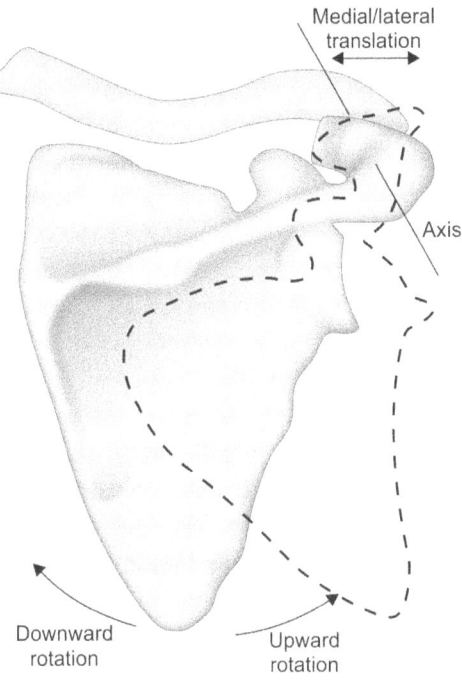

Fig. 6.20: Upward and downward rotation of AC joint

Anterior and posterior tilting: The motion occurs around an oblique coronal axis. During elevation as in shoulder shrug, the scapula moves in anterior tilting and during depression the scapula moves in posterior tilting in relation to AC joint to adjust to the contour of thorax. In movements like shoulder flexion or abduction there is posterior tilting observed.

Upward and downward rotation: The motion of course around an oblique A-P axis which is approximately perpendicular to the plane of the scapula. Upward rotation tilts the glenoid fossa upward and on the downward rotation tilts the glenoid fossa downward. During abduction and flexion the scapular moves in upward rotation in relation to acromion about 30°, whereas during adduction and extension the scapular moves in downward rotation in relation to the acromion about 30°. The amount of available passive motion into upward/downward rotation at the acromioclavicular joint is limited by the attachment of the coracoclavicular ligament.

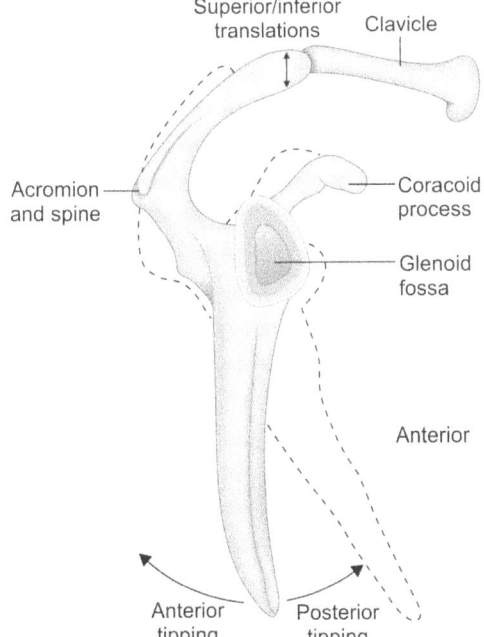

Fig. 6.19: Anterior and posterior tipping of AC joint

Muscles

The clavicle serves as an attachment to many muscles that function at the upper extremity and head
- Pectoralis major (clavicular head)
- Sternocleidomastoid
- Deltoid
- Trapezius

Pathology

The joint is susceptible to both trauma and degenerative changes. The acromioclavicular dislocations are graded based on the displacement between the acromion and the clavicle and the amount by which the displacement occurs. The grades are:

Type 1: Sprain to the acromioclavicular ligament only

Type 2: Injury with the rupture of acromioclavicular ligaments and sprained coracoclavicular ligament

Type 3: Rupture of both ligaments with a 25-100% increase in coracoclavicular space

Type 4: Rupture of both ligaments and posteriorly displaced lateral clavicle often pressing into the trapezius posteriorly

Type 5: Complete rupture of both ligaments, inferior displacement of acromion with the coracoclavicular space 3-5 times greater than the normal

Type 6: Complete rupture of the ligaments, displacement of the distal clavicle into subacromial or subcoracoid position, inferior displacement of clavicle in relation to acromion.

STERNOCLAVICULAR JOINT

The sternoclavicular joint is the only joint that connects the upper limb to the axial skeleton. It is a plane synovial joint with three degrees of freedom that is three rotatory and three translatory degrees of freedom **(Fig. 6.21)**.

Articulating Surfaces

The proximal articulating surface is the notch formed by the manubrium and first costal

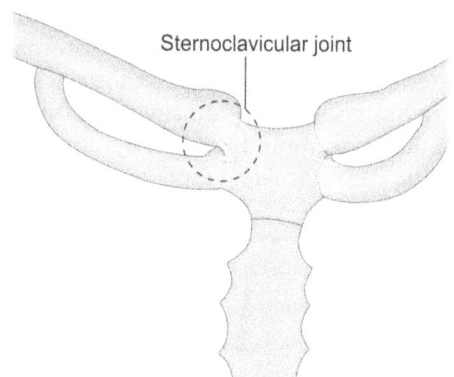

Fig. 6.21: Sternoclavicular joint

cartilage. The distal articulating surface is formed by the medial end of clavicle. The medial end of clavicle and manubrium is incongruent with the superior part of medial clavicle having no contact with manubrium.

Sternoclavicular Disc (Fig. 6.22)

It is a fibrocartilaginous disc. The disc is attached to the posterior surface of the clavicle superiorly at one end and attached to the manubrium, first costal cartilage, and fibrous sternoclavicular capsule. The disc divides the joint cavity diagonally into two separate cavities. The function of the disc is to provide stability and absorb and transmit the forces from the lateral end of the clavicle to the sternoclavicular joint. It also acts like a hinge for the medial clavicle during the shoulder movements. The diagonal attachment of

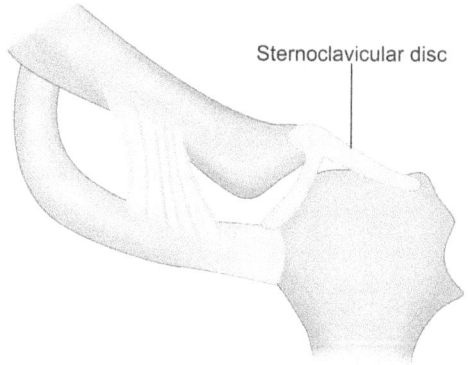

Fig. 6.22: Disc of sternoclavicular joint

the disc limits the medial movement of the clavicle, thus preventing it from overriding the shallow facet of the manubrium. During elevation and depression of the clavicle the medial articulating surface rolls and slides on the stationary disc, whereas during protraction and retraction of the clavicle the disc along with the medial clavicle rolls and slides on the manubrial facet. Thus, the disc is considered as a part of the manubrium during elevation and depression and part of clavicle during protraction and retraction.

Sternoclavicular Joint Capsule and Ligaments (Fig. 6.23)

The static stability of the joint is provided by a strong capsule surrounding the joint and by three ligament complexes.

Ligaments:
1. Anterior and posterior sternoclavicular ligament
2. Bilaminar costoclavicular ligament
3. Interclavicular ligament

The sternoclavicular ligament: It reinforces the capsule and its main function is to prevent excessive anterior and posterior translatory movement of the clavicle.

The costoclavicular ligament: It is attached to the clavicle and first trip and is very strong, it has two segments anterior segment that starts from the first rib, runs laterally and attaches the clavicle and the posterior segment that attaches the first rib, runs medially and then attaches to the clavicle the ligament functions to prevent excessive elevation of the lateral end of the clavicle and also limits superiorly directed forces applied to the clavicle.

The interclavicular ligament: It prevents excessive depression of distal clavicle and superior gliding of medial clavicle on the manubrium. This function is crucial as it protects the brachial plexus, subclavian artery which run between the clavicle and first rib.

Sternoclavicular Motions (Figs. 6.24 and 6.25)

The sternoclavicular joint has three degrees of freedom the rotatory motions are:
1. Elevation and depression
2. Protraction and retraction
3. Anterior and posterior rotation of the clavicle.

The translatory motions are small in magnitude. The translation of the medial clavicle on manubrium occurs in the anterior-posterior, medial-lateral, and superior-inferior direction.

Elevation and depression: The movement occurs in frontal plane and AP axis. During elevation, the convex surface of the clavicle slides inferiorly on the concave manubrium

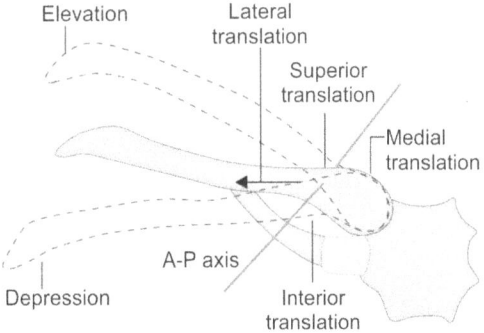

Fig. 6.24: Movements of sternoclavicular joints

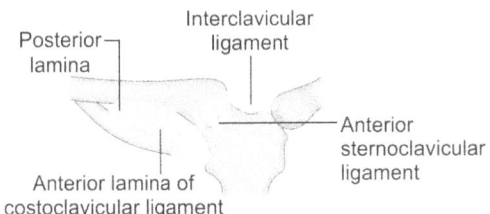

Fig. 6.23: Ligaments of sternoclavicular joint

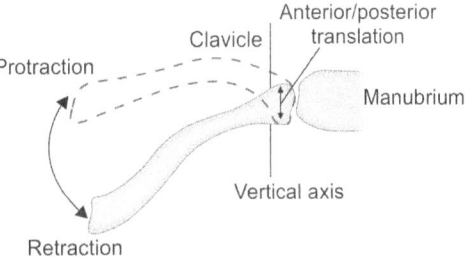

Fig. 6.25: Movements of sternoclavicular joint

and 1st costal cartilage. Elevation is around 48° with the lateral clavicle rotating upward and depression is less than 15° with lateral clavicle rotating downward.

Protraction and retraction: Occurs in the transverse plane and vertical axis. The concave medial clavicle slides anterior on the convex distal articulating surface and during retraction it slides posteriorly. The protraction is around 15–20° and retraction is around 30°.

Anterior and posterior rotation of clavicle: Axis of rotation runs longitudinally through clavicle. The clavicle only rotates in one direction from neutral which is posteriorly and it further returns to neutral by rotating anteriorly. Posterior rotation is around 50°. From neutral a small magnitude of anterior rotation around 10° can be observed.

Muscular Attachments

No muscles are directly attached to the sternoclavicular joint and its movements mimic the reciprocal of scapular movement but a few muscles have an attachment to the clavicle and thus produce clavicular movement. These are deltoid, pectorals major (clavicular head), trapezius, sternocleidomastoid, scalene, and subclavius muscle.

CHAPTER 7

Elbow Complex

Chapter Outline

- True elbow joint
- Ligaments
- Humeroulnar Joint and Humeroradial Joint
- Superior radioulnar joint
- Kinematics
- Kinetics
- Carrying angle
- Pathomechanics

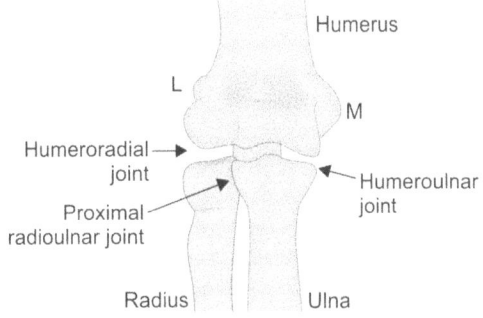

Fig. 7.1: Elbow complex (Anterior view)

INTRODUCTION

The joints at the elbow complex are (**Fig. 7.1**):
- Humeroulnar joint
- Humeroradial joint
- Superior radioulnar joint

All the three joints are enclosed in a single capsule.

HUMEROULNAR JOINT AND HUMERORADIAL JOINT (TRUE ELBOW JOINT)

Type—Hinge type of synovial joint
Degrees of freedom—One
Articulating surfaces—
- **Proximal:** Trochlea and capitulum of humerus (**Figs. 7.2 and 7.3**)
- **Distal:** Trochlear notch of ulna (**Fig. 7.4**)—upper surface of head of radius

Close pack position—Extension
Loose pack position—70° flexion and 10° supination of elbow
Capsular pattern—Flexion > extension
Stability—Factors responsible for the shoulder joint are
- Joint design
- Capsule
- **Ligaments**
  - Ulnar collateral ligament
  - Radial collateral ligament
  - Lateral ulnar collateral ligament
  - Annular ligament
- Muscles (dynamic stability)

Joint Design

The articulating structure is in the form of a hinge. This itself serves as a stable structure and resists traction force. However, in flexion position this design does not protect posteriorly directed force. Therefore, anterior dislocation of elbow is not possible unless there is a fracture and posterior dislocation of elbow is common.

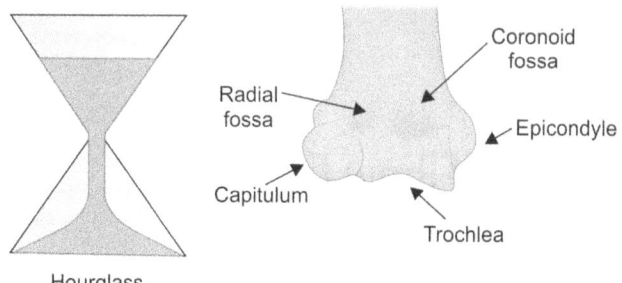

Fig. 7.2: Humerus (Anterior view)

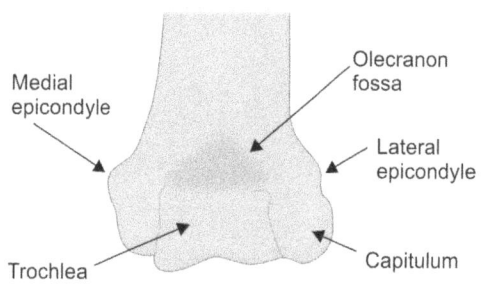

Fig. 7.3: Humerus (Posterior view)

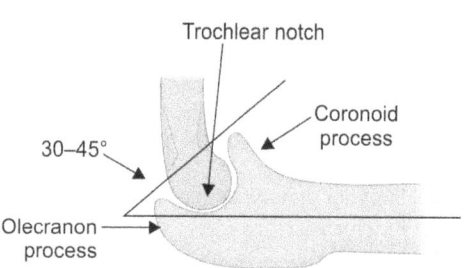

Fig. 7.4: Humeroulnar joint (Lateral view)

Capsule (Fig. 7.5)

All the three joints are covered in one capsule. Distally capsule attaches into ulna along the margins of coronoid process and blends with proximal borders of annular ligament. Medially and laterally capsule is continuous with the collateral ligaments. Posteriorly the capsule is attached to the humerus along upper edge of olecranon fossa and to the back of medial epicondyle. The capsule is large, loose and weak anteriorly and posteriorly it contains folds that are able to expand to allow for a full range of elbow motion.

Ligaments

The ligaments of the elbow joint are
- Ulnar collateral ligament
- Radial collateral ligament
- Lateral ulnar collateral ligament
- Annular ligament **(Fig. 7.6)**

Ulnar Collateral Ligament

- Also called as medial collateral ligament of elbow.
- It is triangular in shape. The apex is attached to medial epicondyle of humerus and base to olecranon and coronoid process of ulna. It has three parts; anterior, posterior, and oblique. The primary function of this ligament is to resist valgus stress.

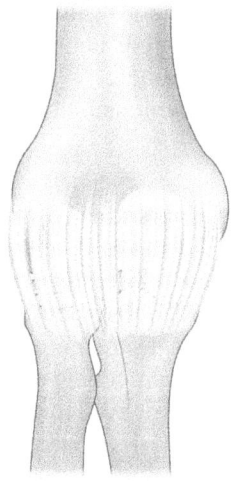

Fig. 7.5: Elbow capsule

Chapter 7 | Elbow Complex

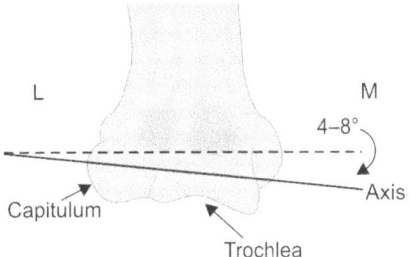

Fig. 7.7: Joint axis of humeroulnar joint

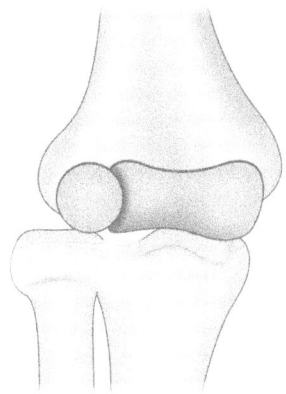

Fig. 7.6: Annular ligament

Radial Collateral Ligament
- It is also called as lateral collateral ligament of elbow.
- It is a fan-shaped structure extending from lateral epicondyle of humerus to annular ligament and to the lateral side of radius. The primary function of this ligament is to resist varus stress.

Lateral Ulnar Collateral Ligament
It attaches from lateral epicondyle of humerus to lateral side of ulna.

Annular Ligament
It surrounds the head of radius and attaches to the superior radioulnar joint.

KINEMATICS

Osteokinematics
The movements available in the elbow joint are
- Flexion
- Extension

Planes and Axes
- Flexion and extension happen in sagittal plane around frontal axis.
- The axis passes through the center of trochlea and capitulum. It is not exactly perpendicular to the longitudinal axis of the humerus but with 4–8° of valgus (**Fig. 7.7**).

Range of Motion

Flexion	145°
Extension	0–5°

- Functional range—30–130°
- Close kinematic chain motion—Push-ups, pull-ups
- Open kinematic chain motion—Biceps curls with a dumbbell.

Factors restricting elbow flexion
- Soft tissue approximation of biceps
- Triceps tightness
- Posterior capsule tightness

Factors restricting elbow extension
- Bony block of ulna to the humerus
- Elbow flexors tightness
- Collateral ligaments
- Anterior capsule tightness

Arthrokinematics (Figs. 7.8A and B)
The arthrokinematic movement is predominantly gliding and very less rolling. The gliding follows the concave-convex rule (**Fig. 7.8 and 7.9**).

In the elbow, the moving surface is trochlear fossa which is concave and nonmoving surface is trochlea which is convex thus the arthrokinematic movement happens in the same direction to that of the osteokinematic movement.

Osteokinematic movement	Arthrokinematic movement	Direction of arthrokinematic movement
Flexion	Gliding	Anterior
Extension	Gliding	Posterior

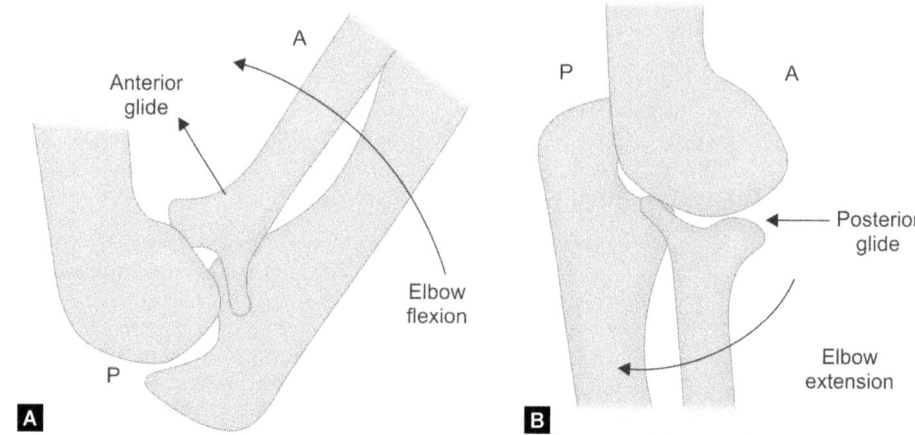

Figs. 7.8A and B: Arthrokinematics of (A) Elbow flexion; (B) Elbow extension

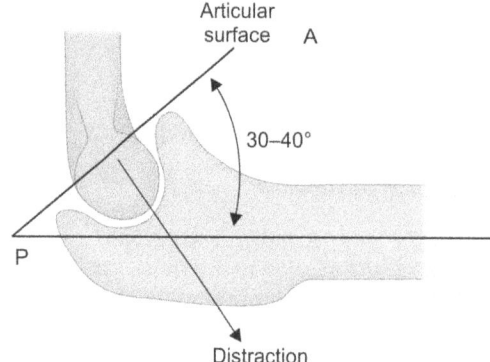

Fig. 7.9: Plane of articulation of humeroulnar joint

KINETICS

Elbow Flexors

- Brachialis
- Biceps brachii
- Brachioradialis

Elbow Extensors

- Triceps
- Anconeus

Biceps brachii is a fusiform muscle having two heads; one short and one long. Long head of biceps is a two joint muscle. It can undergo active and passive insufficiency at the extreme range. The biceps is mainly a phasic type and can undergo fatigue on sustained activity. However, it can perform short bursts of heavy activity like any other phasic muscle. It is not a postural muscle. This muscle is most effective at the mid-range to slightly outer range (90–110°). The lever of this muscle is of 2nd order.

Triceps Brachii

Triceps is a muscle consisting of three heads; medial, lateral, and long head. It undergoes both active insufficiency and passive insufficiency at the extreme range. The medial head is predominantly type 1 fibers and lateral head is type 2b fibers. Thus it has both shunt and spurt properties.

Anconeus

Acts as elbow extensor. Stabilizes elbow during forearm pronation and supination. Acts against valgus stress.

SUPERIOR RADIOULNAR JOINT (FIG. 7.10)

Type—Pivot synovial joint
Degrees of freedom—One
Articulating surfaces—Ulnar radial notch articulates with the head of the radius.
Close pack position—5° supination
Loose pack position—70° of elbow flexion and 35° of forearm supination

Chapter 7 | Elbow Complex

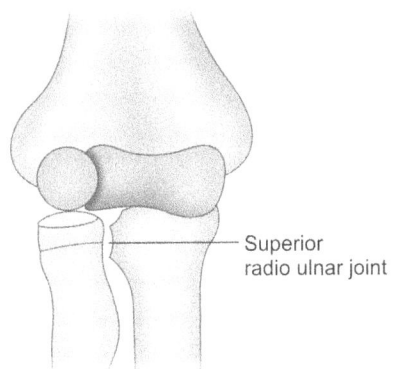

Fig. 7.10: Superior radioulnar joint

Capsular pattern—Supination more restricted than pronation.
Stability—Ligaments are the stabilizing factors.

Ligaments
- Annular ligament
- Quadrate ligament
- Oblique cord ligament

Annular ligament: This ligament is attached to anterior and posterior edges of the ulnar radial notch. It surrounds the radial head in an annual ring shape. It resists anterior or posterior translation of the superior radioulnar joint but it is poor resister of traction force resulting in pulled elbow seen in children.

■ KINEMATICS (FIGS. 7.11 AND 7.12)

Osteokinematics
The movements available in the elbow joint are
- Pronation
- Supination

Planes and Axes
- Pronation and supination happen in transverse plane around vertical axis.
- The axis passes through the center of radial head and distal ulnar head.

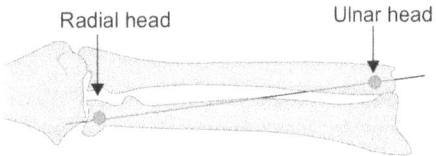

Fig. 7.11: Axis of forearm motions

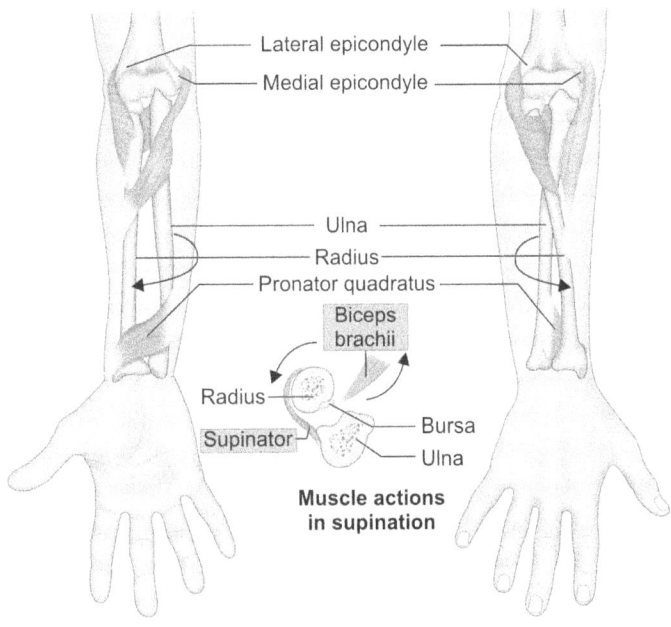

Fig. 7.12: Forearm supination and pronation

ROM

Pronation	90°
Supination	80°

- **Functional range:** Mid prone position
- **Close kinematic chain motion:** No specific movement
- **Open kinematic chain motion:** Screwing unscrewing using a screw driver.

Arthrokinematics

The arthrokinematic movement is predominantly gliding and very less rolling. The gliding follows the concave-convex rule.

In this the moving surface is radial head which is convex and nonmoving surface is notch of ulna which is concave thus the arthrokinematic movement happens in the opposite direction to that of the osteokinematic movement.

Osteokine-matic movement	Arthrokine-matic movement	Direction of arthrokinematic movement
Pronation	Gliding	Posterior
Supination	Gliding	Anterior

KINETICS

- **Pronators**
  - Pronator teres
  - Pronator quadratus.
- **Supinator:** Supinator muscle.

SPECIAL FEATURE OF ELBOW

Carrying Angle

The angle formed between the long axis of arm to the long axis of forearm is called as carrying angle. It is only visible when the elbow is in extension. The elbow loses the angle when the elbow is taken into flexion or pronation (**Fig. 7.13**).

The carrying angle is caused by the bony configuration of the articulating surface. The medial condyle of trochlea extends more distally than the lateral condyle of trochlea resulting in the deviation of the ulna toward lateral. This is results in the carrying angle.

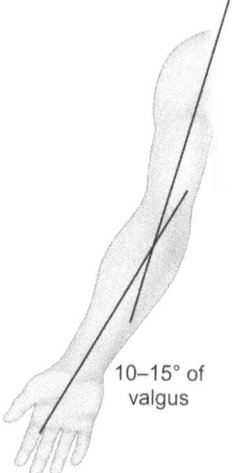

Fig. 7.13: Carrying angle

Technically it is nothing but cubitus valgus. The carrying angle is more in females than males.

Normal value: Females—8–15°
Males—0–5°

The carrying angle is an evolutionary modification for the females which is helpful keeping in view that females have a wider pelvis.

PATHOMECHANICS

- Tennis elbow
- Golfer's elbow
- Student's elbow
- Nurse maid's elbow

Tennis Elbow

- This is also called as lateral epicondylitis
- This is the condition characterized by pain and acute tenderness at the lateral aspect of the elbow related to the common extensor tendon.
- This is because of the overuse or misuse or abuse of the common extensor tendon most commonly extensor carpi radialis brevis during day-to-day activities.
- This is also seen in sports population most commonly in tennis players. When tennis players play backhand shot it create extreme stress to the common extensor tendon.

- Treatment is strengthening of the extensor muscle to make it stronger to take the load. Also tendinitis relieving techniquesand pain relieving modalities.

Golfer's Elbow

- This is also called as medial epicondylitis.
- This is the condition characterized by pain and acute tenderness at the medial aspect of the elbow related to the common flexor tendon.
- This is because of the overuse or misuse or abuse of the common flexor tendon.
- This is also seen in sports population most commonly in golf players. When golfers play their shot it creates extreme stress to the common flexor tendon.
- Treatment is strengthening of the flexor muscle to make it stronger to take the load. Also tendinitis relieving techniques and pain relieving modalities.

Student's Elbow

Olecranon bursitis is commonly referred as student's elbow. This is seen commonly in students or any individual who has the habit of resting elbow on a hard surface like table, bench. This hard table over a period of time and with micro movements at the elbow results in friction between the olecranon bursa and olecranon process. This friction damages the burse gives it inflammation. This is called as olecranon bursitis.

Nurse Maid's Elbow/Pulled Elbow

- Pulled elbow is also called as Nurse maid's elbow.
- Usually seen in children between 2 and 5 years. This happens when the child is lifted holding the child's hand. This results in traction force being exerted to the elbow which will result in the head of the radius coming out of the annular ligament. In the Western world, the nurse maids who handle the children resulting in pulled elbow might have been the reason for it to be popularly referred to it as nurse maid's elbow.
- The treatment of pulled elbow is fairly simple under a professional who reduces the dislocation by fully supinating the forearm and applying direct pressure over the head of the radius. A sudden click is heard indicating it is back into its position.

CHAPTER 8

Wrist and Hand Complex

Chapter Outline

- Wrist complex
  - Osteology
  - Arthrology
  - Joints of wrist
  - Wrist ligaments
  - Kinematics of wrist
  - Kinetics of wrist
  - Pathomechanics
- Hand complex
  - Arches of hand
  - Joints of hand
  - Kinematics and kinetics
  - Prehension

INTRODUCTION

The human hand has been characterized as a symbol of power, as an extension of intellect, and as a seat of will. The symbiotic relationship between mind and hand is, e.g., brain is responsible for design of civilization, but the hand is responsible for its formation. The hand cannot function without the brain to control it likewise the encapsulated brain needs the hand as a primary tool of expression. Any loss of function in upper limb, regardless of the segment, ultimately translates into diminished function of its most distal joints.

THE WRIST COMPLEX

The wrist has eight small carpal bones that act as a flexible "spacer" between the forearm and hand. The wrist has two major articulations other than several small intercarpal joints. Wrist (carpus) comprises of two compound joints—radiocarpal and midcarpal joints together termed as wrist complex. The radiocarpal joint is the articulation between distal end of radius and proximal row of carpal bones. Distal to this joint lies the midcarpal joint that involves the articulation between proximal and distal row of carpal bones. These two joints allow movements, such as wrist flexion, extension, ulnar, and radial deviation. Distal radioulnar joint is considered to be part of the forearm complex as it plays a role in pronation and supination.

Many muscles that control the fingers originate extrinsic to hand with their proximal attachments located in the forearm. Wrist complex plays an important role to control the length tension relationships in multiarticular hand muscles and thus allows fine adjustment of grip. The wrist muscles appear to be designed for balance and control rather than for maximizing torque production. The wrist has been called the most complex joint of the body from both an anatomic and physiologic perspective. The structure and biomechanics of wrist and hand vary from person to person and that even subtle variations can produce differences in how given function occurs.

The wrist complex as a whole is considered to be biaxial with motions of flexion and extension around a coronal axis and radial and ulnar deviation around an anterior posterior axis. Some degrees of pronation and supination are also found at the radiocarpal joint. The ranges of motions are variable and reflect the differences in carpal kinematics due to such factors as ligamentous laxity, shape of

Chapter 8 | Wrist and Hand Complex

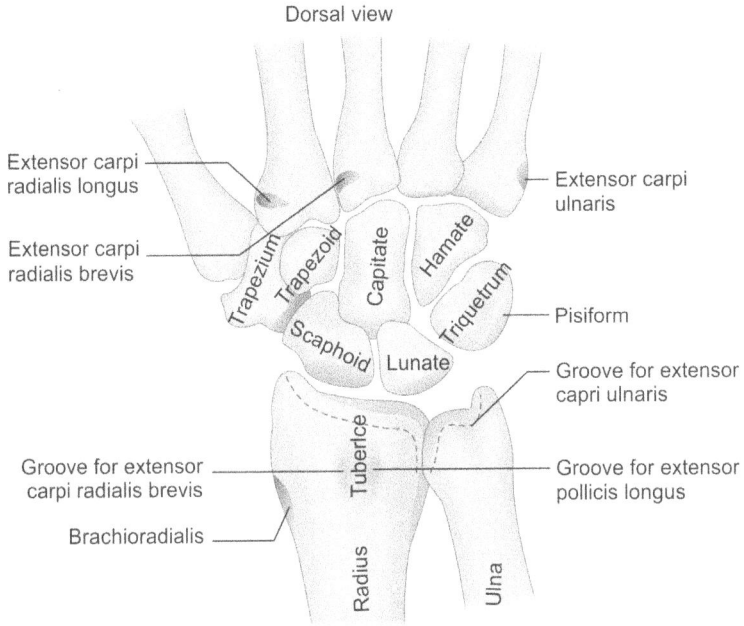

Fig. 8.1: Structure of wrist complex

articular surfaces, and constraining effects of muscles. Normal ranges are 78–85° of flexion, 55–70° of extension, 150–21° of radial deviation and 38–45° of ulnar deviation. Gilford and colleagues proposed that the two joint, rather than single joint, systems of wrist complex: permitted large ROMs with less exposed articular and tighter joint capsules, had less tendency for structural pinch at extreme of ranges, and allowed for flatter multijoint surfaces that are more capable of withstanding imposed pressures.

■ OSTEOLOGY

Distal Forearm
- Dorsal or Lister's tubercle of the radius
- Styloid process of the ulna
- Styloid process of the radius
- Distal articular surface of the radius

Carpal Bones
Proximal row of carpal bones (Fig. 8.1):
- Scaphoid
- Lunate
- Triquetrum
- Pisiform

Distal row of carpal bones (Fig. 8.1):
- Trapezium
- Trapezoid
- Capitate
- Hamate

■ ARTHROLOGY

Joint Structure of the Wrist
The primary joints of the wrist are radiocarpal and midcarpal joint. Many less significant intercarpal joints exist between adjacent carpal bones. Intercarpal joints contribute to wrist motion through gliding motions.

■ JOINTS OF WRIST
- Radiocarpal joint
- Midcarpal joint: Medial and lateral compartment
- Intercarpal joint

Radiocarpal Joint

This joint is formed by the radius and radioulnar disc (as part of the triangular fibrocartilage complex TFCC) proximally and by the scaphoid, lunate, and triquetrum distally. The proximal radiocarpal joint surface has a single continuous biconcave curvature that is long and shallow side-to-side (frontal) and shorter and sharper anteroposteriorly (sagittal plane). The proximal joint surface is composed of (1) the lateral radial facet that articulates with the lunate, (2) the medial radial facet that articulates with the lunate and (3) the TFCC that articulates predominantly with the triquetrum although it has some contact with the lunate in the neutral wrist. The scaphoid and lateral facet of the radius account on an average for slightly more than half the radiocarpal surface contact: The TFCC accounts for only 10%. The TFCC consists of the radioulnar disc, a connective tissue wedge, meniscus homologue, and the various fibrous attachments. The articular disc is a fibrocartilaginous continuation of the articular cartilage of the distal radius. The disc is connected medially via two dense fibrous connective tissue laminas. The upper lamina attaches to ulnar head and ulnar styloid process: the lower lamina has connections to the sheath of the extensor carpi ulnaris and to triquetrum, hamate, and the base of the fifth metacarpal via fibers from the ulnar collateral ligament. The medial connective tissue structures may facilitate ROM because connective tissue is more compressible than fibrocartilage. The ulna does not participate as part of radiocarpal joint other than as an attachment site for segments of TFCC. As a whole the compound proximal radiocarpal joint surface is oblique angled slightly volarly and ulnarly. The proximal carpal row is the distal surface of the radiocarpal joint. The proximal carpal row and ligaments together appear to present a single biconvex joint surface that unlike a rigid segment can change shape to accommodate to the demands of space between the forearm and hand. The pisiform does not take part in the articulation but increases the moment arm of flexor carpi ulnaris that attaches to it. The curvature of distal radiocarpal joint surface is sharper than the proximal making the joint somewhat incongruent. Joint incongruence and the angulations of the proximal joint surface result in a greater range of flexion and extension and greater ulnar than radial deviation. The radiocarpal joint is enclosed by a strong but somewhat loose capsule and is reinforced by capsular and intercapsular ligaments that cross the radiocarpal joint also contribute to stability at the midcarpal joint, similarly muscles of the radiocarpal joint also function at the midcarpal joint.

- **Ulnar negative variance:** Describes as a short ulna in comparison with the radius at their distal ends **(Fig. 8.2)**
- **Ulnar positive variance,** the distal ulna is long relative to the distal radius **(Fig. 8.2)**

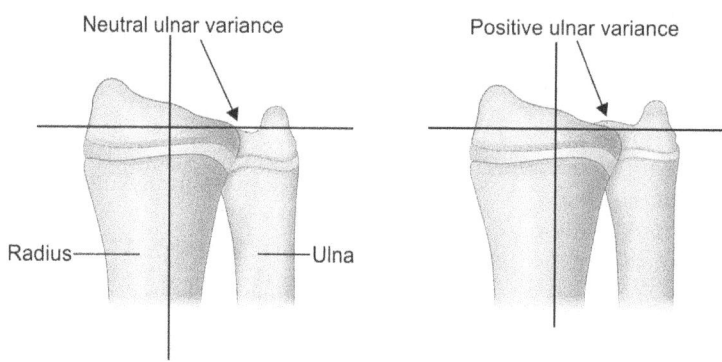

Fig. 8.2: Positive and negative ulnar variance

- **With an ulnar positive variance:** Potential for impingement of the TFCC between the distal ulna & triquetrum
  Palmer et al. Found an inverse relationship between thickness of TFCC and ulnar variance
  - *Positive ulnar variance:* Thinner TFCC
  - *Negative ulnar variance:* Thicker TFCC
- *Ulnar:* Negative variance may result in abnormal force distribution across the radiocarpal joint with potential degeneration at the radiocarpal joint. Avascular necrosis associated with negative ulnar variance

Midcarpal Joint Structure

This joint is the articulation between the scaphoid, lunate, and triquetrum proximally and the distal carpal row composed of the trapezium, trapezoid, capitate, and hamate. It is a functional rather than anatomical joint. It does not have its own capsule, however, it is separated from the radiocarpal joint and has a capsule and synovial lining that is continuous with each intercarpal articulation **(Fig. 8.3)**. The midcarpal joint surfaces have reciprocally concave-convex configuration. Functionally, the carpals of the distal row with move as an almost fixed unit. Together the bones of the distal row of carpals contribute second degree of freedom to the wrist complex. The excursions permitted by the articular surfaces of the midcarpal joint favor the range of extension and radial deviation opposite to radiocarpal joint.

The functional union of the distal carpals with each other and with their contiguous metacarpals not only serves the wrist complex but also the foundation for the transverse and longitudinal arches of the hand. The midcarpal ligament can be divided in to medial and lateral joint compartments. The larger medial compartment if formed by the convex head of the capitate and apex of hamate, fitting in to concave recess formed by the distal surfaces of the scaphoid, lunate, and triquetrum. The head of the capitate fits into this concave recess much like ball and socket joint. The lateral compartment of the midcarpal joint is formed by the junction of the slightly concave proximal surfaces of the trapezium and trapezoid. Shape of lateral is less pronounced than medial compartment. For this reason, subsequent arthrokinematic analysis of the midcarpal joint focuses on the medial compartment.

Axes and Motions

Joint	Axis	Motion	Close-packed position
Wrist • Radiocarpal • Midcarpal	Lateral	Flexion/Extension	Extension
	A-P	Ulnar and radial deviation	

Even though flexion and extension occur at both of the wrist's articulations:
- Most wrist extension occurs around the midcarpal joint's lateral axis.
- Most wrist flexion occurs around the radiocarpal joint's lateral axis.
- Ulnar and radial deviation occurs around an axis that passes through the capitate **(Fig. 8.4)**.
- Two wrist creases on the hand's palmar (or volar) surface are landmarks for the locations of the radiocarpal and midcarpal joints.

Wrist Arthrokinematics

In open chain movement, the convex surfaces of the scaphoid and lunate move on the concave surfaces of the radius and ulna.

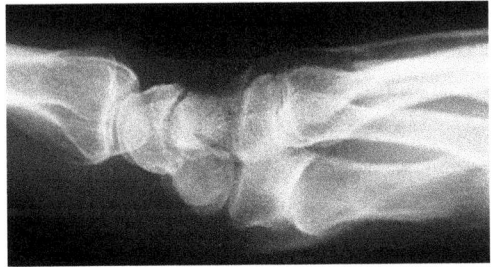

Fig. 8.3: X-ray-lateral view of carpal bones

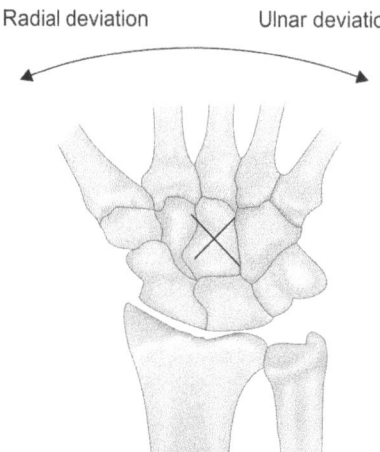

Fig. 8.4: Osteokinematics of wrist radial and ulnar deviation

- **During flexion:** Scaphoid/lunate rolls anteriorly (toward palm) and glide posteriorly (toward dorsum) **(Fig. 8.5B)**
- **During extension:** Scaphoid/lunate rolls posteriorly (toward dorsum) and glide anteriorly (toward palm) **(Fig. 8.5A)**.
- **During ulnar deviation:** Scaphoid/lunate rolls toward ulna and glide toward radius **(Fig. 8.6A)**.
- **During radial deviation:** Scaphoid/lunate rolls toward radius and glide toward ulna **(Fig. 8.6B)**.
  - Most wrist extension occurs around the midcarpal joint's lateral axis.
  - Most wrist flexion occurs around the radiocarpal joint's lateral axis.
  - Ulnar and radial deviation occurs around an axis that passes through the capitate.

Two wrist creases on the hand's palmar (or volar) surface are landmarks for the locations of the radiocarpal and midcarpal joints.

WRIST LIGAMENTS

Many of the wrist ligaments of the wrist are small and difficult to isolate. They are essential to maintaining natural intercarpal alignment and transferring forces through and across the carpus. These are not only important for

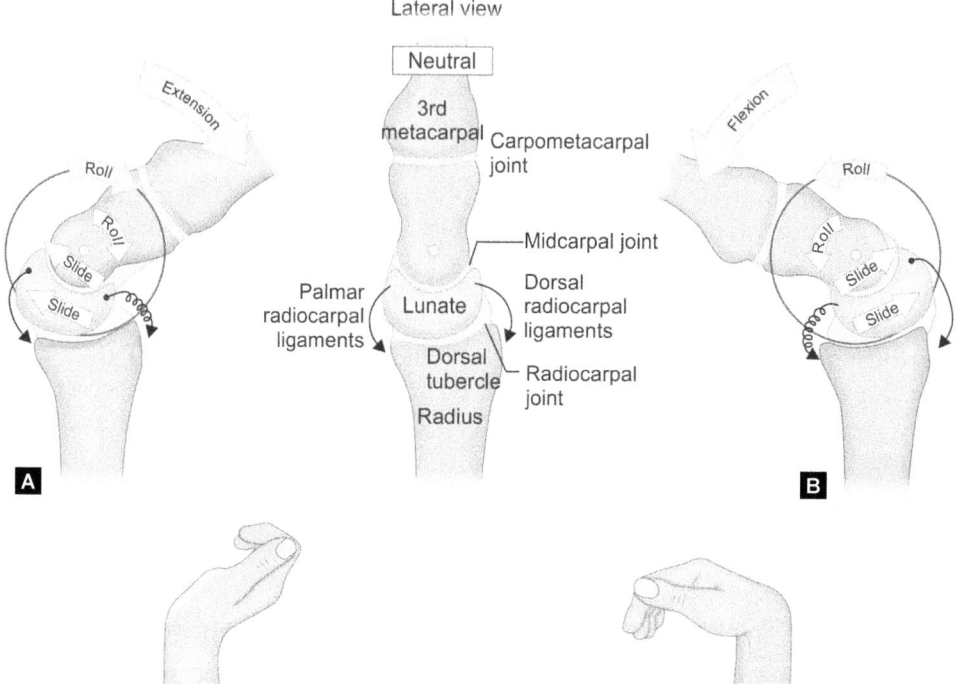

Figs. 8.5A and B: Kinematics of wrist motion: (A) Wrist extension; (B) Wrist flexion

Chapter 8 | Wrist and Hand Complex

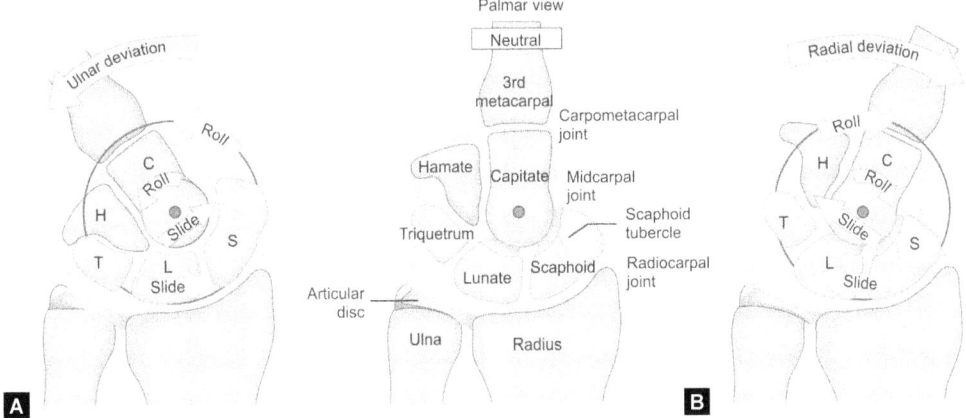

Figs. 8.6A and B: Osteokinematics of (A) Ulnar deviation, (B) Radial deviation

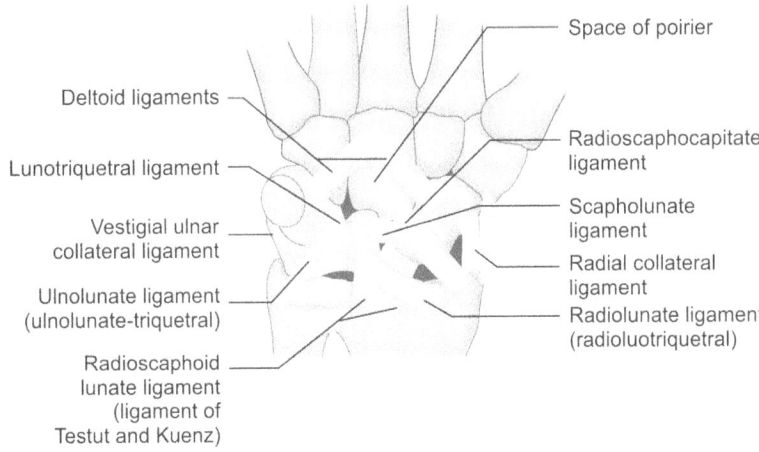

Fig. 8.7: Ligaments of wrist joint

articular stability but also for guiding and checking motion between and among the carpals. Ligaments that are damaged through injury and disease leave the wrist vulnerable to deformation and instability.

Wrist ligaments are classified as extrinsic and intrinsic. Extrinsic ligaments have their proximal attachments outside the carpal bones; intrinsic ligaments in contrast, have both their proximal and distal attachments on carpal bones. The extrinsic ligaments therefore are more likely to fail but also have better potential for healing and help protect the slower to heal intrinsic ligaments by accepting forces first **(Fig. 8.7)**.

Extrinsic Ligaments

A fibrous capsule surrounds the external surface of the wrist and the distal radioulnar joint. Dorsally, the capsule thickens slightly to form ligamentous bands known as **dorsal radiocarpal ligaments**. It reinforces the posterior side of radiocarpal joint becoming taut in full flexion. Another dorsal intercarpal ligament together with dorsal radiocarpal ligament forms a horizontal "v" that contributes to radiocarpal stability.

The lateral part of the wrist capsule is strengthened by fibers called the **radial collateral ligament**. It extends from styloid process to trapezium and adjacent transverse carpal ligament. It provides only part of lateral stability to wrist joint. These fibers are maximally taut when ulnar deviation of the wrist is combined with extension.

On the volar surface of the wrist complex, the numerous intrinsic and extrinsic ligaments are variously described by the composite or separate names and have been described as the **volar radiocarpal ligaments**. These include the radiocapitate, radioscaphoid, and radiotriquetral ligament. Each ligament arises from a roughened area on the distal radius, travels distally in an ulnar direction and attaches to the palmar surface of several carpal bones. These ligaments are much stronger than the dorsal one. These become maximally taut in extension.

A complex set of connective tissues exists near the ulnar border of the wrist known as the **ulnocarpal complex also referred as TFCC** which includes articular disc, the ulnar collateral ligament, and the palmar ulnocarpal ligament. This complex set fills most of the space between distal ulna and carpal bones. This space allows the carpal bones to pronate and supinate with the radius without the interference from the distal end of the ulna.

The **articular disc**, the main feature of the ulnocarpal complex attaches from the ulnar notch of the radius to near the styloid process of the ulna. A meniscal extension of the disc is often called ulnocarpal meniscal homologue. Between the meniscal extension of the disc and the ulnar collateral ligament is the small prestyloid recess a space filled with synovial fluid. This space often becomes distended and painful with rheumatoid arthritis. Tears in the disc may permit synovial fluid to spread from the radiocarpal joint to distal radioulnar joint.

The **ulnar collateral ligament** is a thickening of the ulnar side of wrist capsule. The ligament extends from the styloid process of ulna, crosses the ulnocarpal space, and attaches distally to the ulnar side of the triquetrum and as far as fifth metacarpal base. Full radial deviation of the wrist elongates the ulnar collateral ligament and surrounding capsule.

The palmar ulnocarpal ligament is a thickened band of connective tissue that originates from the anterior margin of the articular disc and extends from lunate to triquetrum, taut in full wrist extension and ulnar deviation.

Intrinsic Ligaments

Classified as short, intermediate, and long ligaments.

Short ligaments within the wrist connect the bones of the distal row by their palmar, dorsal or interosseous surfaces and stabilize and unite the row of bones, permitting them to function as a single mechanical unit.

Three intermediate ligaments exist within the wrist: The lunotriquetral ligaments are a fibrous continuation of the palmar radiolunate ligament which extends and maintain stability between the lunate and triquetrum. Scapholunate interosseous ligament maintains scaphoid stability and therefore much stability of the wrist.

Two long ligaments are present with in the wrist. The palmar intercarpal ligament is firmly attached to the palmar surface of the capitate bone. The ligament bifurcates into two fiber groups that form an inverted "v" shape one end from capitate to scaphoid and other one from capitate to triquetrum.

KINEMATICS OF WRIST

Osteokinematics

The osteokinematics of wrist are limited to two degrees of freedom flexion, extension, radial and ulnar deviation. Wrist circumduction—a full circular motion made by the wrist—is a combination of the aforementioned movements, not a third degree of freedom. The wrist does not rotate about an axis running longitudinally through the radius. This motion is blocked by the bony fir of the radiocarpal joint and the fiber direction of many radiocarpal ligaments. The apparent axial rotation of the palm called as pronation and supination occurs at the proximal and distal radioulnar joints of the forearm. Forearm motion requires hand movement with the radius, not separately from it. The lack of this third degree of freedom at the radiocarpal joint allows the pronator and supinator muscles to transfer torques across the wrist to working hand. Normal ranges are 78–85° of flexion, 55–70° of extension. Total flexion exceeds 10–15°. The wrist rotates in the sagittal plane approximately 45–55° as 15–21° of radial deviation and 38–45° of ulnar deviation. Because of the ulnar tilt of the distal radius maximum ulnar deviation normally is double that of radial deviation. Most natural movements of the wrist use a combination of frontal and sagittal plane motions. The greatest continuous arc of motion at the wrist exists between full extension/radial deviation and full flexion/ulnar deviation.

Arthrokinematics

The proximal carpals therefore are effectively a mechanical link between the radius and the distal carpals and metacarpals to which the muscular forces are actually applied. Gilford and colleagues said the proximal carpal row is an intercalated segment, a relatively unattached middle segment of a three segment linkage. When compressive forces are applied across an intercalated segment the middle segment tends to collapse and move in opposite direction from the segments above and below, e.g., application of compressive muscular extensor forces across the biarticular wrist complex would cause an unstable proximal carpal row to collapse into flexion while the distal row extended.

The axis of rotation for wrist movement is assumed to pass through the head of the capitate. The axes migrate slightly throughout the full range of motion. The wrist is a double joint system with motion occurring simultaneously at both the radiocarpal and midcarpal joints.

- **During flexion:** Scaphoid/lunate rolls anteriorly (toward palm) and glide posteriorly (toward dorsum)
- **During extension:** Scaphoid/lunate rolls posteriorly (toward dorsum) and glide anteriorly (toward palm).

Wrist Flexion and Extension

During flexion/extension, the scaphoid seems to show the greatest motion of the three proximal carpals while the lunate moves the least. The motion begins with the wrist in full flexion. Active extension is initiated at the distal carpal row and the attached metacarpals by the wrist extensor muscles attached to those bones. The distal carpals glide on relatively fixed proximal bones. The distal carpal row effectively glides in the same direction as motion of the hand. When the wrist complex reaches neutral (long axis of the third metacarpal in line with the long axis of the forearm), the ligaments spanning the capitate and scaphoid together into a close packed position. Continued extensor force now moves the combined unit of distal carpal row and scaphoid on relatively fixed lunate and triquetrum. At approximately 45° of hyperextension of the wrist complex, the scapholunate interosseous ligament brings the scaphoid and lunate into close-packed position. This unites all the carpals and causes them to function as a single unit. Wrist complex extension is completed as the proximal articular surface of the carpals move as a solid unit on the radius and radioulnar disc. All ligaments become taut as full extension is reached and the entire wrist complex is close packed.

Wrist motion from full extension to full flexion occurs in the reverse sequence. In this, scaphoid participates at different times in scaphoid-capitate, scaphoid-lunate, or radioscaphoid motion. Crumpling of the proximal carpal row is prevented and full ROM is achieved. Normally in the wrist, the displacement of the bones is minimized by the action of the ligaments especially the scapholunate ligament. Damage to this ligament can occur through traumatic dislocation, chronic synovitis from rheumatoid arthritis, and even from surgical removal of a ganglion cyst. A torn scapholunate ligament may predispose a person to scapholunate joint instability which interferes with the natural kinematics of the wrist.

- **During ulnar deviation:** Scaphoid/lunate rolls toward ulna and glide toward radius.
- **During radial deviation:** Scaphoid/lunate rolls toward radius and glide toward ulna.

Ulnar and Radial Deviation of the Wrist

These also occur through synchronous convex on concave rotations at both the radiocarpal joint and the midcarpal joint. The arthrokinematics of ulnar and radial deviation is slightly more complicated than those of flexion and extension. Radial deviation produces not only deviation of the proximal and distal carpals radially, but simultaneous flexion of proximal carpals and extension of distal carpals. The opposite motions of the proximal and distal carpals occur with ulnar deviation. During radial/ulnar deviation the distal carpals moves as a relatively fixed unit, although the magnitude of motion between the bones of proximal carpal row may differ.

During ulnar deviation, the radiocarpal joints: The scaphoid. Lunate and triquetrum roll ulnarly and slide a significant distance radially. At midcarpal joint, ulnar deviation occurs primarily from the capitate rolling ulnarly and sliding slightly radially. Full range causes triquetrum to contact the articular disc. Compression of the hamate against the triquetrum pushes the proximal row of carpal bones radially against the styloid process of the radius. This compression helps to stabilize the wrist for activities that require large gripping forces.

Radial deviation at the wrist occurs through similar arthrokinematics as for ulnar deviation. The amount of radial deviation is limited because of impingement of styloid process of the radius. Most of this movement occurs at midcarpal joint.

Tension in the inverted V shape ligament during radial and ulnar deviation.

The arthrokinematics of the wrist motion is actively driven by muscles but controlled by the passive tension of ligaments.

During ulnar deviation, tension rises in the lateral leg of the palmar intercarpal ligament and palmar ulnocarpal ligament. During radial deviation tension rises in medial leg of the palmar intercarpal ligament and palmar radiocarpal ligament. There is consensus that wrist extension and ulnar deviation are most important for wrist activities. Wrist extension and ulnar deviation were also found to be the position of maximum scapholunate contact.

KINETICS

Motor Innervation

Radial nerve supplies all the muscles that cross the dorsal side of the wrist. The median and ulnar nerves innervate all the muscles that cross the palmar side of the wrist.

Sensory Innervation

- **Radiocarpal and midcarpal:** C6–7-median and radial nerve
- **Midcarpal:** C8-deep branch of ulnar nerve.

Functions of the Wrist Muscle

The primary role of wrist muscles is to provide a stable base for the hand while permitting positional adjustments that allow for optimal length tension in the finger muscles. The axis of rotation for all wrist motion is located at the base of capitate. No wrist muscle actually crosses directly to this axis. For example, extensor carpi radialis brevis (ECRB) passes dorsally to wrist's medial lateral axis of rotation and laterally to wrist anterior posterior axis of rotation.

Function of Wrist Extensors

Primary: ECRB, extensor carpi radialis longus (ECRL), extensor carpi ulnaris (ECU)

Secondary: Extensor pollicis longus (EPL), extensor digitorum communis (EDC), extensor indicis (EI), abductor pollicis brevis (APB), extensor digiti minimi (EDM)

The EDC is capable of generating sufficient wrist extension torque, but is primarily involved with finger extension. The tendons of the muscles that cross the dorsal and dorsal-radial side of the wrist secured in place across the wrist by extensor retinaculum. Between the extensor retinaculum and the dorsal surface of wrist are six fibro-osseous tunnels that house the tendons along with their synovial sheaths. The extensor retinaculum prevents the tendon from bowstringing up and away from the radiocarpal joint during active extension. The retinaculum and associated tendons also assist the dorsal capsular ligaments in stabilizing the dorsal side of the wrist.

Wrist extensor activity while making a fist: The main functions of the wrist extensors are to position and stabilize the wrist for activities involving the fingers.

Role of wrist extensor muscles and making a fist:

The strong synchronous activities from the wrist extensors can be demonstrated by rapidly tighten and release the fist. The extrinsic finger flexor muscles, namely flexor digitorum profundus (FDP) and flexor digitorum superficialis (FDS) pass a significant distance palmar to the wrist's medial-lateral axis of rotation. Their contraction as primary finger flexors generates a significant flexion torque at the wrist that must be counter balanced by the extensor muscles. As a strong grip is applied to an object, the wrist extensors hold the wrist in about 35° of extension and 5° of ulnar deviation. This position optimizes the length-tension relationship of the extrinsic finger flexors, thereby facilitating maximal grip strength. The most active wrist extensor during light closure is ECRB. As grip increases ECU then ECRL joins ECRB. Activities that require repetitive forceful grasp, such as hammering or playing tennis may overwork the wrist extensors especially the highly active ECRB. A condition known as lateral epicondylitis or tennis elbow occurs from stress and resultant inflammation of the proximal attachment of the wrist extensors.

Grip strength is significantly decreased with wrist in full flexion because of two factors first; the finger flexors cannot generate adequate force because they are functioning at an extremely shortened length on their length tension curve. Second, the overstretched finger extensors, particularly the EDC create a passive extension torque at the fingers which further reduce effective grip force. This combination of physiologic events explains why a person with paralyzed wrist extensors has difficulty producing an effective grip even though the finger flexors remain fully innervated.

Attempts at producing a maximal effort grip when the wrist extensors are paralyzed results in a posture of finger flexion with wrist flexion. Stabilizing the wrist in greater extension enables the finger flexor muscles to nearby triple their grip force. Manually or orthotically preventing the wrist from flexing maintains the extrinsic finger flexors at an elongated length more conducive to higher force production.

Function of Wrist Flexors

Primary: FCR, FCU, PL

Secondary: FDP, FDS, FPL

FCU produces the greatest flexor torque of the three primary wrist flexor muscles based on the internal moment arm and cross sectional area. ECU demonstrates significant EMG activity during active wrist flexor muscles. This EMG activity reflects eccentric activity from the muscle as it produces a force to assist the ulnar collateral with stability of ulnar side of wrist. The ulnocarpal space is inherently fragile due to its lack of bony reinforcement. The FCR and FCU work synergistically to flex the wrist. Muscles that flex the wrist have a cross-sectional area twice that of the muscles that extend the wrist and so as the strength. Many activities that require a powerful grip, such as lifting and pulling objects, also require isometric wrist flexor torques; coactivation of wrist toward extension in order to maintain the favorable activation length of the finger flexors.

Function of Radial and Ulnar Deviators

Radial deviators: ECRL, ECRB, EPL, EPB, FCR, APL and FPL.

Ulnar deviators: ECU and FCU.

The radial deviator muscles generate about 15% greater isometric torque than the ulnar deviator muscles. For example, striking a nail with a hammer both ulnar and radial deviators will work. The axis of rotation will be capitated and internal moment arm will be FCU, ECU, ECRB, and ECRL.

There is strong functional association between FCU and ECU because of which injury to either muscle can incapacitate the overall kinetics of ulnar deviation. For example, RA often causes inflammation and pain in the extensor carpi ulnaris tendon near to its distal attachment. Attempts at active ulnar deviation with minimal to no activation in the painful extensor carpi ulnaris causes the action of flexor carpi ulnaris to remain unopposed. The resulting flexed posture of the wrist is thereby not suitable for an effective grasp.

PATHOMECHANICS

Carpal Instability

Essentially all types of carpal instability lead to a loss of function due to a loss of normal anatomic alignment. Two common types are:
1. Rotational collapse of wrist
2. Translocation of the carpus

Rotational Collapse of Wrist

Mechanically, the wrist consists of a mobile proximal row of carpal bones intercalated or interposed between two rigid structures: The forearm and distal carpal row. Like derailed freight of train, the proximal row of carpal bones is prone to a rotational collapse in a zig-zag fashion when compressed from both the ends. In healthy persons, the collapse and joint dislocation are prevented by resistance from ligaments, tendons, and intercarpal articulations. The lunate is the most frequently dislocated bone as no muscles attach directly to it and it has to depend on the ligamentous stability and scaphoid. The scaphoid functions as a mechanical link between lunate and rigid row of carpal bones. When injury to one or more ligament attached to scaphoid unlinks the lunate from the stabilizing influence of the scaphoid, the lunate is left to act as an intercalated segment. When ligamentous constraint on the scaphoid is reduced or removed, the scaphoid tends to follow its natural tendency to collapse into flexion on the volarly inclined radius. The flexed scaphoid slides dorsally on the radius and subluxes. Released from scaphoid stabilization, the lunate and triquetrum follow their natural tendency to extend, and the muscular forces applied to the distal carpals cause them to flex on the extended lunate and triquetrum. The flexed distal carpals glide dorsally on the lunate and triquetrum accentuating the extension of lunate and triquetrum. The zig-zag pattern of the three segments is known as DISI. For example, a fall over an outstretched hand with resulting fractures of scaphoid and tearing of scapholunate ligament. Disruption of this mechanical link leads to lunate dislocation. The lunate most often dislocates so its distal articular surface faces dorsally called as **dorsal intercalated segmental stability** (DISI) **(Fig. 8.8B)**. With sufficient ligamentous laxity, the capitate may sublux dorsally off the extended lunate and migrate in to the gap between the flexed scaphoid and extended lunate. At this point, the deformity has been termed scapholunate advanced collapse or **SLAC.** Injury to other ligaments, such as lunotriquetral ligament may cause a lunate and scaphoid together fall into flexion and the triquetrum and distal carpal row extend and distal articular surfaces of lunate faces volarly called as **volar intercalated segmental instability (VISI) (Fig. 8.8A).** Changes in natural arthrokinematics of the wrist may create regions of high stress, eventually leading to joint destruction, and joint morphology changes. A painful and arthritic wrist may fail to provide a stable platform for the hand.

Wrist Joint Fractures

It accounts for 6% of all fractures and dislocations in the body, with the bones of the proximal row the most common site of debilitating injury. The scaphoid is the most frequent fractured bone. It is also involved in the most common carpal instability.

Carpal tunnel syndrome: The "structure" that maintains the tunnel's shape is the flexor retinaculum, also called the transverse carpal ligament or the volar carpal ligament (**Fig. 8.9**).

This ligament connects the scaphoid and trapezium on the hand's radial side with the hamate on the ulnar side.

The carpal tunnel contains (from radial to ulnar side):
- FCR tendon
- FPL tendon
- Median nerve.
- Tendons of FDS and FDP
- Also contains vascular structures.

Repetitive motion can produce a tenosynovitis in the tendon sheaths of the long flexor muscles. This, in turn, can increase hydrostatic pressure in the tunnel, causing compression damage to median nerve. Carpal tunnel syndromes impairments include pain and paresthesia in the distribution of the median nerve. They also include weakness of muscles innervated by the median nerve, the thenar muscles, and the first and second lumbricals.

The tunnel's contents are also prone to compression injury due to trauma, congenital stenosis, acromegaly, or hormonal changes.

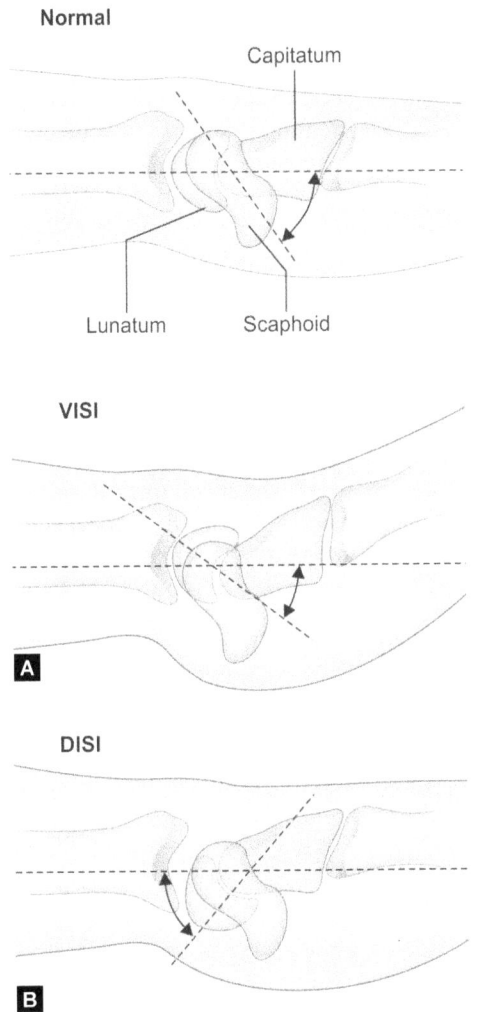

Figs. 8.8A and B: (A) Volar intercalated segmental instability; (B) Dorsal intercalated segmental instability

Translocation of the Carpus

The distal end of radius is angled from side to side so that its articular surface is sloped ulnarly about 25°. Ulnar tilt of the radius creates a natural tendency for the carpus to slide (translate) in an ulnar direction. This sliding force is naturally resisted by passive forces from various extrinsic ligaments. A disease, such as rheumatoid arthritis significantly weakens the wrist ligaments.

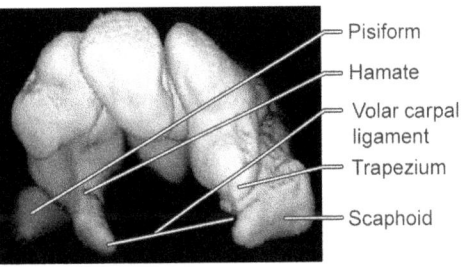

Fig. 8.9: Carpal tunnel

THE HAND COMPLEX

Introduction

The hand serves as important sense organ for the perception of the surroundings. It is also the primary effector organ for most complex motor behaviors and also, the hand helps for gesture, touch, craft, and art. There are 19 bones and 19 joints with in the hand driven by 29 muscles. Because of its enormous biomechanical complexity, the function of the hand involves a disproportionately large region of cortex of the brain. A hand totally incapacitated by rheumatoid arthritis or nerve injury, for instance, can dramatically reduce the functional importance of the other upper limb joints.

Terminology

The hand has five digits; each one contains a set of phalanges. The thumb contains two phalanges and one interphalangeal joint where as other four fingers contain three phalanges and two interphalangeal joints one proximal and other distal interphalangeal joint. The articulation between the metacarpals and phalanges is called as metacarpophalangeal joint (MCP). And the articulations between the metacarpals and carpals is called ac carpometacarpal joint (CMC). A ray describes one metacarpal bone and its associated phalanges.

External Anatomy of Hand

Palmar creases function as dermal "hinges" markings where the skin folds upon itself during movement and to increase palmar friction to enhance the security of grasp.

Osteology

Metacarpal: The first metacarpal is the shortest and the stoutest. Each metacarpal has an elongated shaft with articular surfaces at each end. The palmar surface is slightly concave longitudinally and distal end has a large convex head with the hand at rest in the anatomic position, the thumb's metacarpal is oriented in a different plane from the other digits. The second through the fifth metacarpals are aligned generally side by side, with their palmar surfaces facing anteriorly. The position of the thumb's metacarpal is rotated 90° medially relative to other digits. Optimum prehension depends on flexion of the thumb occurring in a plane that intersects, versus parallels, the plane of flexing fingers. The position of the metacarpal and trapezium is caused by the distal pole of the scaphoid.

Phalanges: The hand has 14 phalanges. The phalanges within each finger are referred to as proximal, middle, and distal. The thumb has only two phalanges. The proximal and middle phalanges of each finger have a concave base and convex head. The distal phalanx of each digit has a concave base. At its distal end is a rounded tuberosity that anchors the fleshy pulp of soft tissue to the terminus of each digit.

ARCHES OF HAND (FIG. 8.10)

The palmar concavity of the hand allows the hand to securely hold and manipulate objects of many and varied shape and sizes. The natural palmar concavity of the hand is

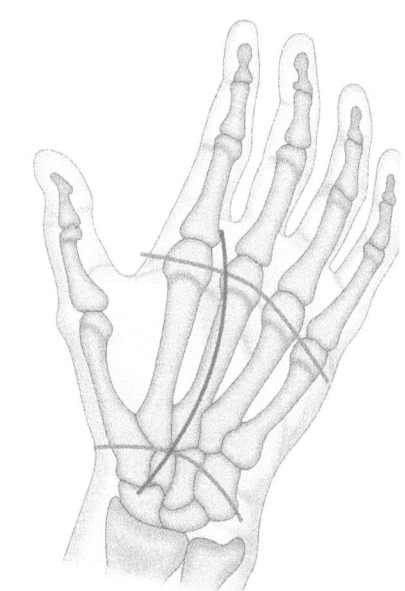

Fig. 8.10: The proximal and distal transverse arches and longitudinal arch

supported by three integrated arches: Two transverse and one longitudinal:

Proximal Transverse Arch

- A stable bony arch that forms the posterior border of the carpal tunnel.
- The arch's integrity is maintained by a soft tissue "strut" formed by the flexor retinaculum or transverse carpal ligament (also called the volar carpal ligament). This ligamentous strut connects the scaphoid and trapezium on the arch's radial side with the hamate on its ulnar side, and forms the anterior border of the carpal tunnel.

Distal Transverse Arch

Hertling and Kessler call this the metacarpal arch, because it is formed by the metacarpal heads; metacarpals 2 and 3 are stable while 4 and 5 are relatively mobile. You can observe the arch's combination of "radial" stability and "ulnar" mobility by loosely closing your fist, then squeezing more tightly, when you will observe movement in the more mobile fourth and fifth metacarpals. The keystone of distal transverse arch is formed by the MCP joints of (2nd and 3rd) these central metacarpals.

Longitudinal Arch

The longitudinal arch of the hand follows the general shape of second and third rays. Observe this arch's behavior as you loosely close your fist. Tighten the fist and watch the fourth and fifth metacarpals.

The arches provide a balance between stability and mobility for grasping. For instance, we produce the so-called "chuck grasp" by using the more stable second and third metacarpals, instead of the more mobile fourth and fifth metacarpals.

Therapeutic splints must support these three arches. All the three arches are interlinked. A structural failure at any joint may weaken other, e.g., destruction of MCP joint by rheumatoid disease, as this joint is the common keystone for both the longitudinal and transverse arches, its destruction will lead to flattening of hand. The carpal arch is created not only by the curved shape of the carpals but also by the ligaments that maintain the concavity. The ligaments that maintain the arch are the transverse carpal ligament (TCL) and the transversely-oriented intercarpal ligaments. The TCL is the portion of the flexor retinaculum that attaches to the pisiform and hook of the hamate medially and the scaphoid and trapezium laterally. The TCL and intercarpal ligaments that link the four distal carpal bones forms the carpal tunnel.

Three arches balance stability and mobility in the hand.

The proximal transverse arch is rigid, but the other two arches are flexible, and are maintained by activity in the hand's intrinsic muscles.

Functional Position of the Hand (Norkin and Levangie; Hertling and Kessler)

- **Wrist:**
  - Extended 20°
  - Ulnarly deviated 10°
- **Digits 2 through 5**
  - MP joints flexed 45°
  - PIP joints flexed 30–45°
  - DIP joints flexed 10–20°
- **Thumb**
  - First CMC joint partially abducted and opposed
  - MP joint flexed 10°
  - IP joint flexed 5°

When therapists immobilize a patient's hand, they often position it this way. During a period of immobilization, the resting lengths of the hand's ligaments and muscles change. This hand position places both the collateral ligaments and extrinsic extensor muscles in a relatively elongated and taut position. This position may prevent subsequent shortening of these tissues and provides the best balance of resting length and force production so the hand can function when the patient mobilizes it again. **Table 8.1** summarizes tabular overview on metacarpophalangeal, proximal interphalangeal and distal interphalangeal joint.

▲ Table 8.1: Tabular overview on metacarpophalangeal, proximal interphalangeal and distal interphalangeal joint.

Joint	Structure	Axis	Motion	Close-packed position
Metacarpophalangeal (MP)	Biaxial (condylar)	Lateral A-P	Flexion/extension abduction/adduction	First: Extension 2nd–5th: Flexion
Proximal interphalangeal (PIP)	Uniaxial	Lateral	Flexion/extension	Extension
Distal interphalangeal (DIP)	Uniaxial	Lateral	Flexion/extension	Extension

JOINTS OF THE HAND

Carpometacarpal Joint

The CMC joint is composed of articulations between the distal carpal row and the bases of five metacarpals. The function of the CMC joints allows the concavity of the palm to fit around many objects. Without this ability, the dexterity of the hand is reduced to a primitive hinge-like grasping motion.

Second Through Fifth Carpometacarpal Joints

- **II MC:** Trapezoid, trapezium, capitate, III MC
- **III MC:** Capitate, II MC, IV MC
- **IV MC:** Hamate, capitate, III MC, V MC
- **V MC:** Hamate, IV MC

All CMC joints are surrounded by articular capsules and strengthened by dorsal, palmar, and interosseous ligaments. All finger CMCs are supported by strong transverse and longitudinal ligaments volarly and dorsally. The deep transverse metacarpal ligament spans the heads of the second through fourth metacarpals volarly.

Joint Structure and Kinematics

- **II-IV CMC:** Plane synovial joints with one-degree freedom-F/E
- **V CMC:** Saddle, with two-degree freedom-flexion/extension, abduction/adduction. The immobile second and third metacarpals provide a fixed and stable axis about which the very mobile first metacarpal and the 4th and 5th metacarpals can move. The irregular and varied shapes of these joint surfaces prohibit standard arthrokinematic description.
- **Ligaments:** Intermetacarpal-strong.
- Volar/dorsal longitudinal carpometacarpal ligament-weak.

Carpometacarpal Joint of the Thumb

- Saddle variety of the synovial joint
- Articular surfaces
- Distal surface of the trapezium
- Proximal surface of the base of the first metacarpal bone
- Two degrees of freedom along with these movements also perform axial rotation, which occurs concurrently with other motions. The net effect at this joint is a circumduction motion commonly termed as opposition. It permits the tip of the thumb to oppose the tips of the fingers.
  - *Capsular ligament:* Most taut in abduction, extension, and opposition
  - *Lateral ligament:* Abduction, extension and opposition
  - *Anterior ligament:* Abduction and opposition
  - *Posterior ligament:* Abduction and opposition
  - *Radial collateral:* All movements to varying degrees except extension.

Saddle Joint Structure

The characteristic feature of saddle joint is that each articular surface is convex in one dimension and concave in another direction. The longitudinal diameter of the articular surface of the trapezium is generally concave from palmar to dorsal direction. The corresponding transverse diameter on the articular surface of the trapezium is generally convex from medial to lateral direction. The contour of the proximal articular surface of the thumb metacarpal has the reciprocal shape of that described for the trapezium. The longitudinal diameter of the articular surface of the metacarpal is generally convex from palmar to dorsal direction. The corresponding transverse diameter on the articular surface of the metacarpal is generally concave from medial to lateral direction.

KINEMATICS AND KINETICS

The primary motions at the CMC joint occur in 2 degrees of freedom. Abduction and adduction occurs in sagittal plane and flexion and extension in coronal plane. Opposition and reposition of the thumb are mechanically derived from the two primary planes of motion at the CMC joint.

Abduction and adduction at the thumb CMC: In abduction, the thumb lies within the plane of the hand. Maximum abduction occurs anterior to plane of the palm. Full abduction opens the web space of the thumb, forming a wide concave curvature used for forceful grasping of objects. During abduction, the convex articular surface of the metacarpal rolls primarily and slides dorsally on the concave surface of the trapezium and there will be palmar roll and dorsal slide and in adduction opposite occurs.

Flexion and extension at thumb CMC: During flexion, the metacarpal rotates slightly medially and during extension, the metacarpal rotates slightly laterally. The axial rotation is evident by watching the orientation of the nail of the thumb between full flexion and full extension. During flexion, the concave surface of metacarpal **rolls and slides** in **ulnar** direction. A shallow groove in the transverse diameter of the trapezium helps guide the slight medial rotation of the metacarpal and elongates radial collateral ligament. During extension of the CMC joint, the concave surface of metacarpal **rolls and slides in radial** direction across the transverse diameter of the joint. A shallow groove in the transverse diameter of the trapezium helps guide the slight lateral rotation of the metacarpal and elongates anterior oblique ligament.

Opposition of thumb carpometacarpal joint: Divided into two phases, in phase one the thumb metacarpal abducts and in phase two the abducted metacarpal flexes and medially rotates across the palm toward the little finger. Muscle force, especially from the opponens pollicis, helps guide the metacarpal to extreme medial side of the transverse articular surface of the trapezium. Abducted thumb increases tension in posterior ligament promotes the medial rotation (spin) of the metacarpal shaft. Full opposition is the close packed position of the thumb and CMC joint. Many of the ligaments in this position are twisted taut. **Reposition** of the CMC joint returns the metacarpal from full opposition back to anatomic position. This motion involves arthrokinematics of both adduction and extension-lateral rotation of thumb metacarpal.

Metacarpophalangeal joints: Synovial joint of the condylar variety of 2 degrees of freedom.

Fingers: Each of four MCP joints of the fingers is composed of convex metacarpal head proximally and the concave base of the first phalanx distally. Mechanical stability at the MCP joint is critical to overall biomechanics to hand. MCP joints serves as keystones for support of the mobile arches of the hand. The joint is surrounded by a capsule that is generally considered to be lax in extension. Imbedded within the capsule of each MCP joints is pair of radial and ulnar collateral ligaments and one palmar ligament or plate.

Volar plate: Volar ligament or plate is a unique structure that increases joint congruence. It is composed of fibro cartilage and is firmly attached to base of proximal phalanx. The plate becomes membranous proximally to blend with the capsule. The four volar plates of the MCP joints of the finger blend with and are interconnected superficially by the deep transverse metacarpal ligament. The connections of each volar plate to the

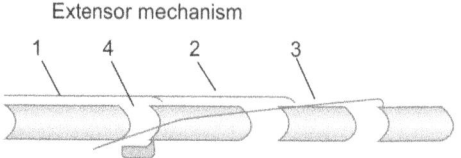

1. Extensor digitorum tendon
2. Central tendon
3. Lateral bands
4. Hood region

Fig. 8.11: Extensor mechanism of finger

collateral ligaments of the MCP joint and the extensor expansion help stabilize the volar plate on the four metacarpal heads. **Fibrous digital sheaths** which form tunnels or pulleys for the extrinsic finger flexors are anchored immediately anterior to palmar plates. The primary function of the palmar plates is to strengthen the MCP joint and resist hyperextension **(Fig. 8.11)**.

The concave component of the MCP joint is formed by the articular surface of the proximal phalanx, the collateral ligaments, and the dorsal surface of the palmar plate. This structure adds joint stability and increases the area of articular contact. Attaching between the palmar plates is three deep transverse metacarpal ligaments. These help to interconnect the second through fifth metacarpals

The collateral ligaments: Slack in extension. Provide stability throughout the MCP ROM with parts of the fibers taut at various points in the range. Studies proposed that the bicondylar shape of the volar surface of the metacarpal head provided a bony block to abduction and adduction at about 70° of MCP flexion, rather than collateral ligamentous testing.

Osteokinematics: Range increases from radially to ulnarly. For example, index finger 90° of MCP flexion and the little finger 110° of flexion. The range of abduction and adduction is maximal in MCP extension: The index and little finger have more frontal plane mobility than the middle and ring fingers. Abduction and adduction occurs 20° on either side of midline. Hyperextension 30–45°.

Arthrokinematics: This is based on the concave articular surface of the phalanx moving on the convex metacarpal head. During active extension, the base of the proximal phalanx rolls and slides in a dorsal direction under the power of extensor digitorum communis muscle. At about 60–70° of flexion, the collateral ligaments are maximally taut. At 0° of extension the collateral ligaments slacken while the palmar plate unfolds and make total contact with the head of metacarpal. Full hyperextension is limited by the stretch placed in the palmar plate. And during flexion roll and glide occur in a palmar direction. During abduction, the proximal phalanx rolls and slides in a radial direction and ulnarly during adduction.

Thumb: Articulation between convex metacarpal with concave proximal phalanx. The only difference with fingers is in osteokinematics. Active and passive motions of thumb are significantly less than of fingers.

Interphalangeal (IP)
- Uniaxial hinge joints
- Supported by two collateral ligaments, and by smaller versions of a volar plate.
- Like MP joint, proximal joint surface is convex and distal surface is concave
- Roll and glide occur in same direction.

Anterior with flexion and posterior with extension
- Close-packed in extension
- Pip flexion is 100–120°
- Dip flexion is 70–90° and 30° of hyperextension

Mechanism for Finger Flexion

Optimal function of the FDS and FDP depends not only on the wrist musculature, but also on the gliding mechanisms. It consists of retinacula, ligaments, bursae, and digital tendon sheaths. As the tendon passes through the carpal tunnel, friction between the tendons themselves and friction of the tendons overlying the transverse carpal ligament are prevented by the radial and ulnar bursae that envelop the flexor tendons at this level. The FPL, FDS, and FDP through the carpal tunnel are encased in radial and rest all tendons are in ulnar bursa. The FDS and FDP tendons of each finger pass through as many as five fibro-osseous tunnels formed by what are known as annular pulleys or vaginal ligaments. These pulleys are tethered by three cruciate ligaments. The synovial fluid contained in each of the digital sheaths permits gliding of the tendons beneath their ligamentous constraints and between each other. Although the FDP is deep to the FDS over most of its course, it attaches to the skeleton more distally, because it passes through a "split" in the FDS tendon known as Camper's chiasma. The function of the annular pulleys is to keep the flexor tendons close to the bone, allowing only a minimum amount of bowstringing and migration volarly from the joint axes and to maintain a near constant moment arm length of the flexor tendons. Trigger finger can occur because of repetitive trauma to a flexor tendon results in formation of nodules on the tendon and thickening of annular pulley. Finger flexion may be prevented completely of unable to reextend.

Mechanism for Finger Extension

- We can extend the PIP and DIP joints without also extending the MP joints.
- But we cannot extend the PIP joint without extending the DIP joint at the same time.
- Flexing only the DIP joint without also flexing the PIP joint is difficult.
- Full (active or passive) flexion of the PIP joint prevents active extension of the DIP joint.

We can understand these finding by learning the structure of the extensor mechanism, also known as the:
- Extensor expansion
- Extensor assembly
- Extensor apparatus
- Dorsal aponeurosis
- Aponeurotic sleeve

The extensor mechanism is an elaboration of the EDC tendon on the dorsum of each phalanx. The EI and the EDM insert into the extensor mechanisms of the second and fifth digits, respectively.

Several tendinous structures comprise the extensor mechanism:
1. The *EDC tendon* attaches by a tendinous slip to the proximal phalanx, through which it extends the MP joint.
2. The *central tendon* (or "slip") proceeds dorsally to attach to base of middle phalanx, where tension can extend the PIP joint.
3. The *lateral bands* proceed on either side of dorsal midline and rejoin before attaching to the distal phalanx. Tension in the lateral bands extends the DIP joint.
4. The *extensor hood* surrounds the MP joint laterally, medially, and dorsally, and receives tendinous fibers from the lumbricals and interossei.
5. Fibers of the *oblique retinacular ligament* (ORL) attach at the sides of the proximal phalanx and digital tendon sheaths, and proceed to distal portion of lateral bands. Thus, the ORL's line of application is volar to the PIP joint's lateral axis and dorsal to the DIP joint's lateral axis.

PIP extension (produced by other tissues in the extensor mechanism) elongates the ORL, creating passive tension that extends the DIP. The DIP extension helps open the hand.

DIP flexion (produced by the FDP) elongates the ORL, creating passive tension that flexes the PIP. The PIP flexion assists in finger closure.

Muscles that transmit force to the otherwise noncontractile extensor mechanism:
1. **Dorsal interossei (DI)**
   - The dorsal interossei attach proximally between adjacent metacarpals.
   - They attach distally either to bone (proximal phalanx) or to soft tissue (extensor mechanism).
   - Apply resistance as you attempt to abduct the second and fourth MP joints. Abduction is stronger at the second MP joint because the most of the first DI's muscle fibers attach directly to the

second proximal phalanx. Abduction of the fourth MP joint is relatively weak because the fourth DI attaches largely to the extensor mechanism itself.
- The dorsal interossei produce MP abduction and in certain instances MP flexion. Because they attach to the extensor mechanism, they also produce PIP and DIP extension.

2. **Palmar interossei (PI):**
   - Four palmar interossei (anatomists often include the ulnar head of flexor pollicis brevis in this group) attach proximally to a metacarpal, and distally to the same digit's proximal phalanx and/or its extensor mechanism.
   - They produce MP adduction and, in certain instances, MP flexion. They also produce PIP and DIP extension when they introduce tension into the extensor mechanism.

3. **Lumbricals:**
   - The four lumbricals attach proximally to the tendons of the flexor digitorum profundus, and distally to the extensor mechanism on its radial side at the level of the lateral bands. The muscles pass on the volar side of the transverse metacarpal ligament.
   - If they act alone, they produce MP flexion. They also produce PIP and DIP extension when they introduce tension into the extensor mechanism.
   - The lumbricals permit a dynamic interaction between flexors and extensors. Their attachments transmit their force to both the FDP tendon and the extensor mechanism. Especifically, lumbricals activity:
   - Increases passive tension in the extensor mechanism.
   - Decreases passive tension in FDP tendon's distal portion.
   - Many of the hand's intrinsic muscles attach to the extensor mechanism. Activity in any of these muscles produces force that the extensor mechanism communicates to its distal attachments.

- The extensor mechanism develops passive tension whenever it is elongated. Hand movements that passively elongate either the extensor mechanism or a structure that attaches to the extensor mechanism produce force in the extensor mechanism itself.

The extensor mechanism's fibers have lines of application that are always dorsal to the lateral axes of the PIP and DIP joints. Therefore,
- Activity in the intrinsic muscles that attach to the extensor mechanism always produces DIP and PIP extension.
- Passive flexion of the MP joint (try it yourself!) elongates the extensor mechanism and extends the PIP and DIP joints.

The fibrous lines of application in the hood and lateral bands pass very near the MP joint's lateral axis. Whether these structures move the MP joint in the sagittal plane depends on whether the MP joint is already flexed or extended.

Extensor mechanism influence on MCP joint function: At each MCP joint, EDC tendon passes dorsal to MCP joint axis. An active contraction of the muscle creates tension on the hood, pulls the hood proximally over the MCP joint, and extends the proximal phalanx. The other active forces that are part of the extensor mechanism are the dorsal interosseous, volar interosseous, and lumbrical muscles. Each of these muscles passes volar to the MCP joint axis and, therefore, creates a flexor force at the joint. When the EDC, lumbrical, and interossei contract simultaneously, the MCP joint will extend because the torque produced by the EDC at the MCP exceeds the MCP flexor torque of the intrinsic muscles. If the intrinsic muscles are inactive, the EDC will hyperextend the MCP and cause passive flexion of IP joints. This position of fingers is called as clawing of hand which is seen with an intercalated segment. The unstable proximal phalanx extends on the metacarpal below while the middle and distal phalanx flex over it. Normally, the collapse is prevented by active tension in the lumbricals or interossei that cross the MCP joint anteriorly. When these muscles are not present as in ulnar nerve injury, the EDC is unopposed and the finger claws also known as an intrinsic minus position.

1. **In MP flexion:**
   - MP flexion occurs when activity in the FDS or FDP flexes the MP joint.
   - The extensor mechanism is not "stretchy." When the digits flex (at the MP, PIP, or DIP joints), passive tension in the lateral bands and central slip pull the hood distally.
   - When the MP joint is already flexed, the lines of application of the interossei fall on volar side of the MP joint, and so produce MP flexion.
   - The distal shift in the extensor hood also increases the lumbricals moment arm so they can produce a greater flexor moment at the MP joint. However, text describes EMG studies which show quite consistently that the lumbricales do not act at the same time as the FDP! The lumbricales' function evidently does not include closure of the hand.

2. **In MP extension:**
   - Action in the extensor digitorum extends the MP joint, and also pulls the extensor mechanism (including the hood) proximally.
   - In this position, the interosseous muscles' lines of application are very close to the MP joint's lateral axis.
   - With such small moment arms, these muscles have little effect on MP joint movement in the sagittal plane. However, they still produce MP abduction/adduction when the MP joint is extended.

Extensor mechanism influence on IP joint function: The PIP and DIP joints are joined by both active and passive forces in such a way that DIP extension and PIP extension are interdependent: when PIP is actively extended, the DIP will also extend. Similarly, active DIP extension will create PIP extension. As per attachments EDC, interossei, and lumbricals are each capable of producing some tension in the central tendon, the lateral bands and the terminal tendon that will simultaneously create some extensor force at both the PIP and DIP joints. An EDC contraction alone will not produce IP extension. An active contraction of DI, VI, and lumbrical muscle is capable of extending the IP joints. However, if one or more of the intrinsic muscles contract without a contraction of the EDC, the MCP will simultaneously flex because each passes volar to the MCP joint axis. Two sources of tension in the extensor expansion appear to be necessary to fully extend the IP joints. Source I is normally provided by an active contraction of one or more of the intrinsic finger muscles. Source II may be provided by either by an active contraction of the EDC or by passive stretch. When the intrinsic musculature is paralyzed, the EDC may be able to extend the IP joints, but only if the MCP joint is maintained in flexion by some external force. The ability to use the EDC to extend the IPs with passively maintained MCP flexion is known as Bunnell's sign. Tension in the lateral bands distal to the PIP and some of the linkage between PIP and DIP may be contributed by passive action of the ORL. The ORLs pass just volarly to the PIP joint axis and attach distally to lateral bands. Tension will increase in the ORLs as the PIP is extended if the lateral bands and their terminal tendon are already tensed by DIP flexion. Consequently PIP extension through passive tension in the ORLs may contribute to DIP extension. The ORLs are significant only during 90° to 45°. Flexion of DIP joint produces flexion of the PIP joint by a similar combination of active and passive forces that link extension of these joints. When the DIP I flexed by FDP a simultaneous flexor force is applied over both joints it crosses. When the DIP begins flexing the terminal tendon and its lateral bands are stretched over the dorsal aspect of the DIP joint. The stretch in the lateral bands pulls the extensor hood distally. The distal migration in the extensor hood causes the central tendon of the extensor expansion to relax, facilitating flexion of the PIP. The bands migrate volarly by the elasticity of the interconnecting triangular ligament. Through the combination of active and passive mechanisms, both active and passive DIP flexion ordinarily results in simultaneous PIP flexion.

Functional coupling of PIP and DIP

When PIP is fully flexed actively by the FDS or flexed passively by some outside force, the DIP cannot be actively extended. When the PIP joint is flexed, the dorsally located central tendon is increasingly stretched. The tensed central tendon pulls the extensor hood distally. This distal movement of the hood releases some of the tension in the lateral bands. Relaxation of the lateral bands relaxes the terminal tendon on the distal phalanx. As 90° of PIP flexion is reached, loss of tension in the terminal tendon completely eliminates any extensor force at the DIP joint. Although the DIP joint can be actively flexed by the FDP when the PIP is already flexed, it cannot be actively re-extended as long as the PIP remains flexed.

- Active extension of the PIP joint will be accompanied by extension of PIP joint.
- Active or passive flexion of the DIP joint will normally be accompanied by flexion of the PIP.
- Full flexion of the PIP joint will prevent the DIP joint from being actively extended.

PREHENSION

These activities involve grasping and taking hold of an object between any two surfaces of the hand: The thumb participates in most but not all prehension activities.

Types of Grip

It is classified broadly into:
- Power grip
- Precision grip

Power Grip

The adductor pollicis stabilizes an object against the palm; the hand's position is static.

- **Cylindrical grip (Fist grasp is a small diameter cylindrical grasp) (Fig. 8.12A):** It almost uses flexors to carry the fingers around and maintain grasp on an object. The function is largely performed by FDP but in static phase FDS also assist to a good level. Recent studies have indicated considerable interosseous activity in cylindrical griping as they are MCP flexors and adductors/abductors. In strong grip, the magnitude of force of the interossei in metacarpal flexion has been found to nearly equal that of the extrinsic flexors. Although the location of the lumbricals indicates a possible contribution to MCP flexion in power grip, their lack of EMG activity, regardless of strength grip is consistent with their role as IP extensors. It is typically performed with the wrist in neutral flexion and extension and slight ulnar deviation. The heavier the object is the more likely it is that the wrist will ulnarly deviate. For example, holding a door handle.
- **Spherical grip (Fig. 8.12B):** This is similar in most respects to cylindrical grip. The extrinsic finger and thumb flexors and the thenar muscles follow similar patterns of activity and variability. The main distinction is greater spread of fingers which encompasses more interosseous activity. Apart from the role of flexors, the extensors not only provide a balancing role but are also essential for smooth and controlled opening and release of the object. Opening the hand during object approach and object release is primarily an extensor function, calling in the lumbricals, the EDC, and the thumb exercises.
- **Hook grip (Fig. 8.12C):** It is a specialized form of prehension. It is a function primarily of the fingers. MP extended with flattening of transverse arch; the person may include the palm but never includes thumb in this grasp. For example, carrying a briefcase. The major muscular activity is provided by FDP and FDS.
- **Lateral prehension (Fig. 8.12D):** It is a unique form of grasp. Contact occurs

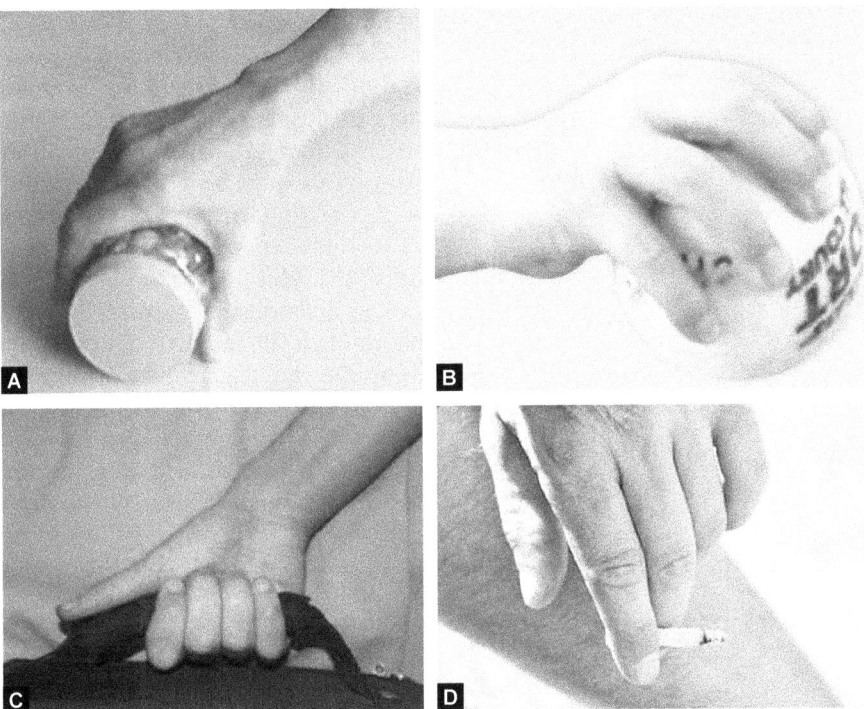

Figs. 8.12A to D: Power grip. (A) Cylindrical; (B) Spherical; (C) Hook grip; (D) Lateral prehension

between two adjacent fingers. The MCP and IP joints are usually maintained in extension as the contiguous MCP joint simultaneously abduct and adduct. This is the only form in which the extensor musculature plays a part in maintenance of posture. This can be a power grip if the thumb is adducted, a precision grip if the thumb is abducted. For example, holding a cigarette.

Precision Handling

These require much finer motor control and are more dependent on intact sensation.
- **One jaw:** Thumb
- **Two-jaw chuck:** Thumb and distal tip or pad or the side of the finger.
- **Three-jaw chucks:** When two fingers oppose the thumb it is called as three-jaw chuck.

(Muscles are active that abduct or oppose the thumb; the hand's position is dynamic.)
- **Pad-to-pad (Fig. 8.13B), palmar prehension (pulp to pulp), includes "chuck" or tripod grips:** Involves opposition of the pad or pulp of the thumb to the pad or pulp of the finger. In the pad of the distal phalanx of each digit that the greatest concentration of tactile corpuscles are found. The finger used in two-jaw chuck is index and in three-jaw is index plus middle. The MCP and PIP joints are partially flexed, with the degree of flexion depends on the object being held. The DIP may be slightly flexed or extended. When DIP is extended, the FDS alone performs the function without assistance of FDP. When DIP is flexed FDP becomes active. The thumb is held in flexion, abduction, and rotation. The first MCP and IP joints are partially flexed to fully extended.
- **Tip-to-tip (with FDP active to maintain DIP flex) (Fig. 8.13A):** Although this is as same as pad-to-pad, there is a significant difference. In tip-to-tip prehension, the IP joints of the finger and thumb must have the range available force to create nearly full joint flexion. As the most precise form

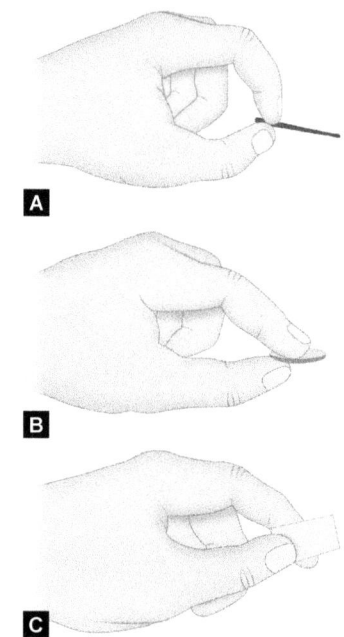

Figs. 8.13A to C: (A) Tip-to-tip; (B) Pad-to-pad; (C) Pad-to-side

of grasp, it is easily disturbed. Tip-to-tip has all the same muscular requirements as pad-to-pad. Additionally, however, tip-to-tip prehension requires activity of the FDP, FDL, and interossei.

- **Pad-to-side; key grip (Fig. 8.13C):** In this, rest all are same, only difference is that thumb is more adducted and less rotated. The activity level of FPB increases and that of OP decreases as compared with tip-to-tip prehension. It is the least precise forms of precision handling, it can actually be performed by a person with paralysis of all hand muscles, e.g., in spinal cord injury above C7 level, active wrist extensors can cause this type of grip.

Muscular function of hand: Extrinsic and intrinsic muscles

Biomechanics of a ruptured flexor pulley: Function of flexor pulleys is to maintain a near constant moment arm length of the flexor tendons. In a damaged or ruptured pulley, the force of contracting muscle causes the tendon to pull away from the joint's axis of rotation, a phenomenon called bowstring of the tendon. Bowstringing of the tendon significantly increases the internal moment arm of the tendon and in turn, increases the mechanical advantage of the muscle. A muscles mechanical advantage has two effects on joint mechanics (1) Amplification of the torque produced per level muscle force, and (2) Reduction of the angular rotation of the joint per linear distance of muscle shortening. The negative clinical implications of a ruptured flexor pulley primarily involve the second factor, for example, assume that with intact A2, A3, and A4 pulleys the moment arm of flexor digitorum profundus tendon is about 0.75 cm at pip joint. A muscle contraction of 1.5 cm would theoretically produce about 115° of PIP joint flexion. A finger with ruptured pulleys may cause a two-fold increase in the moment arm of the FDP across the PIP joint. Consequently, a muscle contraction of 1.5 cm, in theory, produces only about 58° of joint rotation about half the motion produced with intact pulleys. Assuming that the maximal shortening range of FDP is about 2 cm, the finger with a ruptured pulley fails to flex fully, regardless of effort. This loss in contraction-to-rotation efficiency tends to be most profound in rupture of A4 pulley. A ruptured pulley often requires surgical correction.

Passive finger flexion via tenodesis action of digital flexors: The position of the wrist significantly alters the length of the extrinsic digital flexors. One implication of this arrangement can be appreciated by actively extending the wrist and observing the passive flexion of the fingers and thumb. The force responsible for the digital flexion is generated by the stretch placed on the extrinsic digital flexors, such as FDP. The stretching of a polyarticular muscle across the joint, which generates a passive movement at the other, is referred to as a tenodesis action of a muscle, for example, a person with C6 level quadriplegia using tenodesis action to grasp a cup of water.

CHAPTER 9

Hip Joint

Chapter Outline

- Stability
- Ligaments
- Osteokinematics
- Arthrokinematics
- Kinetics
- Pathomechanics
- Angles in the hip

HIP SEGMENT AND THE PARTS

The hip joint or coxofemoral joint forms an articulation between femoral head that is spherical in shape and the hollow acetabulum of the pelvis **(Fig. 9.1)**. The main function of the hip joint is to bear the weight of the head arm and trunk in either static or dynamic postures such as walking, running, and ascending or descending stairs. However, it also provides stability during activities of daily living. Hip musculature generates torque that is needed either to accelerate or decelerate the body.

Anatomy of the Hip Joint

- **Innominate (Fig. 9.2):** Each innominate is the fusion of three bones: the ilium, pubis, and ischium.
  - *Relations to the pelvis:* Right and left innominate—anteriorly fused at pubis symphysis.
  - Posteriorly at the sacrum, forming a complete osteoligamentous ring.
  - Acetabulum is a hollow, hemisphere concave socket that lodges the femoral head.
  - Ilium, pubis, and ischium unite in Y shape to contribute for acetabulum. Pubis comprises one-fifth of the acetabulum (anterior aspect), ischium forms two-fifths (posterior), and the ilium forms the three-fifth (superior aspect or roof). However, hip mobility is influenced by the orientation of the acetabulum and location of weight bearing forces on femoral head. Acetabulum faces laterally, inferiorly, and anteriorly. The peripheral portion of the acetabulum that resembles a

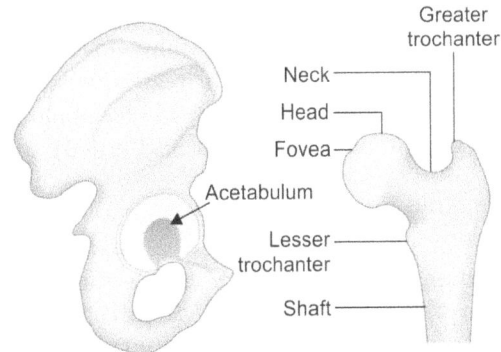

Fig. 9.1: Hip segment and the parts

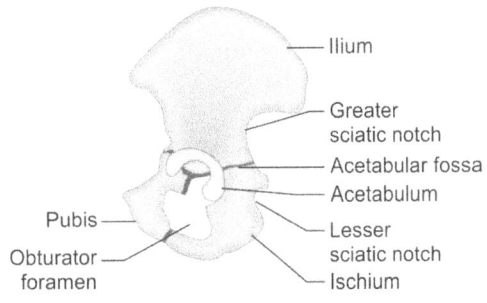

Fig. 9.2: Innominate

horseshoe-shaped articulates with the head of femur. It is covered with hyaline cartilage that thickens at the superior anterior region of dome. Studies have shown that the inferior pole of the rim of the acetabulum is incomplete thus forming an acetabular notch. Acetabular notch is traversed by transverse acetabular ligament. The ligament creates a fibro-osseous tunnel, called the acetabular fossa that provides a passage for blood vessels to communicate with the innermost portion of the acetabulum.

- **Femur:** It is composed of a head, neck and shaft, which ends in distal femoral condyles. It is a long and strong bone in the human body. The femur has slight anterior convexity thus the posterior part of the femur, because of concavity gets compression stress and the anterior part because of convexity gets tensile stress. This bowing allows greater load.

  Femoral head is rounded (unlike the irregularly shaped acetabulum), the surface of the femur is covered by hyaline cartilage. The sphere of femoral head is slightly larger than a hemisphere. Femoral head is located inferiorly to the middle one-third of inguinal ligament.

  Femoral head is smaller in women compared to men. Fovea or fovea capitis is a small roughened pit on the femoral head.

Type of the Joint
Synovial joint—ball-and-socket variety.

Degrees of Freedom
Three degrees of freedom.

Articulating Surfaces
- **Proximal articulating surface:** Horseshoe-shaped area of the acetabulum covered by hyaline cartilage ilium, ischium, and pubis combine together to form the acetabulum.
- **Distal articulating surface:** Head of the femur covered with hyaline cartilage.

Close Pack Position
Full extension and medial rotation.

Loose Pack Position
30° flexion, 30° abduction and slight lateral rotation.

Capsular Pattern
Medial rotation > Flexion > Abduction.

STABILITY

Static:
- Articular congruence
- Negative intra-articular pressure
- Capsule
- Acetabular labrum
- Ligaments

Dynamic: Muscles

Articular Congruence
The hip joint is most congruent joint.

Neutral position, femoral head is oriented anteriorly and superiorly which is covered by thick anterior capsular ligament and iliopsoas tendon in order to provide support. Subjects with excessive acetabular anteversion exposes the femoral head even further thus increasing the risk of anterior dislocation.

In the neutral hip joint, articular cartilage from femoral head is exposed anteriorly. Also to a lesser extent superiorly. (b). Maximum articular contact of the femoral head with the acetabulum is obtained as the femur is flexed, abducted, and laterally rotated slightly.

In nonweight bearing hip position, example frog-leg position wherein the hip is in flexion, abduction, and slight lateral rotation. It is said that in this position the femur and acetabulum are in extreme contact **(Figs. 9.3A and B)**.

Capsule
Capsule of hip joint is a strong stabilizing structure attached proximally to the bony rim of acetabulum and distally to the intertrochanteric line. Fibers of the capsule are parallel along the length from acetabulum to

Chapter 9 | Hip Joint

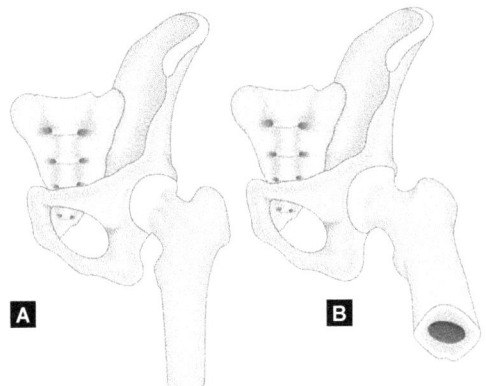

Figs. 9.3A and B: Complete contact between femoral head and acetabulum during femoral flexion, abduction and lateral rotation

femur. It also has circumferential fibers around the neck of femur interiorly. This bundle is known as zona orbicularis, some refer to it as arcuate ligament. The capsule is thick anterosuperiorly, thin, and loosely attached posteroinferiorly. Femoral neck lies inside the capsule thus it is intracapsular, but the greater and lesser trochanter lie outside the capsule thus they are extracapsular.

Acetabular Labrum

The acetabulum labrum is a rim-like structure along the periphery of the acetabulum, which acts like a gasket (sealing ring in pressure cooker). This deepens the socket. Close to acetabular notch, labrum widens leading to the formation of transverse acetabular ligament. The acetabular labrum gradually fuses with the articular cartilage. Labrum has an enormous supply of afferent nerves that are highly capable of providing proprioceptive feedback and when injured provides sensation of pain.

Uses of Acetabular Labrum

- Acetabular labrum provides stability to hip joint
- Maintains a negative intra-articular negative pressure
- Holds the synovial fluid within joint
- Protects the articular cartilage.

Ligaments

- Iliofemoral ligament
- Pubofemoral ligament
- Ischiofemoral ligament
- Ligamentum teres
- Transverse acetabular ligament

Iliofemoral Ligament (Fig. 9.4)

It is the strongest ligament which has the shape of an inverted Y. Thus, it is also called as Y ligament of Bigelow. With its attachments to anterior inferior iliac spine (AIIS) proximally and intertrochanteric line of the femur distally. The fibers divide into two medial and lateral on the either end of intertrochanteric line. Ligament resists extension.

Studies have stated that during bipedal stance with hips fully extended, femoral head (anterior surface) presses firmly against the iliofemoral ligament and superimposed iliopsoas muscle. Iliofemoral ligament develops passive tension thus resisting further hip extension. Subjects with paraplegia rely on passive tension of iliofemoral ligament to assist with standing.

Pubofemoral Ligament (Fig. 9.4)

Pubofemoral ligament is attached to anterior and inferior rim of the acetabulum proximally and superior pubic ramis distally. The iliofemoral ligament along with pubofemoral ligament forms the shape of Z, contributing to

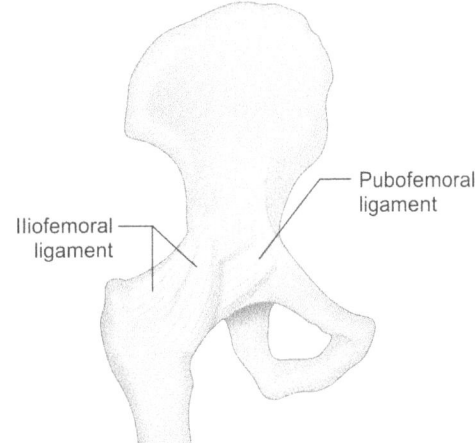

Fig. 9.4: Iliofemoral and pubofemoral ligaments

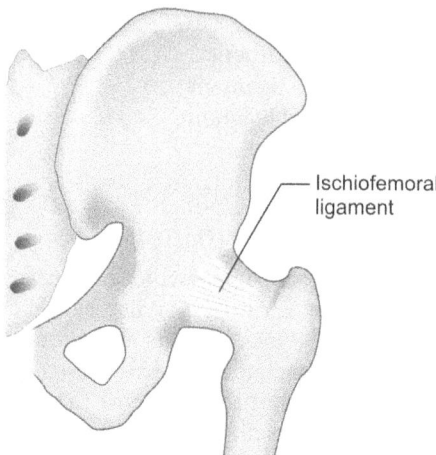

Fig. 9.5: Ischiofemoral ligament

the stability of the joint. This ligament resists extension.

Ischiofemoral Ligament

Ischiofemoral ligament **(Fig. 9.5)** is attached posteriorly and inferiorly of acetabulum proximally and ischium distally. Ischiofemoral fibers join with circular fibers of the capsule to enhance stability of hip joint. This ligament resists flexion.

Ligamentum Teres

Ligamentum teres is a triangular band attached proximally to the acetabular notch and distally to the fovea of the femur; Also named as ligament of head of femur. This ligament is an intra-articular and extrasynovial structure. The ligament passes beneath the transverse acetabular ligament. This ligament does not communicate with the synovial cavity. However, its main function is to allow passage of the obturator artery and nerves to reach the head of the femur. Slightly this ligament helps in resisting tensile stretch of the joint **(Figs. 9.6A and B)**.

KINEMATICS

Osteokinematics

Kinematics at the hip can be described in twofold:

1. **Femur on pelvis osteokinematics:** Rotation of the femur about a relatively fixed pelvis.
2. **Pelvis on femur osteokinematics:** Rotation of the pelvic and superimposed trunk over a relatively fixed femur

Femoral on Pelvic Osteokinematics

Movements

The possible movements at the hip joint are flexion, extension, abduction, adduction, medial rotation, and lateral rotation.

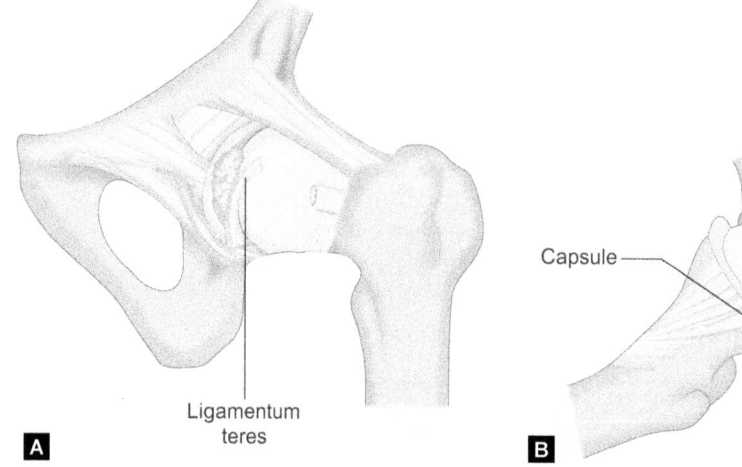

Figs. 9.6A and B: Ligament teres. (A) Anterior view of a right hip; (B) Oblique view

Planes and Axis

- Flexion and extension happen in the sagittal plane around frontal axis.
- Abduction/adduction in frontal plane around A-P axis
- Medial and lateral rotation in the transverse plane around vertical axis.

Range of Motion

Movement	ROM (degrees)
Flexion	110–120
Extension	15
Abduction	30–50
Adduction	20–30
Medial rotation	45
Lateral rotation	50

Pelvis on Femur Osteokinematics

In weight-bearing position such as standing, femur is fixed, and movement is produced when the pelvis moves on femur. Distal end of axial skeleton is articulated to the pelvis at the sacroiliac (SI) joint. Any movement of the pelvis over the fixed femur leads to an alteration of lumbar spine. This kinematic relationship is known as lumbopelvic rhythm.

Two contrasting types of lumbopelvic rhythm are there:
1. Ipsidirectional
2. Contradirectional

Ipsidirectional Lumbopelvic Rhythm

Pelvic and lumbar spine rotates ipsilateral in order to gain maximum angular displacement of the trunk in accordance to lower limb. This provides an effective way for increasing the reach of upper limbs. For example:

- **Bending forward and reaching the floor:** A normal kinematic strategy used to flex the trunk from a standing position incorporates nearly 40° of lumbar spine flexion and 70° of hip (pelvic on femur) flexion. Movements of lumbar spine and pelvis are performed nearly simultaneously. Kinematic strategies that deviate significantly from this pattern may help distinguish pathology affecting lower spine from those affecting the hip

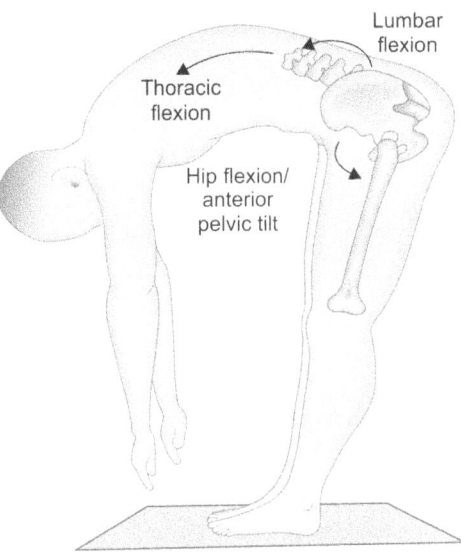

Fig. 9.7: Lumbopelvic rhythm

joint. The lumbar spine had a greater contribution to early forward bending, hips and lumbar spine contributed almost equally to middle forward bending, and the hips had a greater contribution to late forward bending.

From limited hip flexion (e.g., Hamstring tightness) bending trunk toward the floor requires greater flexion in the lumbar and lower thoracic spinal regions.

When lumbar spine flexion is limited, reaching forward toward the floor requires disproportionally greater flexion of the hips.

- **Lumbopelvic rhythm during trunk extension from a forward bent position (Fig. 9.7):** When a subject performs trunk extension with knees in fully extended position, his primary movement initiated is hip extension. This is usually followed after a short delay by extension of the lumbar spine.

Contradirectional Lumbopelvic Rhythm

Here pelvis and lumbar motions are in opposite direction, as the pelvis rotates in one direction, lumbar spine rotates in the opposite direction. The supralumbar trunk remains stationary as the pelvis rotates on the fixed femur. This is mostly used during walking. Lumbar spine

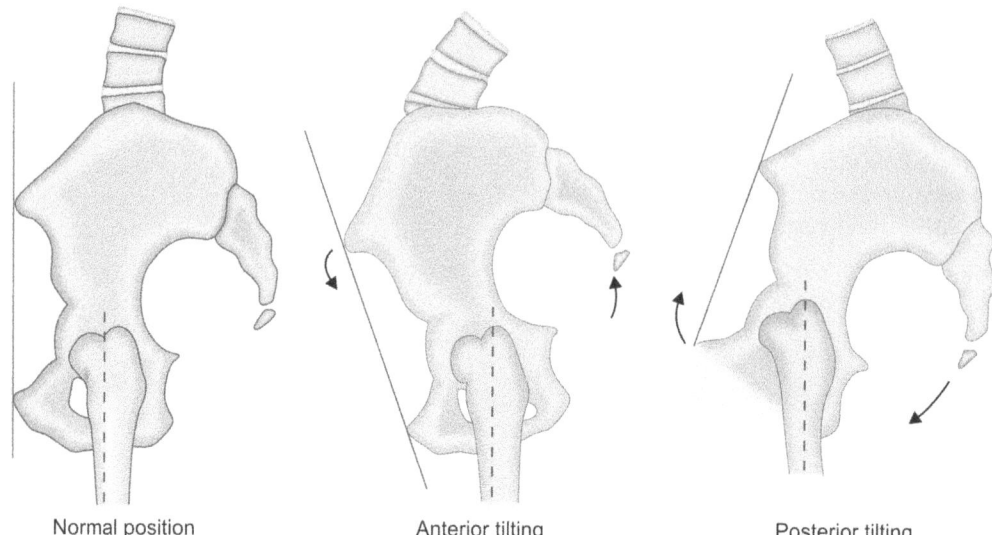

Normal position   Anterior tilting   Posterior tilting

Fig. 9.8: Pelvic rotation in saggital plane

functions like a mechanical decoupler by allowing pelvis and supralumbar spine to work independently. However, if the subject has a fused lumbar spine, there would be no rotation motion at the pelvis and supralumbar trunk.

Pelvic Rotation in the Sagittal Plane (Fig. 9.8)

Anterior and posterior pelvic tilt

Pelvic tilt occurs in the sagittal plane in relation to stationary femur. The direction of tilt is stated on the direction of rotation of a point on the iliac crest.

- **Anterior tilt:** Anterior tilting occurs in the medial-lateral axis of rotation. During hip flexion the pelvis tilts anteriorly wherein ASIS moves anteriorly and inferiorly.
- **Posterior tilt:** During hip extension pelvis tilts posteriorly wherein the symphysis pubis goes superiorly and the sacrum of the pelvis moves closer to the femur. However, it increases the length of rectus femoris and iliofemoral ligament.

Pelvic Rotation in Frontal Plane

- **Lateral pelvic tilt:** It takes place in frontal plane around anteroposterior axis. Individuals with normally aligned pelvis, a line through the ASIS is horizontal.

  In pelvic lateral tilt during unilateral stance, one hip acts as an axis for the motion in the opposite hip as it elevates (pelvic hiking) or pelvic drop. When a subject stands on right limb and hike the pelvis, the right hip joint will be abducted because the angle between femur and line through ASIS increases.

  If a person is standing on right limb and hike the pelvis, the right hip joint will be abducted because the angle between femur and line through ASIS increases. Due to this, mild concavity of lumbar spine can be seen on the adducted side of the hip **(Figs. 9.9 and 9.10)**.
- **Lateral shift of the pelvis:** In bilateral stance, lateral pelvic tilt can be seen. This will happen when one limb is flexed at the hip and knee. In this, the nonflexed opposite limb is weight bearing. And is the same as in unilateral stance. Lateral tilt of the pelvis will lead to pelvic shift. The shift can be on either side. Because of this pelvic shift there will be no hike, but only pelvic drop. There is a close chain between the two weight-bearing feet and pelvis. As the pelvic shift occurs both hip move in frontal plane. If the pelvis is shifted left in the bilateral stance, the right side of the pelvis will drop. Thus, left hip will go for adduction and right hip for abduction **(Fig. 9.11)**.

Pelvic Rotation in Transverse Plane

Pelvic rotation is nothing but the transverse movement of the pelvic ring around the

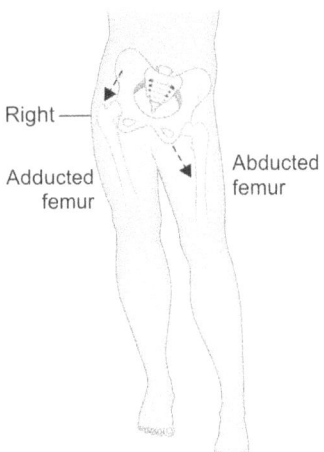

Fig. 9.11: Lateral shift of the pelvis

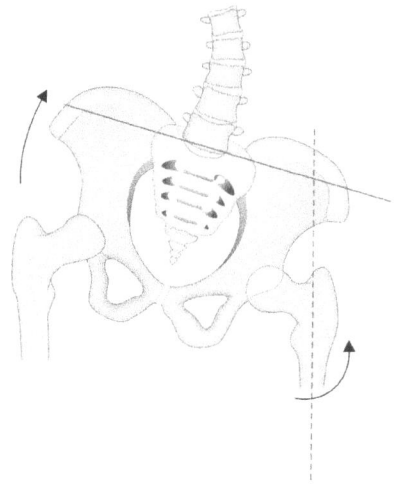

Fig. 9.9: Abduction of the supported limb

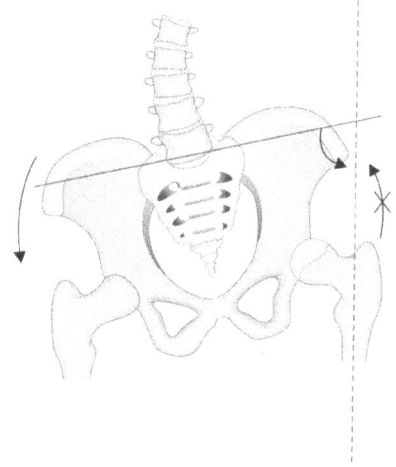

Fig. 9.10: Adduction of the supported limb

vertical axis. The rotation can happen in bilateral stance and the vertical axis is in the middle of the pelvic ring. But, it is more important in single limb support. Forward rotation of pelvis during unilateral stance results in medial rotation of the weight bearing joint. In this, as the name suggests the pelvis moves anteriorly. In backward rotation, the opposite pelvis of weight bearing hip moves posteriorly. This results in lateral rotation of weight bearing hip joint. Due to limited axial rotation in lumbar spine, the exaggerated movement of the weight bearing hip is also limited **(Figs. 9.12A to C)**.

As the pelvis rotates beneath a relatively fixed trunk, there should be simultaneous rotation of the lumbar spine in opposite direction.

Arthrokinematics

Predominant arthrokinematic movement in the hip joint is gliding.

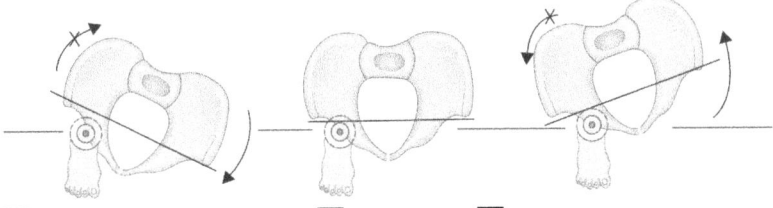

A Left forward rotation **B** Normal **C** Left backward rotation

Figs. 9.12A to C: Pelvic rotation in transverse plane. (A to C) Right limb is supported

Concave–Convex Rule

As the convex femoral head moves on concave acetabulum according to concave–convex rule the arthrokinematic movement is opposite to that of osteokinematic movement.

Movement	Direction of the glide
Flexion	Posterior
Extension	Anterior
Abduction	Inferior
Adduction	Superior
Medial rotation	Posterior
Lateral rotation	Anterior

Kinetics

Hip Flexors
- Iliopsoas
- Sartorius
- Tensor fascia lata
- Rectus femoris

Hip Extensors
- Gluteus maximus
- Hamstrings

Hip Abductors
- Gluteus medius and minimus
- Tensor fasciae latae

Hip Adductors
- Pectineus
- Gracilis
- Adductor longus, brevis, and magnus

Hip Medial Rotators
Force couple of:
- Gluteus medius, minimus, tensor fasciae latae
- Adductor longus and brevis, pectineus

Hip Lateral Rotators
- Obturator internus
- Obturator externus
- Gemellus superior
- Gemellus inferior
- Quadratus femoris
- Piriformis muscles

Hip Joint Flexors

The flexors of the hip joint function primarily as mobility muscles in open-chain function. Hip flexors primarily resist hip extension forces that occur while the body passes over the weight bearing foot.

Primary flexors are the:
- Iliopsoas
- Sartorius
- Tensor fascia lata
- Rectus femoris
- Adductor longus and pectineus
- Adductor brevis, gracilis, and anterior fibers of gluteus minimus are the secondary hip flexors muscles.

Iliopsoas is a potent hip flexor from both femoral on pelvis and pelvis on femoral point of view. It produces force that crosses the lumbar and lumbosacral regions as well as hip joint. It provides excellent vertical stability to lumbar spine when hip in extension. Psoas minor has no ability to flex the hip. Isolated bilateral contraction of it tilts the pelvis posteriorly. Sartorius muscle plays an important role when both hip and knee need to be flexed simultaneously (as in climbing stairs). Tensor fascia lata, from the anatomic position fascial lata is primary flexor and abductor of the hip. Rectus femoris produces one third of total isometric torque at the hip. The rectus femoris is a two-joint muscle that causes hip flexion and knee extension.

Hip Adductor Muscles

The primary hip adductors are:
- Pectineus
- Adductor longus, brevis and magnus
- Gracilis

Secondary hip adductors are biceps femoris (long head), lower fibers of gluteus maximus, and quadrates femoris.

Adductor magnus (posterior fibers) are powerful extensors of the hip, similar to hamstrings. Within an arc of about 40–70° of hip flexion, line of force of muscles tends to run through or close to medial-lateral axis of rotation of hip joint. Due to this the adductor muscles lose its potential to generate any torque in sagittal plane. However, beyond 40–70° flexed position, adductor muscle gain leverage as significant hip flexors or extensors.

Hip Extensors

The primary hip extensors are:
- Gluteus maximus
- Hamstrings
- Gluteus medius (posterior fibers) and adductor magnus (anterior fibers) are secondary extensors. With hip flexed to 70° most adductors are capable of assisting with hip extension.

Hip extensors performing posterior pelvic tilt with supralumbar trunk held stationary, hip extensors, and abdominals posteriorly tilt the pelvis. Posterior tilt extends the hip joint and reduces the lumbar lordosis.

Forward leaning while standing is a very common activity, wherein muscular support is provided by hamstrings. When a subject goes for a minimal forward lean, his/her body weight gets displayed slightly anterior to the mediolateral axis of rotation of the hip joint. This flexed posture is restrained by the minimum activity of gluteus maximus and hamstrings. In this posture marked activity of hamstrings is required; gluteus maximus remains relatively inactive during this position.

Hip Abductor Muscles

Primary hip abductor muscles are:
- Gluteus medius and minimus
- Tensor fasciae latae

Piriformis and sartorius are secondary hip abductors.

The gluteus medius has three functional sets of fibers: Anterior, middle, and posterior. Regardless of the hip position, all fibers of muscle abduct the hip. Anterior fibers play an important role during hip flexion and posterior fibers during hip extension. At neutral hip position, posterior portion produces a lateral rotator moment, and middle and anterior fibers create a slight medial rotatory moment. When the hip is in flexion position, all its fibers medially rotate the hip. Deep to the gluteus medius is the gluteus minimus. Gluteus minimus primarily helps in hip abduction and flexion, with its rotator function dependent on hip position. Gluteus minimus is a medial rotator when hip is flexed. Gluteus minimus has a tendinous insertion as it passes through the greater trochanter and inserts into the joint capsule. Studies have hypothesized that this attachment leads to retraction of capsule when the hip is abducted thus preventing entrapment or capsule tightness. This adds to the primary function of gluteus minimus of stabilizing femoral head within acetabulum.

Hip Abductor Mechanism

Pelvic control in frontal plane during walking
Hip abductor muscle produces a relevant abduction torque that is necessary to control frontal plane motions, i.e., pelvic on femoral kinematics during walking. It plays a vital role during single limb support phase where the opposite leg is off the ground and swings forward. However if the stance limb is devoid of abduction torque, the pelvis and trunk tend to drop uncontrollably toward the side of the swinging limb.

Clinical Relevance

Trendelenburg test is the commonly performed screening procedure for hip abductor weakness. The test is positive for abductor weakness if the subject leans excessively towards the stance limb or presence of pelvic drop on the unsupported side.

Maximal Abduction Force Varies According to Hip Joint Angle

Adductor muscles produce their peak torque when elongated. The maximal torque is produced during slight hip adduction or neutral hip position (as in single limb support phase of walking). Hip abduction torque potential is least at nearly full shortened muscle length that is 40° of hip abduction.

Hip Internal Rotators

In the anatomic position, there are no primary internal rotators of hip. Secondary internal rotators include anterior fibers of gluteus medius and minimus, tensor fascia latae, adductor longus, brevis, and pectineus. With hip approaching 90° of flexion, the internal rotation torque potential of the internal rotators increases dramatically. Even some external rotators like, piriformis, gluteus maximus (anterior fibers) and gluteus minimus (posterior fibers), switch action, and become internal rotators beyond about 90° of flexion.

Hip External Rotators

- Obturator internus and externus
- Gemellus superior and inferior
- Quadratus femoris
- Piriformis muscles

Gluteus medius and minimus (posterior fibers) and gluteus maximus may produce external rotation along with primary action of the muscle.

PATHOMECHANICS

- Trochanteric bursitis
- Femoroacetabular impingement
- Labral tears
- Piriformis syndrome
- Osteoarthritis
- Fracture

Labral tears are the common cause for chronic hip pain. The mechanisms of labral tears could be trauma or activities that involve repeated twisting or pivoting motions. Soccer or golf players are particularly susceptible. Clinical diagnosis is difficult. However, pain with active or passive hip flexion, medial rotation, and adduction and clicking during hip movements could be positive findings. Labral tears destabilize the joints and increases stress on articular cartilage leading to degenerative changes within the joint.

Piriformis syndrome: It refers to pain due to tightness or spasm of piriformis muscle that exerts pressure on sciatic nerve. This causes radicular symptoms that are aggravated by stretching or contracting the muscle. Clinician uses passive or resisted movement to elicit the patient's symptoms and the condition.

ANGLES IN THE HIP SEGMENT

- Angle of inclination
- Angle of torsion
- Angle of anteversion and angle of retroversion
- Central edge angle

Angulation of the Femur: Namely angle of inclination and torsional angle.

Angle of Inclination

Angle of inclination (**Fig. 9.13**) is formed between femoral neck and medial side of femoral shaft that is in the frontal plane. At birth, it is about 140–150° as a result of loading across the femoral neck during walking. However, the angle reduces to about 125° as one attains adulthood, thus optimizing the alignment of the joint surfaces.

Angle of inclination in women is smaller as compared to men, due to the greater width of the female pelvis. Pathologic increase in medial angulation between neck and femoral shaft is termed as coxa valga (**Fig. 9.14A**) and a pathologic decrease is termed coxa vara (**Fig. 9.14B**).

Abnormal angles can significantly affect the biomechanics of the hip joint as the articulation between the spherical head of femur and shallow acetabulum is altered.

Angle of Torsion (Fig. 9.15)

Femoral torsion is defined as the relative rotation (twist) between shaft of the femur and femoral neck.

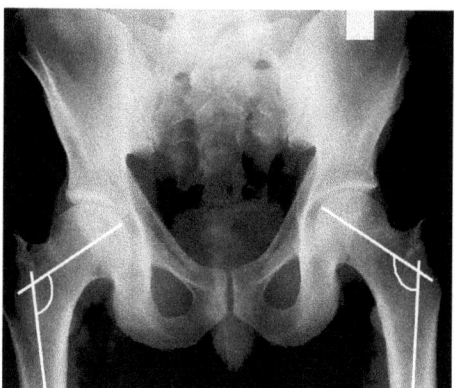

Fig. 9.13: Angle of inclination

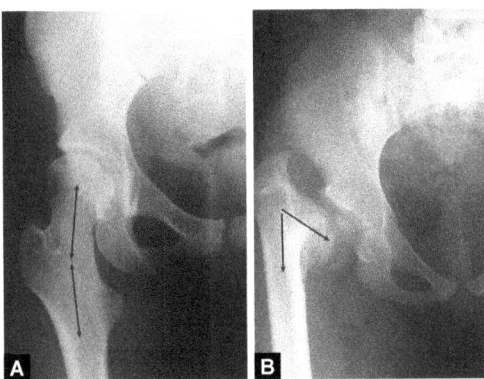

Figs. 9.14A and B: (A) Coxa valga; (B) Coxa vara

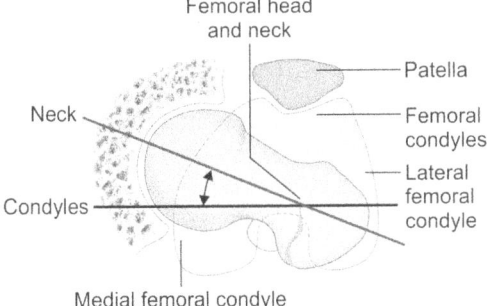

Fig. 9.15: Angle of torsion

When viewed from above, an approximate 15° of femoral neck projection can be observed anterior to the medial-lateral axis through the femoral condyles. This degree of torsion is called normal anteversion.

The angulation formed is the medial rotatory migration of lower limb that took place during fetal development. Upper and lower extremity undergoes significant axial rotation during prenatal development. Fifty four days postconception, the lower extremities have rotated internally about 90°, thus positioning the kneecap anteriorly. Lower extremity became permanently pronated. That's why extensor muscles face anteriorly and the flexors muscles face posteriorly after birth.

Anteversion is defined as the pathologic increase in the angle of torsion whereas pathologic decrease in the angle or reversal of torsion is known as retroversion **(Figs. 9.16A and B)**.

In newborn, angle of torsion is approximately 40° and a substantial decrease is noted during the first 2 years. Children with both normal and exaggerated angles of anteversion show a considerable decrease of approximately 1.5° per year until cessation of growth. As one attains 16 years of age, angle decreases to about 15° due to bone growth, increased weight bearing, and muscle activity. Excessive anteversion places the femoral head further anteriorly in the acetabulum than normal. Excessive anteversion is compensated by medial rotation of the hip within the acetabulum. Bipedal stance, such as compensatory rotation leads to in-toes posture. A correlation is present between amount of in-toeing and femoral anteversion. These subjects typically display increased in medial hip rotation ROM and reduce in hip lateral rotation. Children with excessive femoral anteversion walk with in-toeing. As age advances, improvement is gait pattern is noticed due to normalization of the anteversion or combined structural compensation in other parts of the lower limb, most commonly the tibia. Tibia laterally rotates (lateral tibial torsion), which turns the foot laterally with respect to knees. As a result in-toeing disappears.

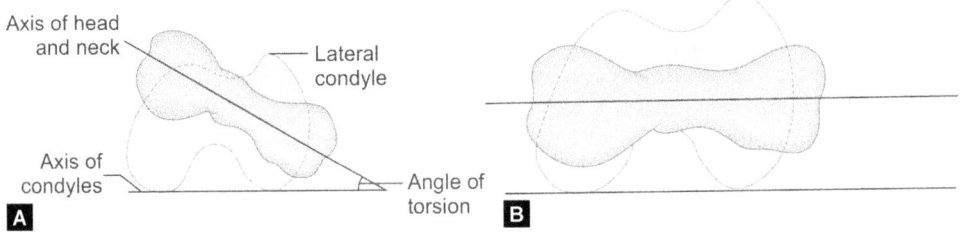

Figs. 9.16A and B: (A) Anteversion; (B) Retroversion

Clinical relevance: Angle of anteversion is measured clinically by Craig's test.
Patient position: Subject lies prone with 90° of knee flexion

Examiner palpates posterior aspect of greater trochanter. Examiner passively rotates testing limb medially and laterally until the greater trochanter is parallel with the examining table or until attains the most lateral position. Degree of anteversion can be estimated based on the angle of lower limb with vertical. This test helps in measuring anteversion and retroversion and named as Ryder method.

Retroversion results in considerable increase hip lateral rotation ROM, decrease in medial hip rotation, and excessive out toeing.

Acetabular Alignment

In anatomic position acetabulum faces laterally combined with inferior and anterior tilt. Congenital and developmental condition may be the predisposed factors that can cause a mal-shaped acetabulum that exposes the femoral head thus leading to chronic dislocation and increased stress. Center edge angle and acetabular anteversion angle are commonly used to describe the extent to which the acetabulum covers and helps secure the femoral head.

Center Edge Angle (Angle of Wiberg)

Radiograph is commonly used to assess the magnitude of inferior orientation by drawing a line connecting the lateral rim of the acetabulum and center of the femoral head. The line forms an angle with the vertical called as the center edge (CE) angle or angle of Wiberg **(Fig. 9.17)** and it helps in quantifying the amount of inferior tilt of the acetabulum. It is vital to measure the inferior tilt as we can state the amount of coverage or "roof" there is over the femoral head. Adult men CE angle is about 38° and 35° in women.

A significantly lower CE reduces acetabular coverage of the femoral head. An angle of 15° reduces the normal contact area by 35%. During single limb stance, reduced

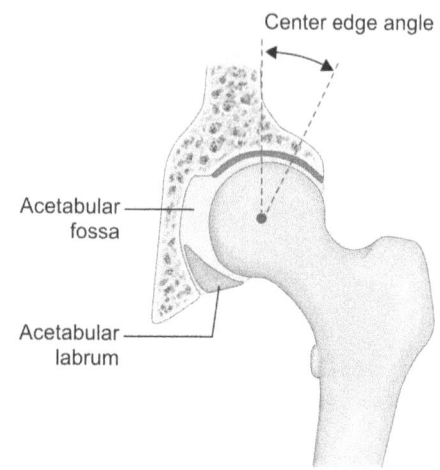

Fig. 9.17: Center edge (CE) angle or angle of Wiberg.

surface area would considerably increase joint pressure (force/area) by about 50%. CE angle tends to increase from childhood until skeletal maturity.

Acetabular Anteversion

Angle of acetabular anteversion is basically the anterior orientation of acetabulum, average value in men is 18.5° and 21.5° in women.

The acetabulum is abnormally retroverted when it projects directly laterally, or even slight posteriolaterally within the transverse plane.

Trabecular System

Compact and Cancellous Bone

Throughout life, proximal femur sustains enormous tension, compressive, bending, shear, and torsion forces during gait cycle. Proximal femur absorbs and resists these repetitive forces without sustaining any injury. This is accomplished by the presence of compact and cancellous bone. Compact bone has a thick cortex, or outer shell, of the lower femoral neck and shaft. They sustain large shear and torsion forces. Cancellous bone is porous, consisting of spongy and three-dimensional trabecular lattice. Elasticity property in cancellous bone is ideal for absorbing external forces. Cancellous bone tends to concentrate along the line of stresses, forming trabecular networks. The medial trabecular and arcuate trabecular network are visible within the femur. Over an extended time the trabecular network pattern changes from proximal femur as subjected to abnormal forces.

Both femoral head and acetabulum have large amount of spongy, trabecular bone that facilitate the distribution of forces absorbed by the hip joint. The pelvic trabeculae that pass through the acetabulum form two major systems within the femur: the medial trabeculae and the lateral trabeculae system. There are also two minor accessory systems of trabeculae, the medial and lateral accessory system. The epiphyseal plates are at right angles to the trabeculae of the medial system. This is perpendicular to the joint reaction force (JRF).

Zone of weakness is the area in the femoral neck where the trabeculae are relatively thin and do not intersect each other. It is more potential to injury.

With aging, the cortical bone is thinned and cancelled and trabeculae are slowly reabsorbed.

HIP JOINT FORCES AND MUSCLE FUNCTION IN STANCE

Bilateral Stance

In the frontal plane during bilateral stance, two-thirds of the body weight of head, arm, and trunk is distributed equally so that each femoral head receives about half of superincumbent weight. Joint axis of each hip lies at equal distance from the line of gravity of head, arm and trunk, where the gravitational moment arm for right and left hip are equal. As the weight borne by each femoral head is same, magnitude of gravitational torques at each hip is also identical (WR × DR = WL × DL).

Where WR: weight of right leg
       WL: weight of left leg
       DR: gravitational moment arm of right hip
       DL: gravitational moment arm of left hip.

Gravitational torques on right and left hips takes place in opposite directions. Body weight acting around the right hip tends to drop the pelvis down on the left (right adduction moment). Both the opposing gravitational moments of equal magnitude balance each other and the pelvis is maintained in equilibrium in the frontal plane without the assistance of active muscles.

However, Bergmann et al. quoted that hip joint is subjected to compressive forces in bilateral stance of 80–100% of body weight. The slight activity in the iliopsoas.

It has been said that the muscles and capsule ligamentous tension accounts for more compressive forces to the hip joint. During bipedal stance, the contralateral hip abductors and adductors act as synergists to control frontal plane motions of the pelvis. However, when bilateral stance is asymmetrical frontal plane muscle activity plays an important role to either control the side-to-side motion or to return the hips to symmetrical stance.

Unilateral Stance

Unilateral stance, the supported limb has to bear whole burden of the superimposed body. Weight of the nonweight bearing limb that is hanging on the side of the pelvis must be supported. The magnitude of body weight (W) compressing the stance hip joint in unilateral stance is:

> Stance hip joint compression: [2/3 weight of HAT] + [1/6 × weight of HAT] that is 5/6 weight of HAT

Body weight is generating a torque around the hip joint **(Figs. 9.18 and 9.19)**.

Suppose person is standing on right limb, with left lower limb hanging over side.

Force of gravity acting on head, arm, and trunk (HAT), and left lower extremity, nonweight bearing (HATLL) will create an adduction torque around the supporting hip joint. The hip musculature controls the abduction counter torque. This results in joint compression or joint reaction force which involves combination of body weight and abductor muscular compression.

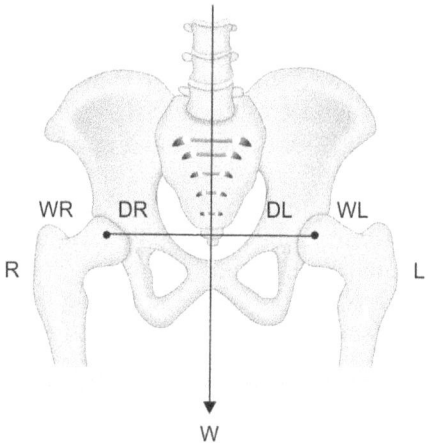

Fig. 9.18: Hip joint forces in bilateral stance

reaction force on the hip in order to avoid pain. Several options are available when there is a need to reduce abductor muscle force requirements.

Compensatory Lateral Lean of the Trunk

When a subject performs a unilateral stance on the painful limb with lateral trunk lean over the pelvis toward the side of pain or weakness, there will be a reduction in the moment arm (MA) of the gravitational force **(Fig. 9.20)**. Compensatory trunk lateral lean on the painful stance limb brings the line of gravity (LoG) nearer to the hip joint, thereby reducing the gravitational MA and thus gravitational torque. Thus, there will be a proportional reduction in abductor counter torque.

Extreme motions/movements require high-energy expenditure subjecting the lumbar spine to constant wear and tear.

Use of a Cane Ipsilaterally

When a cane is held on the painful side or hip with muscle weakness, sum weight of HATLL would pass from the arm to the cane rather than arriving on the sacrum and weight bearing joint. Inman et al. quoted that it is realistic to expect that someone can push down on a cane with approximately 15% of his total body weight. Total hip joint compression is greater when the cane is used ipsilaterally

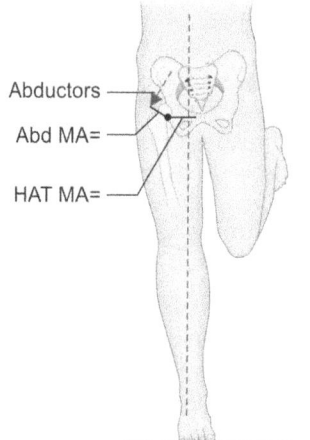

Fig. 9.19: Hip joint forces in unilateral stance

Total hip joint compression/Joint reaction force:

> Force produced by abductor muscle of stance limb + Weight of the HATLL

Unilateral stance, the hip is subjected to compressive forces or joint reaction forces that are 2.5 to 3 times body weight.

Reduction of Muscle Forces in Unilateral Stance

If the hip joint undergoes osteoarthritic changes with symptoms such as pain during weight bearing. It is better to reduce the joint

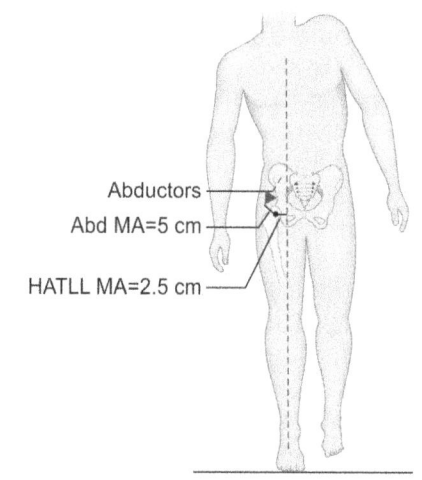

Fig. 9.20: Compensatory lateral lean of the trunk

is greater, than the total joint compression found with a compensatory lateral trunk lean. Although a cane used ipsilaterally provides some benefits in energy expenditure and structural stress reduction, it is not as effective in reducing hip joint compression as the undesirable lateral lean of the trunk.

Use of a Cane Contralaterally

The reduction in HATLL is the same whether the cane is held on the nonaffected side of the painful or weak hip joint or on the affected side. As it is on the nonaffected side, it can alleviate some of the superimposed body weight and can assist abductor muscle in providing a counter torque to the torque of gravity.

The torque around the right stance hip produced by a cane in the left hand exceeds the torque produced by the remaining weight of HATLL.

The total hip joint compression forces in unilateral stance when a cane is used in the opposite hand would be:

> 0 N abductor joint compression + body weight (HATLL-cane) compression.

Role of Latissimus Dorsi

The force that is added on to the cane through the pelvis is due to the contraction of the latissimus dorsi muscle. Latissimus dorsi is described as a "crutch walking" muscle as it primarily depresses the humerus. The latissimus dorsi is very active as the downward thrust on the cane is through shoulder depression. Activation of latissimus dorsi results in an upward pull on the iliac crest on the side of the cane. Upward pull on the side of the pelvis opposite the supporting hip joint axis (hip hiking force) creates an abduction torque around the supporting hip joint. This abduction torque can offset the gravitational adduction torque around the same hip joint.

Presuming the subject is using a cane in the left hand, the line of pull of left latissimus dorsi muscle should lie twice that distance from the right weight-bearing and impaired hip joint. Krebs et al. stated that the use of cane on the unaffected side could relieve load on the affected hip to about 40% and reduce activation of gluteus medius to about 45%.

CHAPTER 10

Knee Joint

Chapter Outline

- Structure of tibiofemoral joint
- Menisci
- Joint capsule
- Ligaments
- Tibiofemoral joint function
- Role of cruciate ligament and menisci in flexion and extension
- Patellofemoral joint

INTRODUCTION

Knee complex (**Fig. 10.1**) is composed of tibiofemoral and patellofemoral joints that are enclosed within a single joint capsule. The superior tibiofemoral joint is not considered to be part of knee complex as it does not lie within the knee joint capsule and is functionally related to ankle joint.

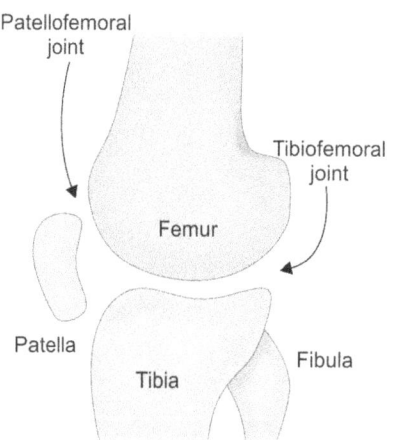

Fig. 10.1: Knee joint (lateral view)

STRUCTURE OF TIBIOFEMORAL JOINT

Tibiofemoral joint is a double condyloid joint that has three degrees of freedom.
1. Flexion/extension movements take place in sagittal plane around coronal axis. The axis passes through epicondyles of distal femur.
2. Medial/lateral (internal/external) rotation movements take place in transverse plane around longitudinal axis. The axis passes through the lateral side of medial tibial plateau.
3. Abduction/adduction motion occurs in frontal plane and around anteroposterior (A-P) axis.

Femur

- The lateral femoral condyle is shifted slightly anteriorly in relation to medial condyle.
- Articular surface of lateral condyle is shorter than medial condyle.
- The two femoral condyles are separated from each other inferiorly by intercondylar notch and joined anteriorly by a shallow groove called patellar groove or surface that engages the patella during early flexion.

Tibia

- A-P diameter of medial tibial plateau is more compared to lateral tibial plateau.
- However, articular cartilage is thicker on the lateral aspect compared to medial.
- Medial and lateral tibial condyles are separated by a roughened area and houses

two bony spines called intercondylar tubercles. During knee extension, the intercondylar tubercles get lodged in the intercondylar notch of femur.
- Menisci improve joint congruency between articulation of femoral condyles and tibial plateaus.

Tibiofemoral Alignment and Weight-bearing Forces

- The longitudinal axis of femur also called as anatomic axis is slightly oblique, that is, it travels inferiorly and medially from its proximal to distal end. The anatomic axis of tibia is almost vertical. The femoral and tibial long axis forms an angle medially at the knee joint of 180–185°, that is, femur is angled up to 5° off vertical, creating slight physiologic (normal) valgus angle at the knee.
- If medial tibiofemoral angle >185°—genu valgum (knock knees)
- If medial tibiofemoral angle is <175°—genu varum (bowlegs)

↓

Knock knees or bow legs can ultimately alter the compressive and tensile forces on the medial and lateral compartments.

Alternative Method

An alternate method to measure tibiofemoral alignment is by drawing a line from the center of femoral head to the center of talus. This line represents the mechanical axis. The mechanical axis or the weight bearing line of lower extremity passes through the joint center and intercondylar tubercles.

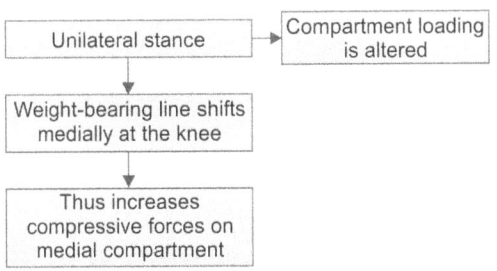

Genu valgum: Weight-bearing line shifts onto the lateral compartment

↓

Increases the lateral compartment—compressive forces
Medial compartment—tensile forces

Genu varum: Weight-bearing line shifts medially

↓

Increases the medial compartment—subjected to compression forces
Lateral compartment—subjected to tensile forces

Genu varum: Genu varum leads to progressive arthritis of medial compartment and leads to excessive medial joint laxity as medial capsular ligaments attachments sites are gradually approximated through the erosion of medial compartments articular cartilage

In bilateral stance: In bilateral stance, the distribution of weight-bearing stresses is equal. In other words, the medial and lateral condyles bear the weight equally.

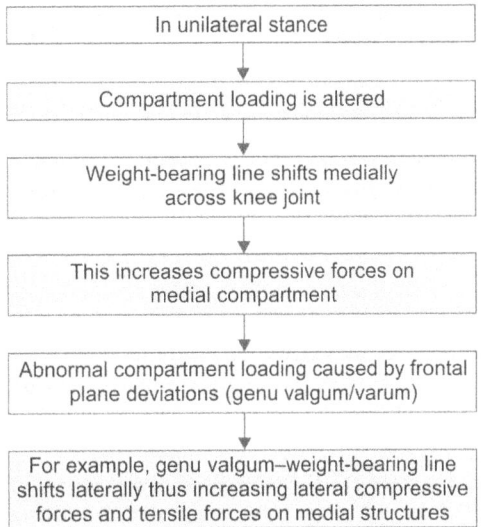

For example, genu varum—weight-bearing line shifts medially. Medial compartment subjected to compressive forces and lateral compartment subjected to tensile forces.

Frontal plane deviations, such as genu valgum and genu varum, result in constant overload of lateral and medial articular cartilage. This ultimately damages the articular cartilage and frontal plane laxity develops.

Genu varum—contributes to progression of medial compartment knee OA and leads to excessive medial joint laxity
↓
As the medial capsular ligaments attachment sites are gradually approximated through the erosion of the medial compartments articular cartilage

MENISCI

- Distribute weight-bearing forces thus reducing friction between tibia and femur
- Serve as shock absorber
- Improve joint congruency
- Medial menisci—C-shaped
- Lateral menisci—forms four fifths of a circle
- Compressive forces in knee reach 1 to 2 times body weight during stair climbing and walking.
- Running increases the compressive forces on the knee to 3-4 times body weight.
- Menisci assume 50-70% of this imposed load

Meniscal Attachments

- One anterior and posterior ends of menisci are called anterior and posterior horns each attached firmly to tibia below.
- Greater ligamentous and capsular restrain of medial meniscus limit its translation to a greater extent than the lateral menisci.
- Greater incidence of injury is reported in medial menisci due to its reduced mobility.
- Menisci are connected to each other anteriorly by transverse ligament.
- Directly or indirectly, both the menisci are attached to the patella via patellomeniscal ligaments.
- At periphery menisci connected to tibial condyles by coronary ligaments.
- Medial menisci motion is restricted by the medial collateral ligament.
- Anterior cruciate and posterior cruciate ligament are attached to anterior and posterior horns of medial menisci
- Tendon of popliteus muscle—attached to lateral menisci
↓
- Helps restrain or control the motion of lateral menisci

Role of Menisci

- Increases congruency of joint
- Menisci—contact at tibiofemoral joint is increased
↓
- Joint stress (force per unit area) is reduced on joint articular cartilage (Fig. 10.2)
- After removal of menisci, contact area in tibiofemoral joint is decreased resulting in increased joint stress.
- Thus, removal of menisci doubles the articular cartilage stress on femur and multiplies the forces by 6 to 7 times on tibial plateau.
- Joint stress increases—contribute to degenerative changes with the tibiofemoral joint.
- Thus, total meniscectomy are rarely done.

Meniscal Nutrition and Innervation

- Peripheral portion of menisci is supplied through blood vessels while the central portion relies on diffusion of synovial fluid. Process of fluid diffusion requires

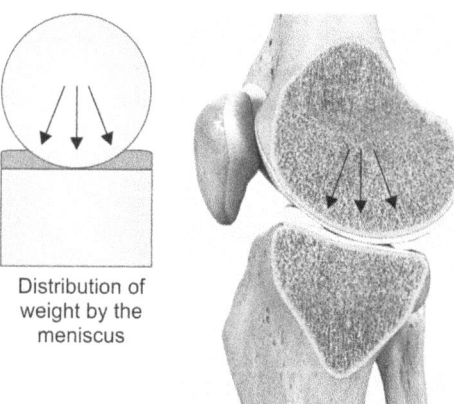

Distribution of weight by the meniscus

Fig. 10.2: Meniscus weight distribution

intermittent loading of the menisci, such as weight-bearing or muscular contractions.
- During periods of immobilization or prolong nonweight-bearing
  ↓
  Menisci do not receive nutrition
- In adults—peripheral vascularized region of menisci is capable of inflammation, repair, and remodeling after an injury.
- Horns of menisci and peripheral vascularized portion of meniscal bodies are innervated by free nerve endings (nociceptors)
- Three different mechanoreceptors (Pacinian corpuscles, Golgi tendon organ, and Ruffini corpuscles) are located within the menisci.
- After meniscal injury, subjects experience alterations in proprioception as a result of injury to mechanoreceptors that lies within the menisci.

JOINT CAPSULE

- Ligament tautness maximum in full extension—closed packed position of knee
- Knee flexion (open packed position)—periarticular passive structures become lax and bony incongruence of joints permits greater anterior and posterior translations and rotations of tibia beneath femur.
- Anteromedial and anterolateral are identified as medial and lateral patellar retinacula or together as extensor retinaculum
- Knee joint capsule and ligaments—resist excessive joint motions to maintain joint integrity and normal function.
- Joint capsule—innervated by nociceptors as well as Pacinian and Ruffini corpuscles
- These mechanoreceptors contribute to muscular stabilization of knee joint by initiating reflex-mediated muscular responses.
- Joint capsule responsible for providing a tight seal—to keep the lubricating synovial fluid within it.

Synovial Layer of Joint Capsule

- Synovial membrane forms the inner lining of joint capsule.

- Synovial tissue secretes and absorbs synovial fluid into the joint. Thus providing lubrication and nutrition to avascular structures such as menisci.
- Anterior cruciate ligament (ACL) and posterior cruciate ligament (PCL) are contained within fibrous capsule (intracapsular) but lie outside of synovial sheath (extrasynovial).
- Infrapatellar fat pad (Hoffa's pad) lies deep to the patellar tendon

Patellar Plicae

- Failure of synovial membrane to become fully absorbed—persistent folds—called patellar plicae
- Frequent locations—inferior (infrapatellar plica), superior (suprapatellar), and medial (mediopatellar plica).
- Plica becomes irritated and inflamed—pain, effusion, and changes in joint structure and function—plica syndrome.
- **Inferior plica** called ligamentum mucosum lies anterior to ACL in intercondylar area, passes through infrapatellar fat pad (Hoffa's pad) and attaches to inferior pole of patella.
- Superior plica—located superior to the patella between suprapatellar bursa and superior portion of the patella
- Medial plica rarely found (25–30%)
- Medial plica—arises from medial wall of the pouch of extensor retinaculum and attach to infrapatellar fat pad.
- Medial and superior plica—plica syndrome
- Medial plica is impinged between medial aspect of patella and medial femoral condyle.
- Attributed to its rich supply of Pacinian corpuscles and free nerve endings

Fibrous Layer of the Joint Capsule

- Anterior portion is called extensor retinaculum.
- Fascia covers quadriceps muscles.
- Medial and lateral retinaculum
- Medial patellofemoral ligament, lateral patellofemoral ligament, and medial and lateral patellotibial ligaments.

LIGAMENTS

- Knee joint stability
- **Resisting or controlling the following:**
  - Excessive knee extension
  - Anterior or posterior displacement of tibia beneath the femur
  - Varus and valgus stresses at the knee
  - Medial or lateral tibial rotation beneath the femur
  - Combination of anteroposterior displacements and rotations of the tibia, together known as rotatory stabilization of the tibia.
- Weight-bearing activities—closed-chain activities—involve motion of femur moving on relatively fixed tibia.
- Nonweight bearing—open-chain activities—tibia moving on fixed femur
- Difference in displacements and rotations of the tibia and femur

For example, anterior displacement of tibia on femur (during nonweight bearing), posterior displacement of femur on tibia (during weight bearing).

Medial Collateral Ligament

- Divided into superficial and deep portion that are separated by a bursa.
- Superficial portion—arises proximally from medial femoral epicondyle and travels distally to insert into medial aspect of proximal tibia distal to pes anserinus.
- Deep portion—continuous with joint capsule from inferior aspect of medial femoral condyle and inserts proximal aspect of medial tibial plateau.
- Superficial portion—restraint to excessive valgus and lateral tibial rotation
- Knee joint—better able to resist a valgus stress at full extension compared to flexion—because MCL is taut in extension (close-packed position).
- Knee flexed—MCL more critical role in resisting valgus stress despite permitted joint gapping.
- MCL—resists anterior translation of tibia on femur
- Thus both partial and complete medial collateral ligament (MCL) tear increase load on anterior cruciate ligament
  ↓
- MCL has a rich blood supply thus has a capacity to heal on its own, when ruptured or damaged.

Lateral Collateral Ligament

- Lateral collateral ligament lies on the lateral side of tibiofemoral joint. It arises from the lateral femoral condyle and travels distally to attach to the fibular head. At the fibular head, it joins with the tendon of biceps femoris.
- Resist varus stress and resist frontal plane motions most successfully with full knee extension.
- Also limit excessive lateral rotation of tibia.

Anterior Cruciate Ligament (Fig. 10.3)

- Attached distally to tibia on the lateral and anterior aspect of medial intercondylar tibial spine
- It extends superiorly, laterally, and posteriorly to attach to the posteromedial aspect of lateral femoral condyle.
- Major blood supply—middle genicular ligament
- Restraints against anterior translation (anterior shear), when tibia moves on femur.
- Knee close to full extension—posterolateral bundle taut
- Knee flexes—posteromedial bundle taut
- ACL—also resists hyperextension of knee.
- ACL—provides rotatory stability of knee during valgus/varus angulations, medial/lateral rotation and combination thereof.
- Isolated quadriceps contraction (knee in near full extension)—generates anterior shear force on the tibia—increases strain on ACL.
- Gastrocnemius muscle—translates tibia anteriorly—strain ACL—because proximal tendon of gastrocnemius wraps around posterior tibia.

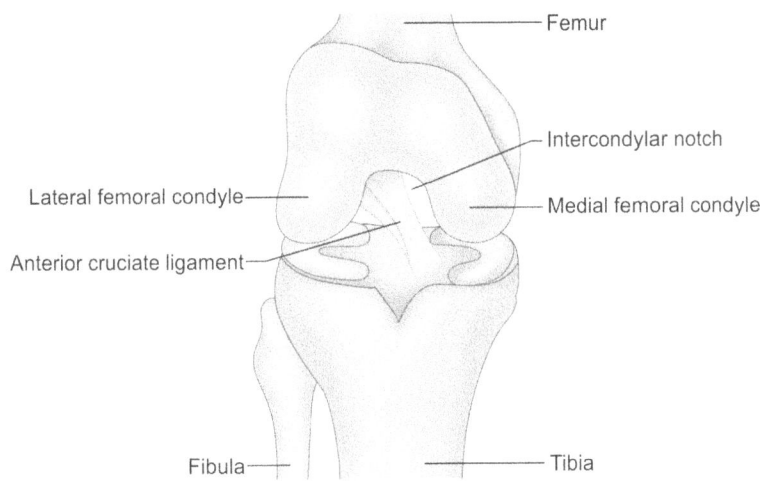

Fig. 10.3: Anterior cruciate ligament

- Throughout knee flexion, hamstring creates a posterior shear force on tibia and thus relieves stress on ACL.
- Soleus muscle has the ability to translate tibia posteriorly and assists the ACL in restraining anterior translation.
- Co-contraction of multiple muscles—influence strain on ACL.
- For example, co-contraction of hamstrings and quadriceps—allows hamstrings to counter the anterior translation imposed by quadriceps—to reduce strain on ACL.
- Activation of gastrocnemius and quadriceps—greater strain on ACL than either muscle alone

  ↓

- Hamstrings are also co-contracted to mitigate the anterior translation imposed by quadriceps and gastrocnemius **(Fig. 10.4)**
- Co-contraction will reduce the anterior shear force on tibia—but increases compressive loads.

Clinics: Quadriceps exercises performed with knee flexed beyond 60°—minimize ACL strain **(Fig. 10.5)**

Posterior Cruciate Ligament

- Posterior cruciate ligament arises distally from the posterior tibial surface between posterior horns of two menisci and then travels superiorly and anteriorly to attach to lateral aspect of medial femoral condyle.
- Posteromedial and anterolateral bundle
- Knee full extension—posteromedial bundle taut
- Knee flexion (80-90°)—anterolateral bundle taut
- Restrains posterior displacement or posterior shear of tibia beneath femur
- Restrains varus and valgus at the knee
- Popliteal muscle shares role of PCL in restraining posterior translation of tibia on femur.
- Isolated hamstring contraction—destabilizes the knee in absence of PCL.
- Contraction of gastrocnemius muscle—strains posterior cruciate ligament at flexion angles greater than 40°, whereas quadriceps contraction reduces the strain in posterior cruciate ligament at knee flexion between 20 and 30°.

Ligaments of the Posterior Capsule

- Posterior oblique ligament and arcuate ligament—taut in full extension and assist in checking hyperextension of knee.
- It also checks valgus and varus forces respectively.
- Meniscofemoral ligaments

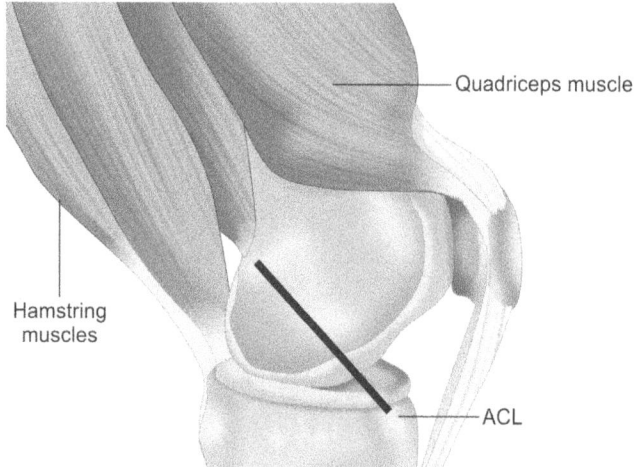

Fig. 10.4: How the hamstrings protect the Anterior cruciate ligament (ACL)

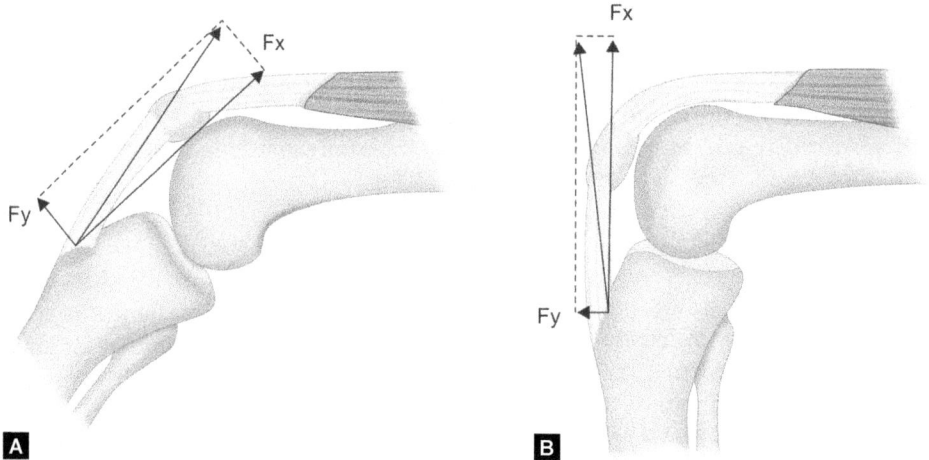

Figs. 10.5A and B: (A) With the knee close to full extension, a forceful quadriceps contraction is capable of inducing an anterior tibial translation; (B) Once the knee is flexed to greater than 60°, little to no anterior translation occurs

Iliotibial Band

- Iliotibial band or tract is formed proximally on the fascia investing tensor fascia lata, the gluteus maximus, and gluteus medius muscle.
- Inserts into anterolateral tibia Gerdy's tubercle **(Fig. 10.6)**
- Iliotibial band moves anteriorly to the knee joint axis as knee is extended and moves posteriorly as knee is flexed.
- As knee moves from full extension to 30° of flexion, compression of highly vascularized and richly innervated adipose tissue increases between the ITB and lateral epicondyle.
- Adipose tissue is less compressed in full extension—thus patients complaints of pain in 30° of knee flexion.

Bursa (Fig. 10.7)

- Suprapatellar bursa, subpopliteal bursa, and gastrocnemius bursa
- Suprapatellar bursa—anteriorly located, lies between quadriceps tendon and anterior femur, superior to the patella

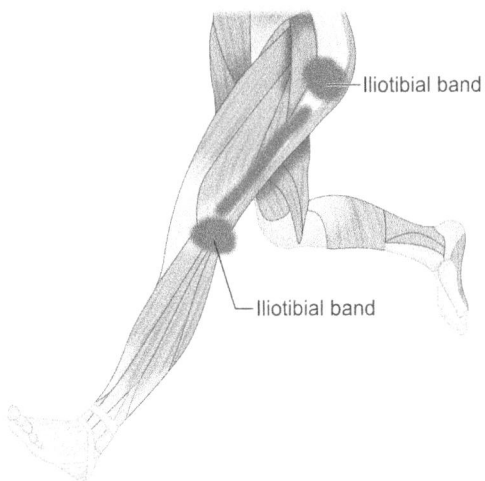

Fig. 10.6: Iliotibial band

- Subpopliteal bursa—posteriorly located, lies between the tendon of popliteus and lateral femoral condyle
- Gastrocnemius bursa—lies between tendon of medial head of gastrocnemius muscle and medial femoral condyle
- Prepatellar bursa—located between the skin and anterior surface of the patella, allows free movement of the skin over the patella during flexion and extension
- Infrapatellar bursa—located inferior to patella, between patellar tendon and overlying skin
- Deep infrapatellar bursa—located between the patellar tendon and tibial tuberosity.
- Reduces friction between patellar tendon and tibial tuberosity.
- This bursa is separated from the synovial cavity of the joint by the infrapatellar (Hoffa's) fat pad.

TIBIOFEMORAL JOINT FUNCTION

Joint Kinematics (Figs. 10.8 to 10.10)

- Primary angular (or rotatory) motions are:
  - Flexion/extension
  - Medial/lateral (internal/external) rotation
  - Varus/valgus (abduction/adduction)
- Translation in anteroposterior direction is common in both medial and lateral tibial plateau.

and

- Less amount of medial and lateral translations occur in response to varus and valgus forces.

↓

Occurs because of joint incongruence

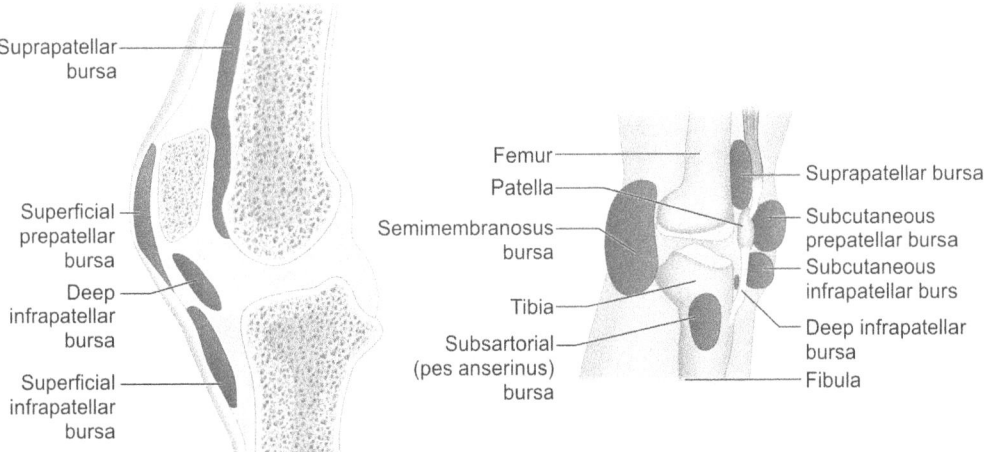

Fig. 10.7: Different bursa in knee joint

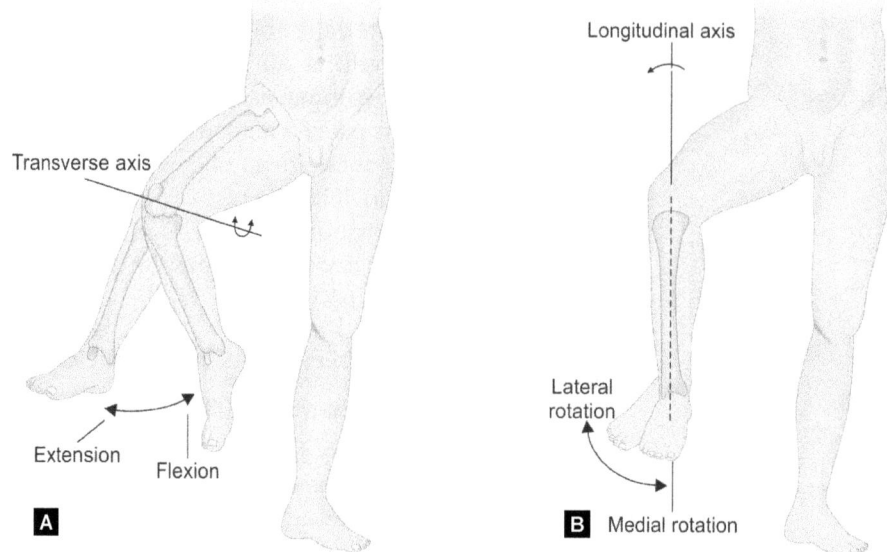

Figs. 10.8A and B: (A) Axis for knee flexion and extension; (B) Axis for tibial rotation

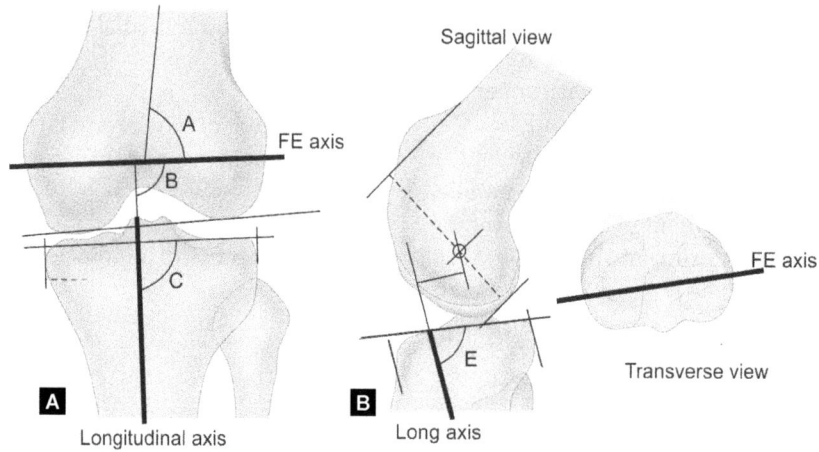

Figs. 10.9A and B: Axis within the knee joint. (A) Flexion and extension—horizontal line passing through femoral condyles; (B) Vertical axis for tibial rotation.

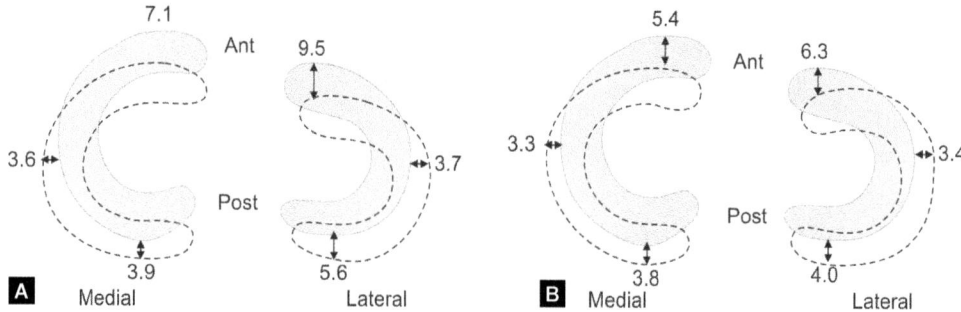

Figs. 10.10A and B: The mean movement (mm) in each meniscus during flexion: (A) Erect and weight-bearing; (B) Sitting, relaxed, bearing no weight. These are not to scale

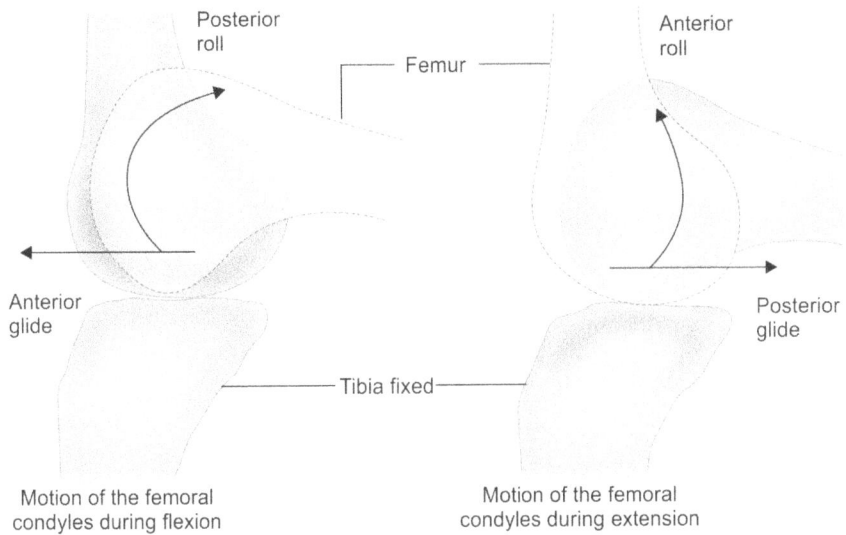

Fig. 10.11: Arthrokinematics during knee flexion and extension in closed kinetic chain

- Excessive motion—indicates ligament incompetence

Flexion/Extension
- **Flexion:** (e.g., during squat)
  - Axis—horizontal line passing through the femoral condyles (**Figs. 10.8** and **10.9**)
  - As femur begins to flex on fixed tibia (Convex-Concave rule)
    ↓
  - Femur condyles roll posteriorly and simultaneously glide anteriorly (**Fig. 10.11**).
  - So, 0–25° of femur on tibia flexion—femur condyles roll posteriorly
  - As flexion continues—rolling of femoral condyles is simultaneously combined with anterior glide.
- **Extension (e.g., during squat) (Convex-Concave rule) (Figs. 10.11 and 10.12)**
  - Extension of the knee from flexion is a reversal of motion
    ↓
  - Tibiofemoral extension occurs initially as an anterior rolling of femoral condyles on tibial plateau
    ↓
  - After that femoral condyles glide posteriorly

- Seated knee extension or swing phase of gait: (Concave-Convex rule) (**Fig. 10.13**)
  ↓
  Tibia moves on fixed femur
  ↓
  Tibia is flexing on fixed femur
  ↓
  Tibia rolls and glides posteriorly on fixed femoral condyles
  - Extension of tibia on fixed femur
  ↓
  Anterior roll and glide of tibial plateau on fixed femur

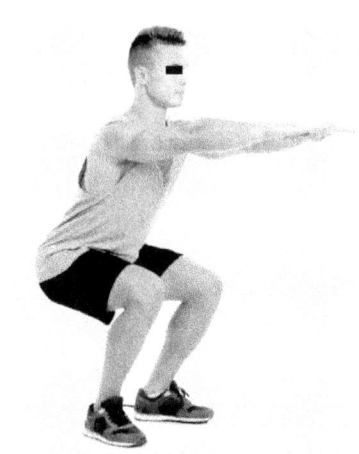

Fig. 10.12: Closed kinetic chain, e.g., squatting

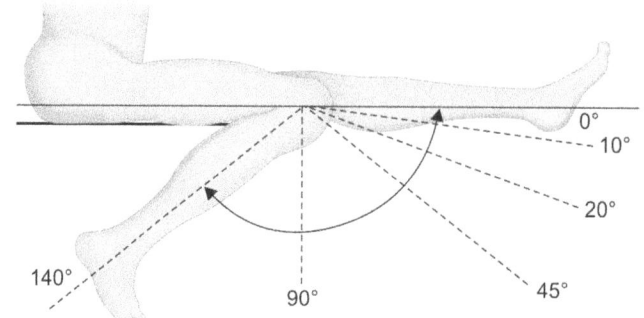

Fig. 10.13: Knee motions in open kinetic chain

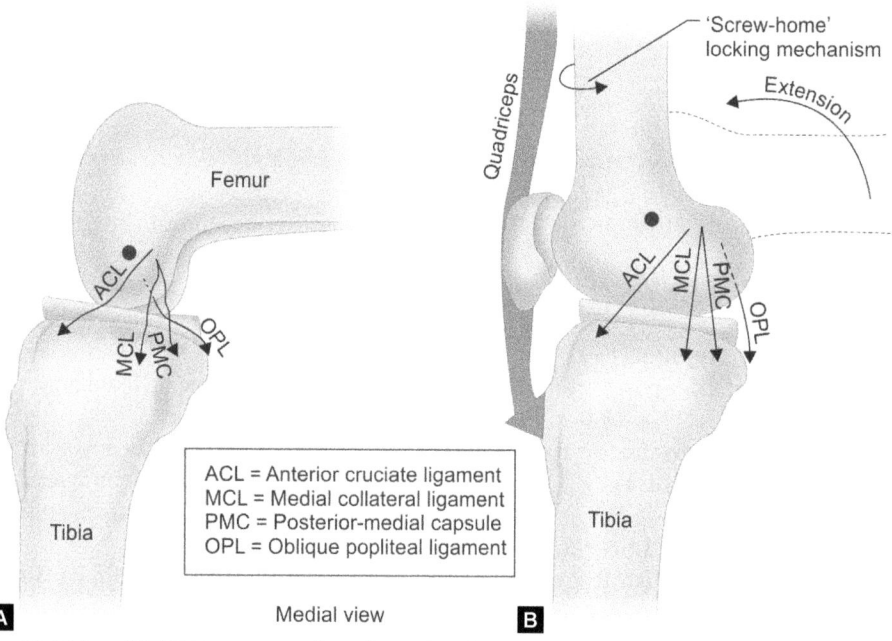

ACL = Anterior cruciate ligament
MCL = Medial collateral ligament
PMC = Posterior-medial capsule
OPL = Oblique popliteal ligament

Figs. 10.14A and B: (A) Ligaments relatively stack in flexion; (B) Ligaments pulled taut in extension

ROLE OF CRUCIATE LIGAMENTS AND MENISCI IN FLEXION AND EXTENSION (FIGS. 10.14A AND B)

- **During knee flexion—femur flexes on tibia (e.g., squat)**
  ↓
  Posterior rolling of femur
  ↓
  Cause ACL to tighten
  ↓
  Continued rolling of femur
  ↓
  Result in taut ACL's simultaneously creating anterior translational force on femoral condyles

- **During knee extension**
  ↓
  Femoral condyles roll anteriorly on tibial plateau
  ↓
  Rigid PCL taut
  ↓
  Further progression of femur
  ↓
  Creates posterior translational force on femoral condyles

- Anterior glide of femur during flexion is because of the shape of the menisci.
- **Wedge-shape menisci**
  ↓
  Posteriorly forces femoral condyles to roll uphill as knee flexes
  ↓
  Oblique contact force of menisci on femur
  ↓
  Helps glide the femur anteriorly
  ↓
  Reaction force of femur on menisci
  ↓
  Deforms the menisci posteriorly on tibial plateau
- **As knee extends**
  ↓
  Posterior margins of menisci return to their neutral position
  ↓
  As extension continues
  ↓
  Anterior margins of the menisci deform

  Thus, motion of menisci is an important component of tibiofemoral flexion and extension.
- Posterior deformation of menisci is assisted by muscular mechanisms to ensure appropriate meniscal motion occurs.
  ↓
- During knee flexion—e.g., semimembranosus exerts a posterior pull on medial menisci
- Popliteus assists with deformation of lateral menisci.

Flexion/Extension Range of Motion

Knee Flexion

- Passive ROM knee flexion—0-130°
- Squatting—knee flexion 0-160° as hip and knee are flexed
- Normal gait on level ground—require approx. 60-70°.
- Sitting down and arising from chair—90° of flexion or more
- Ascending stairs—80°

Knee Extension/Hyperextension

- 5° considered normal
- Excessive knee hyperextension (i.e., beyond 5°)—termed as genu recurvatum
- Two joint muscles around the knee, i.e., cross either hip or ankle joint
- Therefore, hip joint position can influence knee joint ROM.
- Passive insufficiency of rectus femoris limits knee flexion to 120° or less if hip joint is simultaneously hyperextended.
- **Note:** Position of ankle can influence knee position, e.g.,
  - Ankle fixed in dorsiflexion by ski boot, knee cannot be fully extended without the forefoot being lifted from the ground.
  - With fixed plantarflexion deformity of ankle/foot, the knee is forced into hyperextension when foot is flat on ground (**Fig. 10.15**).

Medial/Lateral Rotation

- Here, tibia moved on fixed femur.
- Longitudinal axis runs through the medial tibial intercondylar tubercle. Axial rotations of knee joint occur about longitudinal axis.
- Medial condyle acts like a pivot.
- Lateral condyles move through a greater arc of motion.

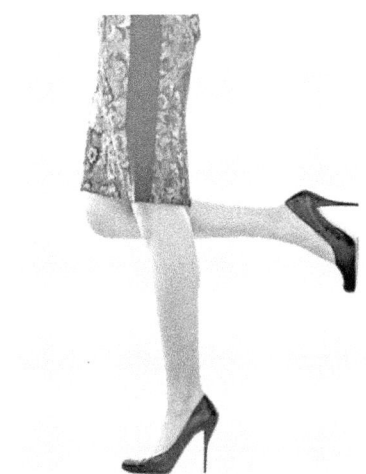

Fig. 10.15: Position of ankle can influence knee joint, e.g., standing with high heels

- When tibia laterally rotates on femur
  ↓
  Medial tibial condyles move anteriorly on fixed medial femoral condyle
  ↓
  Lateral tibial condyles move posteriorly on relatively fixed lateral femoral condyles
- During tibial medial rotation
  ↓
  Medial tibial condyle moves slightly posteriorly
  ↓
  Whereas lateral condyle moves anteriorly through a larger arc of motion

Note: Both medial and lateral rotation, knee joint menisci will distort in the direction of movement

- Axial rotation is permitted by articular incongruence and ligamentous laxity.
- Range of knee joint rotation depends on flexion and extension position of knee.
- Knee fully extended—ligaments are taut, very little axial rotation is possible.
- Knee flexes to 90°—capsular and ligament laxity increases—tibial tubercles no longer in intercondylar notch—maximum rotation is possible.
- Magnitude of rotation diminishes—as knee approaches full extension and full flexion.
- At 90° knee flexion—total medial/lateral rotation is approx. 35° (ROM lateral rotation, 0–20° and medial rotation, 0–15°)

Valgus (Abduction)/Varus (Adduction)

- Minimal motion
- Frontal plane ROM is 8° at full flexion and 13 with 20° of knee flexion.
- Excessive frontal plane motion—indicates ligamentous insufficiency.

Coupled Motion

Medial femoral condyle lies slightly distal to lateral femoral condyle—results in physiologic valgus angle in extended knee.

Automatic or Locking Mechanism of the Knee

- Lateral rotation with knee extension—referred to as automatic or terminal rotation
- During last 30° of knee extension (non-weight bearing)
- Shorter lateral tibial plateau completes its rolling-gliding motion before the longer medial articular surfaces do.
- As extension continues—longer medial plateau continues to roll and to glide anteriorly after lateral side of the plateau has halted.
- **Note:** Knee extension—closed packed position of knee—tibial tubercles become lodged in intercondylar notch
- In closed packed position—menisci tightly interposed between tibial and femoral condyles and ligaments taut
- Automatic rotation—known as locking or screw home mechanism.

To Initiate Knee Flexion

- When the knee goes from full extension to full flexion, knee must unlock first. The tibia medially rotates concomitantly as flexion is initiated.
- This automatic rotation or locking of knee occurs in both weight and nonweight bearing.
- In weight bearing—freely moving femur

Locking—medially rotates on fixed tibia during last 30° extension.

Unlocking—lateral rotation of femur on tibia before flexion

MUSCLES

Muscles that cross the knee—flexors and extensors.

Knee flexor group:
- Seven muscles flex the knee
- Semimembranosus, semitendinosus, biceps femoris (long and short heads), sartorius, gracilis, popliteus, and gastrocnemius muscles **(Fig. 10.16)**
- Exception of short head of biceps femoris, and popliteus—all others are two joint muscles.
- Popliteus, gracilis, sartorius, semimembranosus, semitendinosus—medially rotate tibia on fixed femur

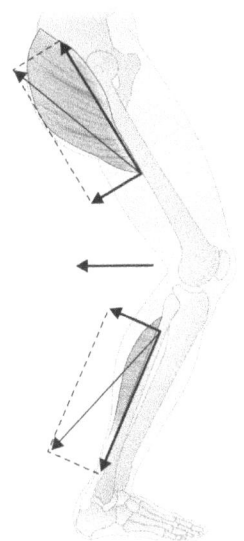

Fig. 10.16: The force systems in the lower limb

- Biceps femoris—capable to laterally rotate tibia on fixed femur
- Hamstrings muscles—semitendinosus, semimembranosus, short and long heads of biceps femoris and adductor magnus.
- Lateral muscles (biceps femoris, lateral head of gastrocnemius, and popliteus)—capable of producing valgus moments at the knee
- Medial side (semimembranosus, semitendinosus, medial head of gastrocnemius, sartorius and gracilis)—generate varus moments
- Greater hamstring force is produced when hip is in flexion, where hamstrings are lengthened.
- Two joint muscles (hamstrings)—when hip extended and knee flexed to 90° or more—hamstrings shorten over both hip and knee

↓

Hamstring weakens as knee flexion proceeds—leading to muscle shortening

and

Muscle group must overcome the increasing tension in rectus femoris muscle that is approaching passive insufficiency.

- Nonweight bearing

↓

Hamstring

↓

Posterior shearing force of tibia on femur increases as knee flexion increases—between 75 and 90° knee flexion

↓

Reduce strain on ACL

- Sartorius muscle—mild knee extensor rather than as a knee flexor
  - Sartorius muscle functions as a flexor and medial rotator of tibia
  - Active during swing phase
- Three muscles of pes anserinus—function as a group to resist valgus forces and provide dynamic stability to the anteromedial aspect of knee joint.
- **Popliteus muscle—medial rotator of tibia on femur:** Role of unlocking the knee
- **Soleus muscle and gluteus maximus—do not cross the knee joint:**
  - Soleus muscle—attaches to proximal aspect proximal posterior aspect of tibia and fibula and attaches distally to calcaneal tendon.
  - Soleus (weight bearing)—assists with knee extension—by pulling the tibia posteriorly.
  - Gluteus maximus muscle—assists knee extension in weight bearing—posterior shear of femur on tibia.

Knee Extensor Group

- The four muscles that are responsible for knee extension vastus intermedius, vastus lateralis, vastus medialis, and rectus femoris. Rectus femoris is a two-joint muscle as it crosses hip and knee joint. Vastus lateralis, medialis, and intermedius arises from femur and joins with rectus femoris muscle into a common tendon called quadriceps tendon.
- Quadriceps tendon inserts into the proximal aspect of patella and continues distally past the patella known as patella tendon (or patella ligament) (**Fig. 10.17**).
- Patella tendon—runs from the apex of patella into proximal portion of tibial tuberosity.

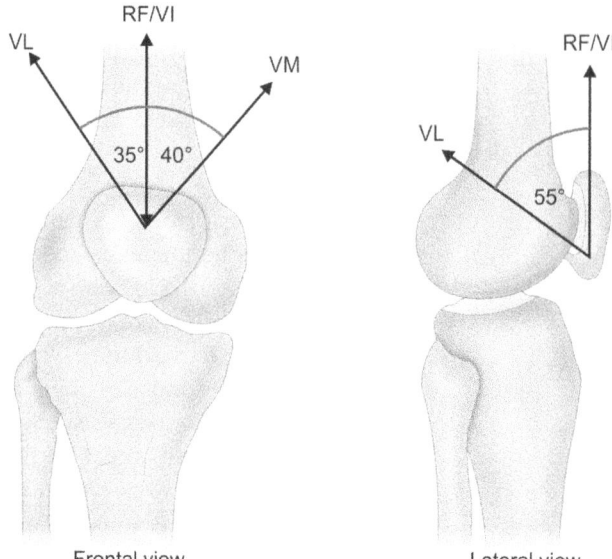

Fig. 10.17: Angle of pull of vastus lateralis, vastus medialis and rectus femoris

- Vastus medialis and lateralis—insert directly into medial and lateral aspects of patella by way of retinacular fibers.
- **Resultant pull of:**
  - Vastus lateralis muscle—35°
  - Vastus medialis muscle—40°
- Because of different orientation of upper and lower fibers of VM muscle

Upper fibers referred to as—vastus medialis longus
Lower fibers—vastus medialis oblique (VMO)

- VMO—patellofemoral pain—causes recruitment of VMO—maximizes medial pull of patella.
- Large vastus lateralis and medialis—posterior attachment site—results in net posterior or compressive forces that averages 55° in extended knee.
- Compressive forces from these muscles is present throughout ROM—but minimized at full extension and increases as knee flexion continues.

Patellar Influence on Quadriceps Function

- Function of quadriceps—influenced by patella
- Patella lengthens the MA of quadriceps by increasing distance between quadriceps and patellar tendon from axis of knee joint.

Stabilizers of Knee

- Passive structures—capsuloligamentous ⎫ Stability of
- Active structures—muscular forces ⎭ tibiofemoral joint
- Injury to posterolateral corner (e.g., posterolateral joint capsule, popliteus, and arcuate ligament)

  Causes posterior instability and excessive lateral tibial rotation
  ↓
  Termed posterolateral instability

- Damage to posterior oblique ligaments, medial hamstrings, MCL and posteromedial joint capsule
  ↓
  Posteromedial instability

- Extensor retinaculum (composed of fibers from quadriceps femoris muscle, fuse with joint capsule)
  ↓
  Dynamic support for anteromedial and anterolateral aspect

Factors Affecting Stability of the Tibiofemoral Joint

- **Bony configuration:** The least important

- **Tension of ligaments or other connective tissues:**
  - *ACL:* Anteromedial stability
    - Prevent anterior displacement of the tibia
  - *PCL:* Anterolateral stability
    - Prevent posterior displacement of the tibia
  - *Lateral collateral ligaments (LCL):* Prevent varus stress
  - *Medial collateral ligament (MCL):* Prevent valgus stress
  - Medial and lateral retinaculum
  - Iliotibial band
  - *Passive tension of muscles:*
    - Quadriceps femoris
    - Hamstrings
    - Pes anserinus
- **Factors affecting patella stability:**
  - *Bony configuration:* Prominent anterolateral aspect of the femoral condyle
  - *Ligaments or connective tissue:*
    - Patellar ligament
    - Medial and lateral retinaculum
    - Iliotibial band
  - *Muscles*
    - Tensor fascia lata muscle
    - Vastus medialis: Contraversial

PATELLOFEMORAL JOINT

- Patella—posterior surface—divided by vertical ridge and covered by articular cartilage
- Ridge divides it into medial and lateral facets
- Medial and lateral facets are flat to slightly convex side to side and top to bottom.
- 2nd vertical ridge—medial border—separates medial facet from extreme medial edge—odd facet
- In extended knee
  ↓
  Posterior surface of patella
  ↓
  Sits on femoral sulcus
- Patella attached to tibial tuberosity by patellar tendon
- Patellofemoral joint is one of the most incongruent joints
- Patella functions as anatomical pulley for quadriceps muscle
- Incongruence of PFJ—patella dependent on static and dynamic structures for stability.

Patellofemoral Articular Surfaces and Joint Congruence

- Fully extended knee—patella lies on femoral sulcus (joint congruency is minimal—greater chances for patellar instability)
- Ratio of length of patellar tendon to length of patella is approximately 1:1—referred as Insall-Salvati index.
- Patellar alta—when the long tendon produces an abnormally high position of patella on femoral sulcus.
- In extended knee—patella sits in femoral sulcus and inferior pole of patella makes contact with femur.
- As knee flexion begins (10-20°)—patella slides down—increasing surface contact area.
  ↓
  Inferior margins of medial and lateral facets
- As flexion progresses—contact area increases—shifts to superior of patella—spreads outward to cover medial and lateral facets
- By 90° knee flexion—all portions of patella are in contact except ODD facet
- As flexion continues beyond 90°—area of contact—inferiorly—smaller odd facet—contact with medial femoral condyle
- During full flexion, the patella gets lodged in the intercondylar groove and the lateral and odd facets are in contact. The medial facet is completely out of contact.

Motions of Patella

- Femur is fixed and knee flexing—patellar fixed to tibial tuberosity via patellar tendon
  ↓
  Patella is pulled inferiorly
  ↓
  Gliding inferiorly and rotating on femoral condyles with distal apex of patella moving posteriorly
  ↓

This sagittal plane rotation as patellar tracks down in the intercondylar groove of femur—patellar flexion

- Knee extension
  ↓
  Patella goes back to original position in femoral sulcus
  ↓
  Apex of patella pointing inferiorly at end of ROM
  ↓
  This motion of patellar gliding superiorly while rotating up and down the femoral condyles—patellar extension
- Patella tilts around longitudinal axis (proximal to distal through the patella)
- Shifts medially and laterally in frontal plane
- Spins and rotates around AP axis (perpendicular to patella)
- **Tilting (medial and lateral tilt):**
  - Lateral patellar tilt—occurs when lateral edge of patella approximates the surface of lateral femoral condyle.
  - Medial patellar tilt—occurs when medial edge of patella moves toward medial femoral condyle.
- Lateral patellar shift—is defined as patella moving toward lateral femoral condyle in frontal plane along medial-lateral axis.
- Rotation of the patella about AP axis (termed medial and lateral rotation)—referred by movement of distal apex of patella.
- Medial rotation—patella spins around perpendicular axis—apex of patella pointing toward medial femoral condyle and base of patella moving closer to lateral femoral condyle.
- Patella situated slightly laterally in femoral sulcus with knee in full extension
  ↓
  As knee flexion initiated
  ↓
  Patella pushed medially by large femoral condyle
  ↓
  As knee flexion proceeds 30°
  ↓
  Patella shifts laterally—engaged within femoral condyles

Patellofemoral Joint Stress

- As knee flexes and extends, the quadriceps tendon pulls the patella superiorly while the patellar tendon resists it inferiorly. Sum of these pull produces posterior compressive force of the patella on femur (varies with amount of knee flexion).
- There is low joint stress at full extension of the knee.
- As knee flexion progresses
  ↓
  Angle of pull between quadriceps tendon and patellar tendon decreases
  ↓
  Increases joint reaction force and produces greater PFJ compression
- During stance phase—peak knee flexion 20° thus—PF compressive force is approximately 25-50% body weight
- During running—greater knee flexion and greater quadriceps activity—PFJ compressive forces reach five and six times body weight.

Note: If patella positioned inferiorly—termed patella baja because of shortened patellar tendon.

Frontal Plane Patellofemoral Joint Stability

- Longitudinal stabilizers of patella—patellar tendon inferiorly and quadriceps tendon superiorly—called as patellotibial ligaments.
- These provide passive increases in patellofemoral compression—in turn help to stabilize patella in medial-lateral direction
- Transverse stabilizers composed of superficial portion of extensor retinaculum—i.e., connect vastus medialis and lateralis directly to the patella.

- Passive stabilizers—i.e., medial and lateral patellofemoral ligament—firmly attach to adductor tubercle medially and ITB laterally.
- Medial patellofemoral ligaments prevent lateral translation of patella.
- Presence of hypermobility—results in patellar subluxation/dislocation
- Hypomobility—greater PF stresses

Asymmetry of Patellofemoral Stabilization

- Q angle—angle formed between line connecting ASIS to midpoint of patella and tibial tuberosity to midpoint of patella.
- 10-15° with knee in full extension
- Alteration in alignment—increases lateral force—thus increases compressive forces
- Women have slightly greater Q angle than do men because of presence of wider pelvis, increased femoral anteversion, and relative knee valgus.

- Pronated foot
  ↓
  Increased medial femoral tibial torsion (femoral anteversion)
  ↓
  Tibial lateral rotation
  ↓
  Larger Q angle and increase lateral force on patella

Prepatellar bursitis (also known as coal miner's knee, housemaid's knee, or nun's knee): It is an inflammation of the prepatellar bursa at the front of the knee. It is marked by swelling, which can be tender to touch, but there will be no range of motion restriction. It is commonly due to trauma either by a single acute instance or by chronic trauma over time. As such, prepatellar bursitis commonly occurs among individuals whose profession requires frequent kneeling.

CHAPTER 11

Ankle and Foot Complex

Chapter Outline

- Introduction
- Joint structure of ankle and foot complex
- Forces in the ankle joint complex
- Pronation and supination twist
- Metatarsophalangeal joint
- Metatarsal break
- Interphalangeal joint
- Plantar fascia
- Arches of foot
- Pathomechanics

INTRODUCTION

A highly intricate and complex joint that bears all the body weight and contributes substantially to bipedal gait is ankle joint. It constitutes of 28 uneven bones, 25 synovial joints and muscles, and numerous ligaments, and therefore referred as ankle and foot complex. Synchronized action of all these structures enables locomotion while maintaining body balance. Being the most distal joint, it is subjected to excessive compressive and tensile load leading to sprains and injuries.

The foot can be classified into three parts as follows (**Fig. 11.1**):

Forefoot	Metatarsals: Phalanges
Midfoot	Navicular: Medial, intermediate and lateral cuneiform: Cuboid
Rearfoot	Talus, calcaneus

Fig. 11.1: Parts of foot

JOINT STRUCTURE OF ANKLE AND FOOT COMPLEX (FIGS. 11.2 TO 11.4)

Talocrural Joint/Tibiotalar and Fibulotalar Joint

Type: Synovial hinge joint

Degree of freedom: One degree of freedom

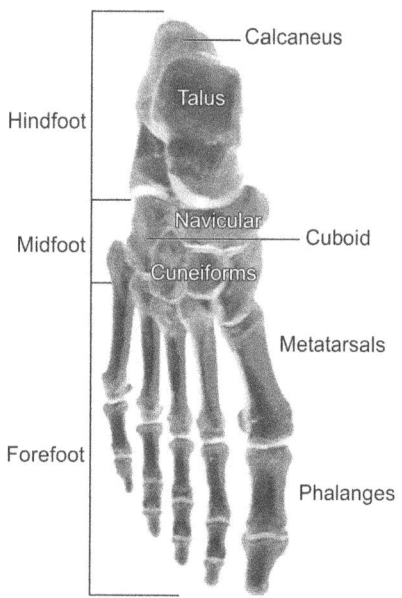

Fig. 11.2: Functional segments and bones of the foot

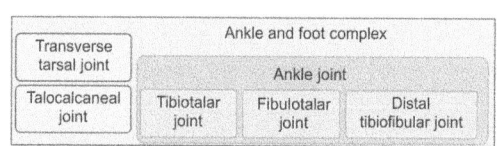

Fig. 11.3: Joints in ankle and foot complex

Chapter 11 | Ankle and Foot Complex

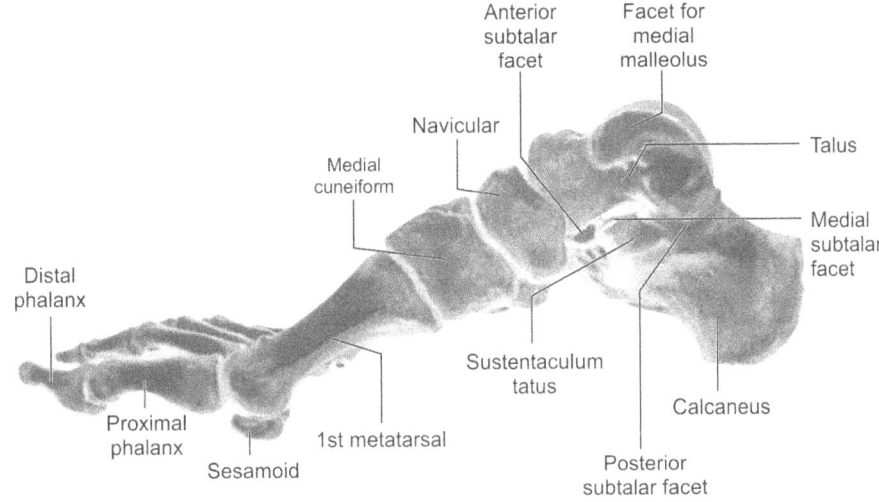

Fig. 11.4: Medial view of the foot, showing the talus sitting on the calcaneus (the subtalar joint)

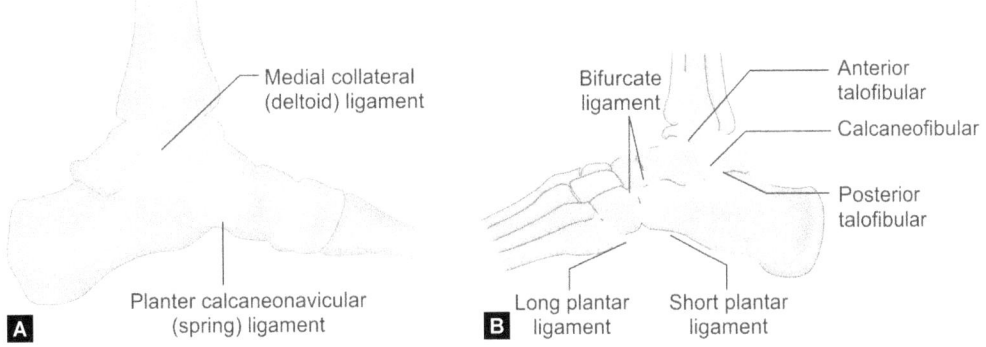

Figs. 11.5A and B: (A) Medial ligaments of the posterior ankle/foot complex; (B) Lateral ligaments of the posterior ankle/foot complex

Articulating surfaces:
- **Proximal:** Distal end of tibia, medial malleolus of tibia, and lateral malleolus of fibula
- **Distal:** Body of talus

Close pack position: Dorsiflexion
Loose pack position: Plantarflexion
Capsular pattern: Plantarflexion; Dorsiflexion

Stability:
- **Joint design:** Proximal articulating surfaces together form a rectangular arch called as *mortise* and talus forms *tenon*. Talus widens anteriorly due to which wedges into mortise during dorsiflexion, therefore improving the joint stability.
- **Capsule:** Weak and thin capsule attached proximally to margins of medial and lateral malleolus, distally to surface of talus. Collateral ligaments reinforce the capsule medially and laterally.
- **Ligaments (Figs. 11.5A and B):** Anterior and posterior talofibular, calcaneofibular, deltoid (tibiocalcaneal, tibionavicular, and tibiotalar), lateral collateral ligaments

Kinematics

Osteokinematics

- **Movements available:** Dorsiflexion, plantarflexion

- **Planes and axis:** Sagittal plane around frontal axis
- **Range of motion (ROM):**

Movement	ROM
Dorsiflexion	0–20
Plantarflexion	0 to 30–50

- **Closed kinematic chain motion:** Squats, lunges.
- **Open kinematic chain motion:** Gait cycle, ankle pumps
- **Factors responsible for restriction of movements:**
  - Passive tension in triceps surae restricts excessive dorsiflexion
  - Excessive plantarflexion is restricted by tension in tibialis anterior, extensor hallucis longus, and extensor digitorum longus.

Arthrokinematics

- **Concave convex rule:** Convex talus moves in a fixed concave mortise
  - Head of talus rolls anteriorly and slides posteriorly during dorsiflexion
  - Rolls posteriorly and slides anteriorly during plantarflexion
- **Movements available:** Sliding is predominant.

Kinetics

- **Movement:** Dorsiflexion, plantarflexion
- **Muscle responsible:**
  - *Dorsiflexion:* Tibialis anterior, extensor digitorum longus, extensor hallucis longus, and peroneus tertius
  - *Plantarflexion:* Gastrocnemius, soleus, plantaris, tibialis posterior, flexor digitorum longus, flexor hallucis longus, and peroneus longus and brevis

Distal Tibiofibular Joint

Type: Syndesmosis
Articulating surfaces
- **Proximal:** Medial surface of distal fibula
- **Distal:** Fibular notch of tibia

Ligaments: Interosseus ligament, anterior, and posterior tibiofibular ligament

Subtalar Joint

Type: Plane synovial joint
Degree of freedom: One
Articulating surfaces:
- **Proximal:** Anterior, middle, and posterior facets of calcaneus
- **Distal:** Anterior, middle, and posterior facets of talus

Close pack position: Supination
Loose pack position: Neutral
Capsular pattern: Limitation of varus movement

Stability:
- **Joint design:** Excessive mobility is prevented due to alternating concave-convex facets
- **Capsule:** A loose capsule enclosing the entire joint, which thickens to form medial, lateral, and posterior talocalcaneal ligament that stabilizes the capsule.
- **Ligaments (Fig. 11.6):** Talocalcaneal ligament (all three parts), talocalcaneal, interosseous ligament, cervical ligament

Kinematics
Osteokinematics

- **Movements available:**
  - *Supination:* Inversion + Adduction + Plantarflexion

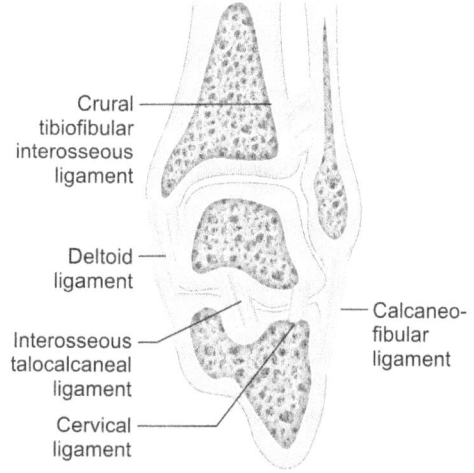

Fig. 11.6: The ligaments of the subtalar joint (in a posterior cross-sectional view)

- *Pronation:* Eversion + Abduction + Dorsiflexion
- **Plane and axis:** Triplanar movements occurring around a unique axis which is obliquely oriented (42° from transverse plane, 16° from sagittal plane)

	Axis	Plane	ROM
Inversion	Sagittal	Frontal	0–30
Eversion	Sagittal	Frontal	0–10
Abduction	Vertical	Transverse	0–30
Adduction	Vertical	Transverse	0–10

Arthrokinematics

- Concave convex rule
- Screwlike movement or complex twisting movement is observed when talus moves over calcaneus. At anterior and middle articulations, talus glides in opposite direction, while it slides in same direction at posterior articulation.
- In frontal plane, tilting of talus → inversion/eversion
- In transverse plane, rotation of talus → dorsiflexion/plantar flexion

	Supination	Pronation
In nonweight-bearing	Calcaneal inversion	Calcaneal eversion
	Calcaneal adduction	Calcaneal abduction
	Calcaneal plantarflexion	Calcaneal dorsiflexion
In weight-bearing	Calcaneal inversion	Calcaneal eversion
	Talar abduction	Talar adduction
	Talar dorsiflexion	Talar plantarflexion
	Tibiofibular lateral rotation	Tibiofibular medial rotation

Kinetics

- **Movement and muscle responsible:**
  - *Inversion:* Tibialis posterior, tibialis anterior
  - *Eversion:* Fibularis brevis, fibularis longus
  - *Supination:* Tibialis anterior, tibialis posterior, extensor hallucis longus, flexor hallucis longus, flexor digitorum longus
  - *Pronation:* Fibularis longus, fibularis brevis, fibularis tertius, extensor digitorum longus, extensor hallucis longus

Transverse Tarsal Joint

	Transverse/Midtarsal/Chopart's joint	
	Talocalcaneonavicular joint	Calcaneocuboid joint
Type	Synovial: Ball and socket	Synovial: Modified saddle
Degree of freedom	One	One
Articulating surfaces		
• Proximal	Anterior surface of talus	Anterior surface of calcaneus
• Distal	Posterior navicular surface, talar facets of calcaneum	Posterior surface of cuboid
Ligaments	Dorsal talonavicular ligament, Spring ligament, Calcaneonavicular part of bifurcate ligament	Calcaneocuboid part of bifurcate ligament, Dorsal calcaneocuboid ligament, Long and short plantar ligaments

Axis: Longitudinal axis—at an upward inclination of 15° from transverse plane, medial inclination of 9° from sagittal plane → predominant supination and pronation

Oblique/transverse axis—medial to sagittal plane by 57°, superior to transverse plane by 52°.

FORCES IN THE ANKLE JOINT COMPLEX

The ankle joint complex bears force that is approximately five times than that of the body weight in a normal bilateral standing or walking and thirteen times of the body weight during running.

The major contribution of this joint is seen in locomotion when the foot is contact with the ground at different phases of gait cycle. The dorsiflexors eccentrically contract to control the movement of foot onto the ground preventing it from slapping in the initial contact. During the loading response, the dorsiflexors contract eccentrically to allow forward progression. And in the midstance the plantar flexors concentrically contract progressing itself to the next phase of gait cycle.

When the speed of walking progresses the kinetic pattern of ankle increases with magnitude. Almost 83% of load is transmitted via tibiotalar joint and the remainder of 17% via fibula. The load is distributed effectively due to the function of ligaments as well as structural impact, while ankle sharing high level of congruency when subjected to stress.

PRONATION AND SUPINATION TWIST

- When the hind foot is unable to compensate the movement, the transverse tarsal joints in turn cannot provide full movement and the tarsometatarsal joints rotates to provide adjustment in forefoot position, and such adjustments are termed as pronation and supination twist.
- These mechanisms occur at tarsometatarsal joints contributing to flattening and hollowing of plantar surface of the foot. The greatest function of tarsometatarsal function is observed in loading phase via primarily augmenting function of transverse tarsal joints regulating the position of metatarsal and phalanges in relation to the load.

Let us learn these adjustments in detail.

Pronation Twist

- It is the combination of outward rotation at ankle, abduction of hind foot, eversion of forefoot, and medial arch depression (**Fig. 11.7**).
- In weight-bearing position, the hind foot and transverse tarsal joints are locked in supination; the forefoot lifts off the ground from the medial side and loads to the ground at the lateral side. The first and second rays maintain the contact with

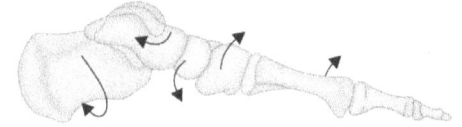

Fig. 11.7: Extreme pronation at the subtalar joint is accompanied by adduction and plantarflexion of the head of the talus, eversion of the calcaneus, and (in some instances) pronation at the transverse tarsal joint as a result of the navicular bone's being forced down by the talus. If the forefoot is to remain on the ground, the tarsometatarsal joints must undergo a counteracting supination twist

the ground due the contraction of plantar flexors. The fourth and fifth rays are forced into dorsiflexion.
- The combined movement of eversion accompanied with plantar flexion of first and second rays and dorsiflexion of fourth and fifth ray along a hypothetical axis. This is termed as *pronation twist*.

Supination Twist

- It is the combination of inward rotation at the ankle, adduction of hind foot, inversion of forefoot, and medial arch elevation (**Fig. 11.8**).
- In weight-bearing position, the hind foot pronates; the transverse tarsal joints supinate to counter rotate and place the plantar aspect of foot on the ground. But, when the transverse tarsal joint is unable to complete the demand imposed while loading results in pronation of the hind foot, the forefoot lifts off the ground from lateral side and loads to the ground at medial

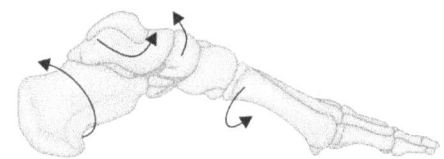

Fig. 11.8: Extreme supination at the subtalar joint is accompanied by abduction and dorsiflexion of the head of the talus, inversion of the calcaneus, and forced supination of the transverse tarsal joint. If the forefoot is to remain on the ground, the tarsometatarsal joints must undergo a counteracting pronation twist

side. The first and second rays are pushed into dorsiflexion due to ground reaction force and the fourth and fifth rays attempt to maintain contact with the ground by plantar flexion of tarsometatarsal joints.
- The combined movement of inversion accompanied with dorsiflexion of first and second rays and plantar flexion of fourth and fifth ray along a hypothetical axis. This is termed as *supination twist*.

Responses of each joint in both the mechanisms		
Joint	Pronation twist	Supination twist
Calcaneum	Inversion	Eversion
Navicular and cuboid bone	Carried along	Pushed downward
Subtalar joint	Supination	Pronation
Talus	Dorsiflexion and abduction	Plantar flexion and adduction
Transverse tarsal joint	Pronation	Supination

Supination Twist

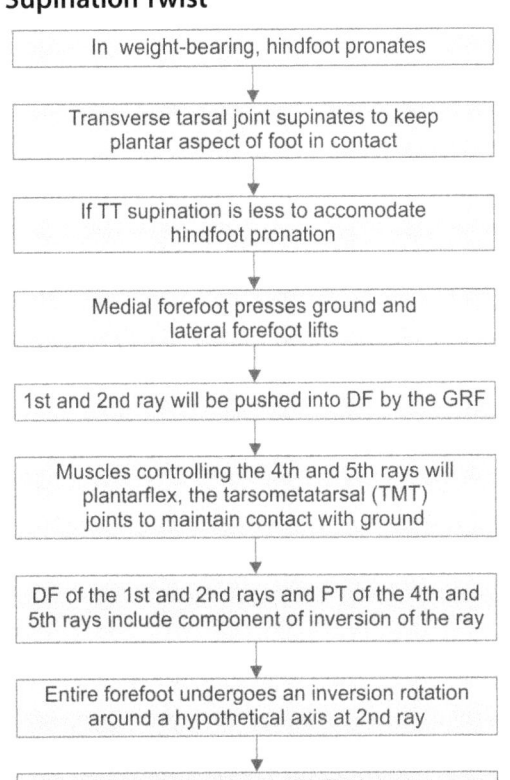

Pronation Twist

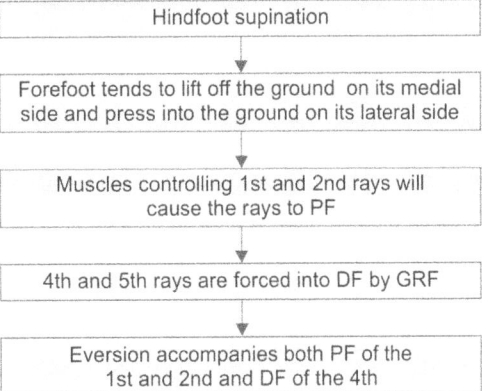

METATARSOPHALANGEAL JOINT

Type: Condyloid synovial joint

Articulating surfaces:
- **Proximal:** Metatarsal heads
- **Distal:** Base of proximal phalanges

Degrees of freedom: Two

Stability:
- Joint capsule,
- Plantar plates,
- Collateral and deep transverse metatarsal ligament

ROM:

	ROM
Flexion	0–30
Extension	0–80

Muscles: Flexor digitorum brevis, flexor hallucis brevis, flexor digiti minimi
- Abductor hallucis, abductor digiti minimi
- Adductor hallucis
- Lumbricals
- Plantar and dorsal interossei

THE METATARSAL BREAK

Metatarsophalangeal extension is known as metatarsal break.

The terminology means hinge or break as the heel rises and the metatarsal heads and toes are in weightbearing. This mechanism occurs along the oblique axis passing through the head of second and third metatarsals. The oblique axis of metatarsal break lies along the coronal axis. The angle is formed laterally between the long axis of foot an oblique axis formed by metatarsal break.

Normal angular range formed is 54–74°.

Schematic Representation of Metatarsal Break

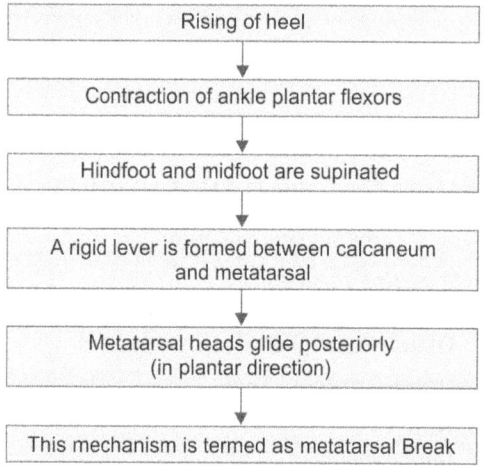

During bilateral stance, the base of support is between the toes and metatarsal heads, and the line of gravity (LOG) passes through the base of support (BOS).

Schematic representation of weight-bearing during a metatarsal break

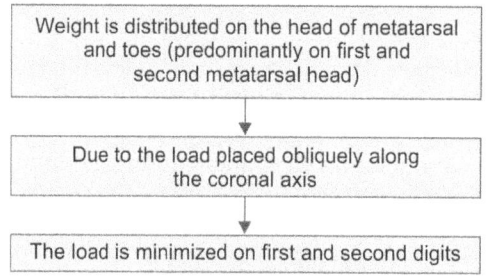

INTERPHALANGEAL JOINT

Type: Hinge synovial joint

Articulating surfaces: Between proximal and distal phalanges

Degrees of freedom: One

Stability: Plantar and collateral ligaments

ROM:

	ROM
Flexion	0–50°
Extension	50–0°

Muscles:
- Lumbricals
- Plantar and dorsal interossei

PLANTAR FASCIA

- Connective tissue covering the sole of the foot which is thick centrally (aponeurosis), thin laterally and medially
- **Attachments:**
  - *Central:* Calcaneal medial tubercle
  - *Lateral:* Abductor digiti minimi
  - *Medial:* Abductor hallucis
  - *Proximal:* Flexor digitorum brevis → divides into five slips near metatarsal heads → At metatarsophalangeal joint, divides into superficial and deep strata
    - Superficial strata: Attaches to skin
    - Deep strata: Subdivides into two segments blends with flexor tendons and deep transverse metatarsal ligament
- **Function:**
  - *Protects deep foot structures:* Nerves and blood vessels
  - Maintains foot's longitudinal arches
  - Acts as site for attachment of muscles
  - Avoids excessive dorsiflexion of foot
  - Equal distribution of plantar pressure during loading

ARCHES OF FOOT

- During weight-bearing, body weight is transmitted down the lower limb to talus → calcaneus → base of metatarsals.
- Two longitudinal and one transverse arch are present between these weight-bearing junctions.
- Being elastic in nature, they flatten and act as a spring—Bears bodyweight and absorbs shock produced during walking and recoil once weight is removed.

Determinants of Integrity of an Arch

- **Bone shape:** Wedge-shaped bones, especially the bone in center of the arch
- **Intersegmental attachments/cement/staples:** Ligaments and plantar aponeurosis connecting articulating bones inferiorly
- **Slings:** Suspending and supporting the arch from above
- **Tie beams:** Connecting ends of interlocking bones to avoid separation of arch

Shape of the bone and staples provides passive support to the arch while muscles form a part of dynamic stability. Description regarding longitudinal and transverse arches has been given in **Tables 11.1 and 11.2**:

Functions of Arches of Foot

- Weight distribution across the weightbearing surface of foot
- Adapting to uneven surface
- Shock absorption
- Protects nerves and blood vessels

Pathomechanics

See **Table 11.3**.

▲ Table 11.1: Longitudinal arch of foot.

	Longitudinal arch	
	Medial longitudinal arch	*Lateral longitudinal arch*
Bones involved	Calcaneum, talus, navicular, three cuneiforms, 1st to 3rd metatarsals	Calcaneum, cuboid, 4th, and 5th metatarsal
Anterior pillar	1st to 3rd metatarsals	4th and 5th metatarsal
Posterior pillar	Calcaneum	Calcaneum
Summit	Talus	Subtalar articulation
Integrity		
Ligaments	• Plantar aponeurosis • Spring ligament • Interosseous	• Plantar aponeurosis • Short and long plantar ligament
Muscles	• Tibialis anterior and posterior • Peroneus longus • Flexor digitorum longus • Flexor hallucis longus • Intrinsic muscles	• Peroneus longus • Flexor digitorum longus • Intrinsic muscles
Cement/staples	• Spring ligament • Tibialis posterior tendon	Short and long plantar ligament
Slings	• Tibialis anterior and posterior • Medial ligaments of ankle	• Peroneus longus • Peroneus brevis
Tie beams	• Plantar aponeurosis • Flexor digitorum longus and brevis • Flexor hallucis longus and brevis • Abductor hallucis	• Plantar aponeurosis • Flexor digitorum longus and brevis • Abductor digiti minimi
Features		
Shape	Very concave, higher arch	Less concave arch, almost flat
Characteristic feature	Resiliency	Rigidity
Mobility	Greater mobility	Less mobility
Function	Responsible for propulsion during gait	During walking and running, it receives and supports body weight

▲ **Table 11.2:** Transverse arch of foot.

	Transverse arch	
	Anterior transverse arch	*Posterior transverse arch*
Articulation	Metatarsal head	Talus and metatarsal
Shape of arch	Complete	Incomplete
Structural differences during weight-bearing	Both ends of the arch meets ground	Lateral half of the arch only meets ground
Muscles	Peroneus longus, tibialis posterior	
Ligaments	Plantar ligament, deep transverse metatarsal ligament	

▲ **Table 11.3:** Pathomechanics.

Pathology	Mechanism
Ankle sprain	• Medial ligament sprain is eversion type of injury • Lateral ligament sprain is inversion type of injury • Occurs due to unstable landing on an uneven surface
Syndesmosis injury	• This is common in footballers • This type of sprain results in persistent pain and dysfunction • Injury to the ligaments interconnecting the tarsal bones and talus to the ankle mortise
Ankle instability	• This presents with symptoms, such as pain, swelling, giving away, and restricted movement • There are two types: Structural and functional instability
Claw toes	• Hyperextension of metatarsophalangeal joint • Callus formation under head of metatarsal • Presents with flexion in proximal and distal interphalangeal joint • Postural sway increases • BOS and stability decreases
Hammer toes	• Hyperextension of MTP joint and DIP joint • Flexion of PIP joint
Pes planus/Flat foot	• Reduced/absence of medial arch • There are two types: Rigid flat foot and flexible flat foot • Rigid flat foot is due to hereditary, medial arch is absent in weight-bearing, nonweight-bearing and toe standing • Flexible flat foot is due to adaptation, the arches appear only during weight-bearing
Pes cavus	• The medial longitudinal arch is unusually high • During walking, unable to adapt to nonsupporting surface

CHAPTER 12

Vertebral Column

Chapter Outline

- Cervical spine
  - Parts of cervical spine
  - Structure
  - Joints
  - Kinetics and kinematics
  - Pathomechanics of cervical spine
- Thorax and chest wall
  - General structure and function
  - Ribs
  - Articulations of rib cage
  - Kinematics of rib cage
  - Muscles associated with rib cage
  - Developmental aspects of rib cage
- Lumbar segment
  - Intervertebral disc
  - Stabilizing structures
  - Ligaments
  - Osteokinematics
  - Arthrokinematics
  - Kinetics
  - Lumbopelvic rhythm
  - Thoracolumbar fascia
  - Lumbosacral joint
  - Pathomechanics
- Sacroiliac joint
  - Stability
  - Joint structure
  - Kinematics
  - Kinetics
  - Pathomechanics
  - Symphysis pubis
  - Sacrococcygeal joint

INTRODUCTION

The vertebral column is a chain of 33 vertebra functioning together as a unit in protecting spinal cord, transmitting the axial load down the vertebral column. It forms the base of movement for trunk and extremities. The head and upper limb weight is evenly distributed over the vertebral column.

Based on the structure and location of the vertebrae, there is a difference in the movements which occur for a single segment. But combination of these movements results in an overall movement of the vertebral column as a single unit. For easier and deeper understanding, the vertebral column is divided into following segments/regions:

- The cervical region
- The thoracic region
- The lumbar region
- The sacral region
- The coccygeal region

The cervical region constitutes seven vertebrae, forming the base of skull and cranial structures. This is followed by 12 vertebrae in the thoracic region, functioning as the posterior articulation of rib cage, which are often stated as upper back. Lower back refers to five lumbar vertebrae that transmit the load down to sacrococcygeal region. Sacrum is formed by fusion of five vertebrae and coccyx, also known as tailbone, by fusion of four vertebrae. The structure and functioning of vertebra in each region are discussed later in this chapter.

Primary and secondary curves

While possessing a vertebral column is a common feature among mammals, presence of curves in the vertebral column is exclusive to humans. These curves increase balance, improve flexibility, enhance load bearing ability, and enable bipedal locomotion in humans. In a fetus, vertebral column presents as a single posteriorly convex curve. During infancy, with the attainment of upright postures, there is development of secondary curves in certain regions of the vertebral column. These secondary curves are opposite in alignment to the original curves, i.e., they are posteriorly concave or "C"-shaped curves.

Thoracic and sacrococcygeal region retain posteriorly convex curve throughout the life and are called as *primary curves*. These curves are also known as *kyphotic curves*. In cervical and lumbar region, there is formation of posteriorly concave curve called as *secondary curves*, also called as *lordotic curves*. It is the presence of these curves which have resulted in an "S"-shaped vertebral column, which is more efficient in stress absorption and distribution. Factors influencing stability and mobility of vertebral column is shown in **Table 12.1**.

Vertebral region	Type of spinal curve	Normal degrees
Cervical	Lordosis	20–40°
Thoracic	Kyphosis	20–40°
Lumbar	Lordosis	40–60°
Sacrococcygeal	Kyphosis	Fused into kyphotic curve

◢ **Table 12.1:** Factors influencing stability and mobility of vertebral column.

Sl. No.	Factors	Reasoning
1.	Structure of vertebral column	• Consists of primary and secondary curves, which are formed due to loading • These curves offer high resistance to compressive forces • Without the stability of vertebral column, the head and the appendicular skeleton cannot move smoothly
2.	Structure of each vertebra	• Each vertebra comprises of body, vertebral arch, vertebral foramen, zygapophyseal facet, spinous and transverse process which structurally vary from cervical to coccyx • This varied segmental design allows sufficient movement of head, trunk, and pelvis
3.	Compressive and axial loading	• Bears weight of head, upper limb, and axial skeleton • Load varies with change in body alignment in different positions
4.	Location of the vertebra	• Regionally, the shape and size of each vertebra varies due to differential loading • Size and thickness of vertebral body increases caudally
5.	Intervertebral disc	About 25% length of the vertebral column is comprised of intervertebral discs. • The disc size increases from cervical to lumbar Comprises: 1. A thick fibrous structure → annulus fibrosus 2. Jelly like structure → Nucleus pulposus 3. Vertebral endplate, above and below 4. As the body moves from bending to standing, the intervertebral disc adds to the mobility and is subjected to compressive loading while standing
6.	Osteoligamentous attachment	• The ligaments being uniaxial, are responsible for tensile forces and rarely contribute to the compressive forces • They massively contribute to the stability with their viscoelastic properties
7.	Muscular attachments	The muscular attachments depict the most complicated arrangement of converging and diverging fascicles. This design of the vertebral column represents first order lever system with considerable mechanical advantage. When weight is balanced with respect to the line of gravity, the muscular activity is minimal

CERVICAL SPINE

INTRODUCTION

The cervical spine, formed by seven structurally unique vertebrae, supports the cranium encasing the central nervous system. As it is the backbone of head-torso transitionary zone, great amount of mobility is allowed. However, the kinematic complexity of cervical spine due to anatomical restraints ensures safety of CNS structures, the adjacent blood vessels, and nerve fibers. Any anatomical or functional alterations in the cervical region can result in symptoms in head, neck, and upper extremity. Thus, knowledge about anatomical supports and functioning of cervical spine vertebra is essential.

PARTS

The cervical spine is further divided into upper and lower cervical regions based upon the structural and functional differences amongst the vertebrae. As C1, C2 and C7 are anatomically different from all the other vertebrae in the human body, they are also called as atypical vertebra while all the other vertebra (C3–C6) are typical vertebra. We will now discuss on anatomical variations of these vertebrae.

STRUCTURE

The first and second cervical vertebrae constitute upper cervical region while the remaining five vertebrae form lower cervical region (C3–C7).

Upper Cervical Region

- **Atlas (C1):** It is a ring like structure with two lateral processes linked by an anterior and posterior arch
  - *Arches:*
    * Anterior arch has a smooth articular facet, fovea dentis, for articulation of odontoid process of atlas
    * Posterior arch thickens toward the center and forms posterior tubercle in the midline
  - *Lateral processes:*
    * Two large oval concave superior facets facing superiorly, medially, and slightly backward
    * Two circular, convex inferior facets facing inferiorly and medially
  - Large transverse process and transverse foramen for blood vessels to pass through
  - Does not have a vertebral body and spinous process.
- **Axis (C2):** It has an odontoid process arising perpendicularly from the superior surface of the vertebral body
  - Anteriorly, body of atlas extends down inferiorly and overlaps with the third vertebra
  - Two convex superior facets facing superiorly, laterally
  - Two inferior facets facing inferiorly, anteriorly
  - Has a bifid spinous process, transverse processes.

Lower Cervical Region

The structure of vertebrae from C3 to C7 is like that of a typical vertebra. The distinguishing features of cervical vertebrae are listed below:
- **Vertebral body:**
  - Saddle like structure as it is concave transversely, convex anteroposteriorly
  - Superior surface has projection posteromedially, called as uncinate process
  - Depression called echancrure or anvil, present inferolaterally
- **Vertebral foramen:**
  - *Size:* Large
  - *Shape:* Triangular
- **Transverse process:** Short and form passage for vertebral artery, and vein and sympathetic nerves
- **Articular facets:**
  - Superior facets facing posteriorly, superiorly, and medially
  - Inferior facets facing anteriorly, inferiorly, and laterally

- **Spinous process:**
  - Faces superomedially and consists of a bifurcated tip
  - Length decreases from C2 to C3, remains constant between C3 and C5, significantly increases toward C7.

JOINTS

The joints present in cervical spine, based on their articular surfaces are
- Disc-vertebral body articulation: Between the intervertebral disc and vertebral body
- Zygapophyseal articulation: Between the inferior facet of upper vertebra and superior facet of lower vertebra
- Nonvertebral articulation: Between two vertebrae, in the absence of intervertebral disc

There are eleven articulations in the cervical segment, of which we will be discussing about Atlanto-occipital and atlantoaxial articulations in **Table 12.2**.

The lower cervical spine consists of disc-vertebral body, zygapophyseal, and uncovertebral articulations. Uncovertebral joints, also called as *joints of Luschka,* are formed by uncinate process of inferior vertebra articulating with echancrure or anvil of superior vertebra. Zygapophyseal joints, which are diarthrodial synovial joints, are formed by two relatively flat superior and inferior facets oriented at an angle of 45° horizontally, 85° sagittally. Also, there is increased laxity of joint capsule posteriorly in lower cervical spine.

Stabilizing Structures

Structures responsible for stability of cervical spine are:
- Ligaments
- Intervertebral disc
- Zygapophyseal joint capsule
- Structure of cervical vertebra

As facet joint capsule and cervical vertebra structure have been discussed previously, we will now be briefing about ligaments and intervertebral disc of cervical spine.

Ligaments (Fig. 12.1)

Ligaments are the anatomical restraints which play a major role in stabilizing and restricting excessive motion at the cervical spine. Most ligaments run down the length of vertebral column while few of them are exclusive to cervical spine. All the ligaments of cervical spine have been listed in **Table 12.3**.

Table 12.2: Atlanto-occipital and atlantoaxial joints.

Features	Atlanto-occipital	Atlantoaxial
Number of joints	Two joints between C0 and C1	Three- one median, two lateral between C1 and C2
Type of joint	Synovial	Synovial
Subtype	Bilateral symmetrical ellipsoid	**Median:** Pivot joint **Lateral:** Plane articulations
Articulating surfaces	Occipital condyles and Superior facets of atlas	**Median:** Atlas and odontoid process of axis **Lateral:** Inferior facet of atlas and superior facet of axis
Degrees of freedom	Flexion, extension lateral flexion	Flexion, extension rotation lateral flexion
Movements	Nodding, turning	
Structures providing stability	• Articular capsule • Anterior and posterior atlantoaxial ligament • Alar ligament • Apical ligament	• Articular capsule • Anterior and posterior atlantoaxial ligament • Transverse ligament of atlas • Alar ligament • Apical ligament • Tectorial membrane

Chapter 12 | Vertebral Column

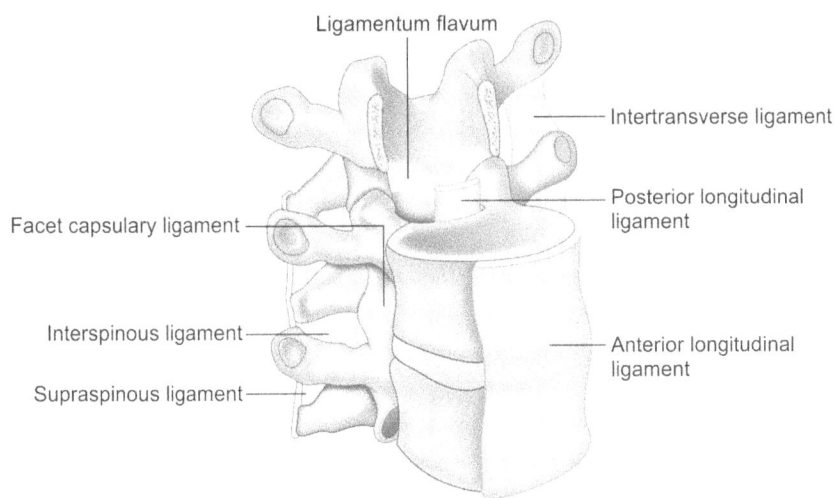

Fig. 12.1: Ligaments of cervical spine

▲ Table 12.3: Ligaments of cervical spine.

Ligaments present throughout the spine	Ligaments of cervical spine
Anterior longitudinal ligament	Anterior atlanto-axial ligament
Posterior longitudinal ligament	Tectorial membrane
Ligamentum flavum	Posterior atlanto-axial ligament
Interspinous ligament	Apical ligament
Supraspinous ligament	Alar ligament
Intertransverse ligament	Ligamentum nuchae
Zygapophyseal joint capsule	Cruciform ligament Transverse ligament

Intervertebral Discs

Vertebral bodies between C2 and C7 consist of intervertebral discs. Discs are thinnest, laterally smaller than vertebral body, thicker anteriorly than posteriorly resulting in wedge shaped disc. This assists in maintenance of cervical spine. Yet, the ratio of thickness of disc to thickness of vertebral body is greatest in this region, i.e., 2:5.

Coupled Motions

Lateral flexion and rotation occur together in cervical spine. Lateral flexion occurs along with same side rotation and rotation occurs with same side lateral flexion.

■ KINETICS (TABLE 12.4)

Due to absence of disc in upper cervical spine, axial stress is transferred to inferior facet joint of axis and adjacent disc. In lower cervical spine, forces are transmitted through three parallel columns—*Anterior column* comprising of vertebral body and discs, two *posterolateral columns* constituting zygapophyseal joints. Muscles of cervical spine are listed in **Table 12.5**.

Pathomechanics has been shown in **Table 12.6**.

THORAX AND CHEST WALL

■ INTRODUCTION

It consists of thoracic vertebrae, ribs, and sternum.
- **Functions:**
  - Protect the heart, lungs and viscera, therefore require inherent stability
  - Role in ventilation

■ GENERAL STRUCTURE AND FUNCTION

- **Rib cage:** Borders (**Fig. 12.2**)
  - Anterior border—sternum

▲ Table 12.4: Kinematics of cervical spine.

Joint	Movement	Osteokinematics			Arthrokinematics	
		Range	Axis	Plane	Direction of roll and slide	Additional features
Upper cervical spine						
Atlanto-occipital	Flexion	5	Frontal	Sagittal	Forward roll and backward slide of occipital condyles over superior facets of atlas	Concavity of articulating surfaces allows nodding motion
	Extension	10			Backward roll and forward slide of occipital condyles over superior facets of atlas	Limited by tension in joint capsule
	Rotation	Minimal	Vertical	Horizontal	-	
	Lateral flexion	5°	Sagittal	Frontal	Lateral rolling and ipsilateral sliding of occipital condyles over superior facets of atlas	
Atlantoaxial	Flexion	5°	Frontal	Sagittal	Anterior tilting of atlas over axis	55 to 58% of cervical rotation occurs here
	Extension	10°			Posterior tilting of atlas over axis	
	Rotation	40°	Vertical	Horizontal	Pivoting of dens Ipsilateral posterior sliding and contralateral anterior sliding of superior facet of axis over inferior facet of atlas	
	Lateral flexion	Minimal	Sagittal	Frontal	-	
Lower cervical spine						
	Flexion	40°	Frontal	Sagittal	• Anterior tilt and translation of superior vertebral body • Inferior facet of superior vertebra glides anteriorly and superiorly over superior facet of inferior vertebra	Flexion range increases from C2-3 to C5-6 and decreases at C6-7
	Extension	60°			• Posterior tilt and translation of superior vertebral body • Inferior facet of superior vertebra glides posteriorly and inferiorly over superior facet of inferior vertebra	
	Rotation	35° to one side, total 75°	Vertical	Horizontal	Ipsilateral posterior and inferior sliding, contralateral anterior and slightly superior sliding of inferior facet of superior vertebra over superior facet of inferior vertebra	Guided by facet orientation
	Lateral flexion	Up to 40°	Sagittal	Frontal	Ipsilateral inferior and slightly posterior sliding, Contralateral superior and slightly anterior sliding of inferior facet of superior vertebra over superior facet of inferior vertebra	

Chapter 12 | Vertebral Column

Table 12.5: Muscles of cervical spine.

Movement	Muscles involved
Flexion	• Rectus capitis • Longus cervicis • Scalene • Suprahyoid • Infrahyoid • Sternocleidomastoid
Extension	• Rectus capitis • Semispinalis cervicis • Levator scapulae • Transverse spinalis • Longissimus cervicis • Longissimus capitis • Trapezius • Spinalis cervicis • Spinalis capitis
Rotation	• Unilateral Sternocleidomastoid • Splenius cervicis • Splenius capitis • Rectus capitis
Lateral flexion	• Levator scapulae • Longus colli • Longus capitis • Iliocostalis cervicis • Rectus capitis

Table 12.6: Pathomechanics.

Sl. No	Pathology	Mechanism
1.	Whiplash injury	• Forceful injury from posterior side • On forced extension followed by forced flexion of the neck • Clinical feature: Hyperextension of C5-C6 and mild flexion at C0 to C4

2.	Facet joint syndrome	• While locking of facet joint, the synovial membrane and the disc gets entrapped between two facet bones
		• Clinical features:
		  – Pain in side flexion and rotation to same side and extension
		  – Coupling movements altered

3.	Cervical spondylosis	• Capsular restriction of the facet joints • Flattening and spurring of vertebral body • Kyphosis of lower cervical spine • Painful side restricted

4.	Fracture	• Most of the cervical fractures occur in hyperflexion:
		  – Anterior subluxation
		  – Simple wedge fracture
		  – Unstable wedge fracture
		  – Unilateral inter facet dislocation
		  – Bilateral inter facet dislocation
		  – Hangman's fracture
		  – Burst fracture

5.	Cervical myelopathy	• A neurological condition caused by stenotic encroachment of the cervical spinal cord • This stenosis occurs secondary to degeneration, causing compression of spinal cord, nerve roots, and blood vessels • Neural ischemia • Tingling and numbness at the affected side

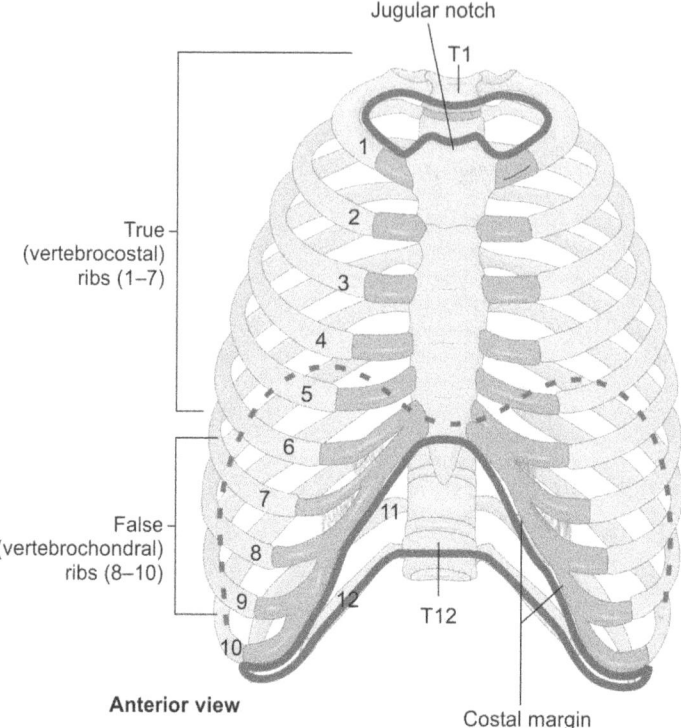

Fig. 12.2: Borders of rib cage

- Lateral border—ribs
- Posterior—thoracic vertebrae
- Superior—jugular notch of sternum, superior border of 1st costocartilage, 1st ribs, and 1st thoracic vertebrae
- Inferior—xiphoid process, 6th to 10th costocartilage, inferior portion of 11th and 12th ribs and 12th thoracic vertebrae.

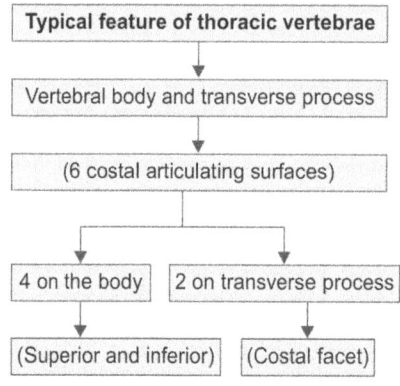

RIBS (FIG. 12.3)

- There are 12 pairs of ribs which increase in length from 1 to 7 and decrease from 8 to 12.
- Ribs 1 to 10 articulate posteriorly to transverse process of thoracic vertebrae and anteriorly have costocartilage that joins directly/indirectly to sternum.
- **Vertebrosternal or true ribs:** 1st to 7th that attach to its costocartilage thus directly attaching to sternum
- **Vertebrochondral or false ribs:** 8th to 10th rib as it indirectly articulates with costocartilages of superior ribs, indirectly articulating with sternum through 7th rib
- **Vertebral or floating ribs:** 11th and 12th rib because of no anterior attachment to sternum.

Chapter 12 | Vertebral Column

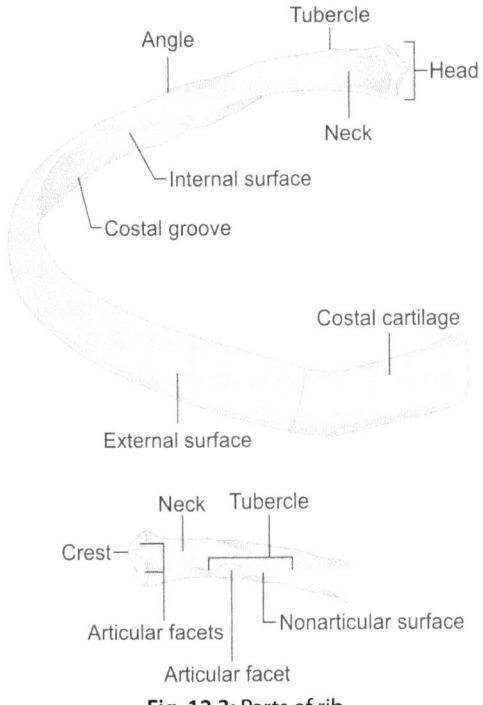

Fig. 12.3: Parts of rib

ARTICULATIONS OF THE RIB CAGE (FIG. 12.4)

It includes:
- Manubriosternal (MS)
- Xiphisternal (XS)
- Costovertebral
- Costotransverse
- Costochondral
- Chondrosternal
- Interchondral

Manubriosternal and xiphisternal joints:
- Manubriosternal joint is the articulation between manubrium and body of sternum. It forms sternal angle/angle of Louis which is about 160°.
- Xiphisternal joint is the articulation between inferior aspects of xiphoid process to the sternal body.
- Both are synchondrosis joint.

Costovertebral joint (CV) (Figs. 12.5 and 12.6):
- It is a synovial joint
- It is formed by articulation of head of rib, two adjacent vertebrae bodies, and interposed intervertebral disc.
- **Ribs:** Articulation—superior and inferior facet of head (demifacet).
- 2nd to 9th costovertebral joints—superior facet of rib articulates with inferior facet of superior vertebrae and inferior facet on superior facet of inferior vertebrae **(Fig. 12.7)**.
- Thus inferior and superior facet of vertebrae—articulate with superior and inferior on head of ribs.
- 1st, 10th, 11th and 12th—atypical ribs (most mobile) articulate with only 1 vertebral body
  - CV joint divided into two cavities by the interosseous or intra-articular ligament that extends from crest of the head

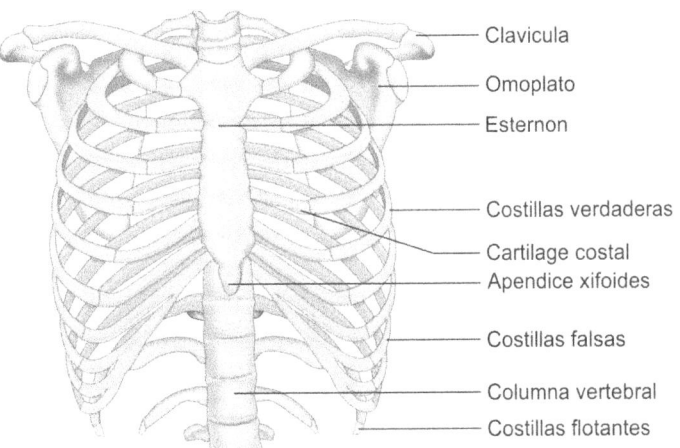

Fig. 12.4: Articulations of rib cage

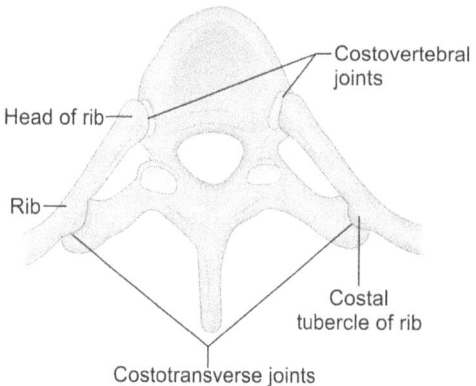

Fig. 12.5: Articulation between rib and thoracic vertebra

of rib to attach to annulus fibrosis of intervertebral disc

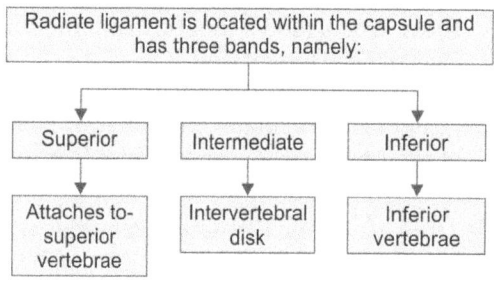

- At the costovertebral joint rotation and gliding movement occurs.
- Costotransverse joint is the articulation of costal tubercle of rib and corresponding transverse process of vertebrae.
  - *Ligaments (Fig. 12.8):*
    - Lateral costotransverse ligament
    - Costotransverse ligament
    - Superior costotransverse ligament

Costochondral and chondrosternal joints:
- Costochondral joint involves articulation of 1st through 10th rib anterolateral with the costal cartilage. It is a synchondrosis joint and has no ligament attachment.
- Chondrosternal joint is the articulation of costal cartilage of 1st to 7th anteriorly with sternum. Anterior and posterior radiate costosternal ligament are attached.
- Costoxiphoid ligament connects anterior and posterior surfaces of 7th costal cartilage to front and back of xiphoid process.

Interchondral joint: 7th through 10th costal cartilage each articulate with the cartilage immediately above them. It is a synovial joint

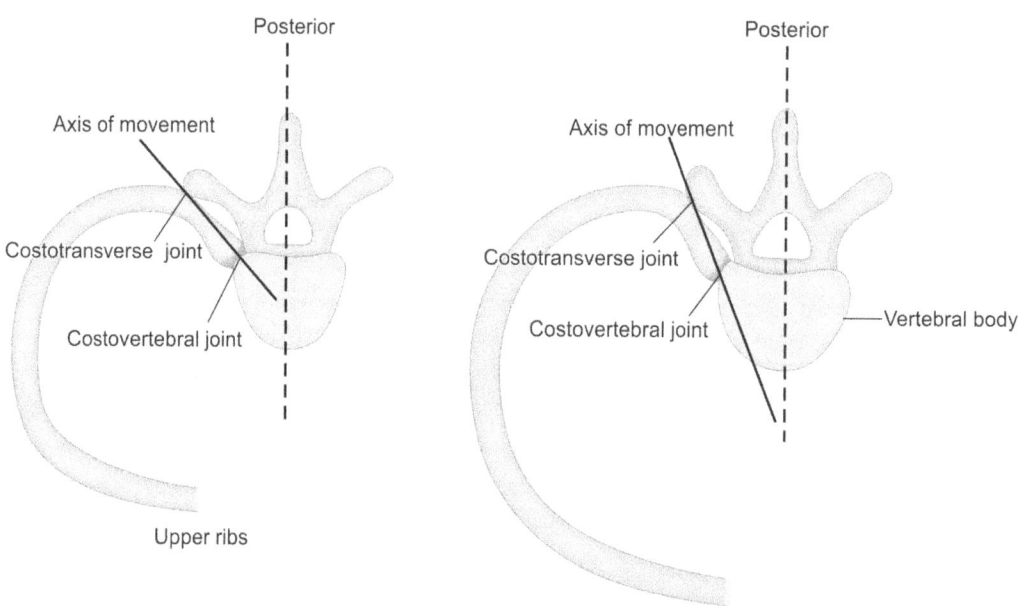

Fig. 12.6: Axis at the costovertebra joint

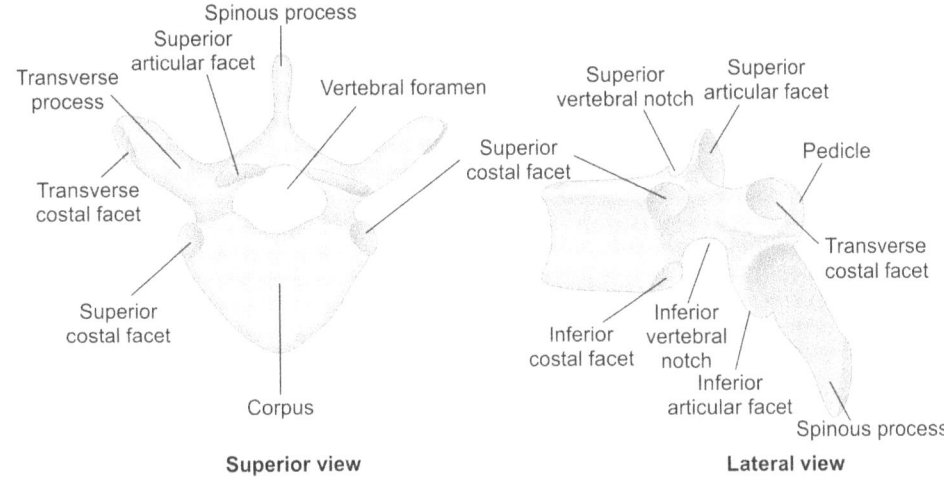

Fig. 12.7: Parts of thoracic vertebra

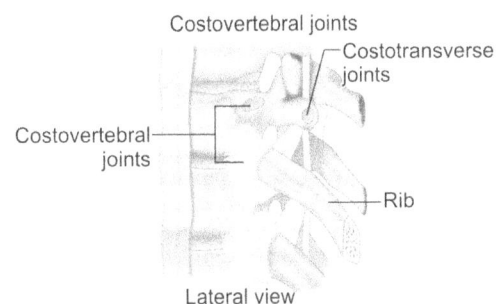

Fig. 12.8: Ligaments of rib cage

which comprises of capsule and interchondral ligaments.

KINEMATICS OF RIB CAGE AND MANUBRIOSTERNUM

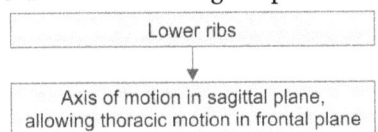

- Axis lies close to frontal plane, allowing thoracic motion in sagittal plane.

```
                 Lower ribs
                      ↓
    Axis of motion in sagittal plane,
   allowing thoracic motion in frontal plane
```

- **11th and 12th ribs:** Axis through costovertebral joint and lies close to frontal plane.

During Inspiration (Figs. 12.9A and B)

- During inspiration, upper ribs elevate and majority of the movement occurs at anterior aspect of ribs. Costocartilage becomes more horizontal and sternum is pushed ventrally and superiorly. Movement of manubrium is less while body of sternum moves more. Thus, increasing anteroposterior diameter of thorax.
- Therefore, combined rib and sternal motion that occurs in sagittal plane is termed as **"Pump-handle"** motion of thorax.
- Elevation of lower ribs occurs in sagittal plane. There is considerably more motion at the lateral aspect of the lower rib cage. Thus, increases transverse diameter of lower thorax. This is termed as **"Bucket-handle"** motion.

Note: 11th and 12th ribs do not participate in closed chain motion of thorax.

MUSCLES ASSOCIATED WITH RIB CAGE

Properties:
- Increased fatigue resistance and greater oxidative capacity
- Muscles contract rhythmically throughout life
- Work against elastic properties of lungs and airway resistance.

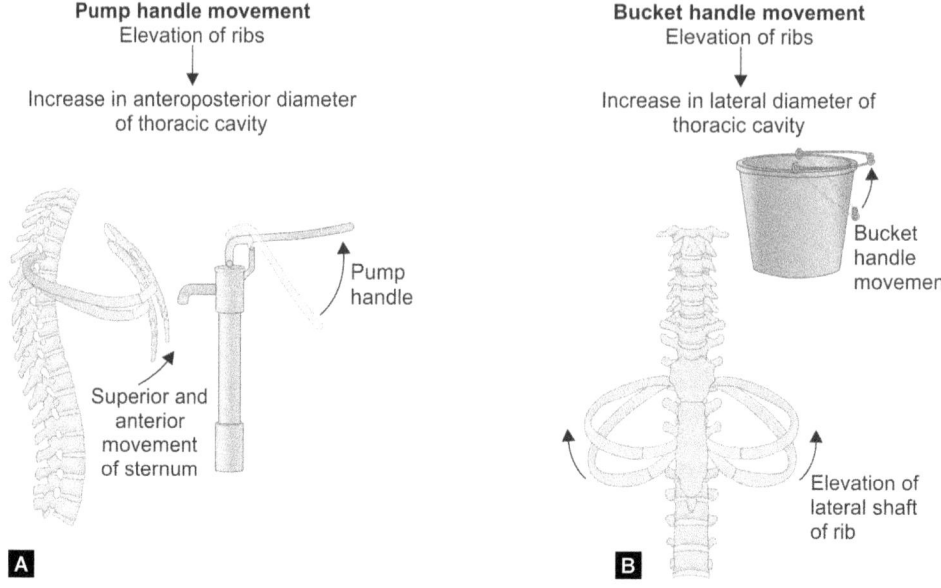

Figs. 12.9A and B: Respiratory movements: Movements of ribs

- Neurologic control—voluntary and involuntary
- Action of muscle are life sustaining.

Recruitment of muscles:
- In quiet breathing (at rest)—primary inspiratory muscles are needed for ventilation.
- Active or forced breathing (increased activity or with pulmonary pathologies)—accessory muscles of both inspiration and expiration.

Primary Muscles of Ventilation

For quiet ventilation. It includes:
- Diaphragm
- Intercostal muscles (parasternal muscles)—inspiration
- **Scalene muscles:** No primary muscles for expiration as expiration at rest is passive.

1. *Diaphragm*: Primary muscle of ventilation
   - Approx. 70-80% of inspiration force during quiet breathing.
   - Arises from sternum, costocartilage, ribs, and vertebral bodies.
   - Fibers travel superiorly to insert into central tendon.
   - Lateral leaflets form the right and left hemidiaphragm.
   - Muscular portion of diaphragm arises from sternum, costocartilage, and ribs.
   - Crural portion from vertebral bodies.
   - Costal portion of diaphragm attaches by muscular slips to the posterior aspect of xiphoid process and inner surface of lower six ribs and their costal cartilage.
   - The vertical fibers, lie close to the inner wall of lower rib cage termed as **Zone of apposition.**

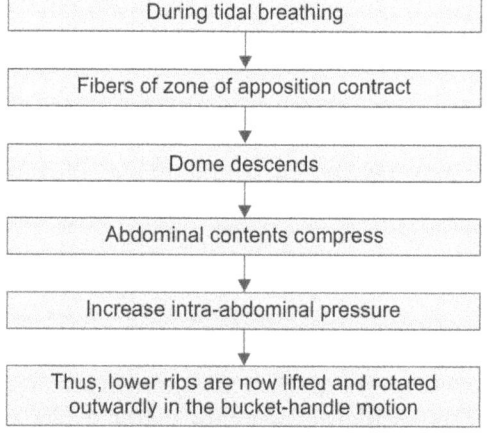

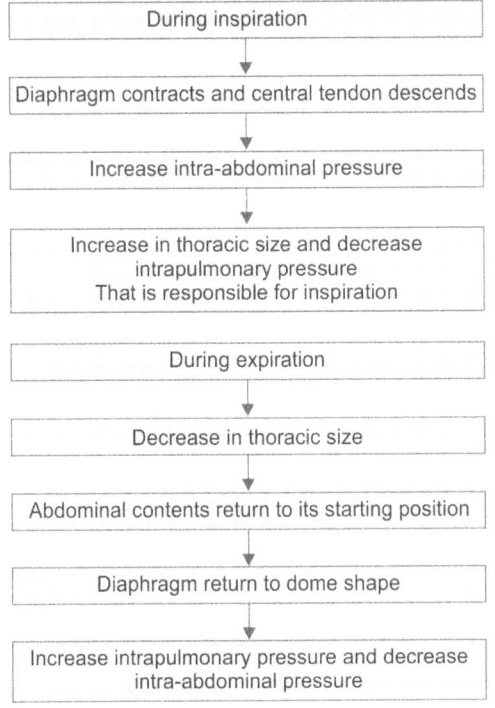

2. *Intercostal muscles*
   External and internal
   ↓   ↓
   During inspiration expiration
   Parasternal muscles
   ↓
   Primary inspiratory muscle during quiet breathing
   - **Action:** Elevation of rib and anterior movement of sternum
   - **Stabilization of ribs:** Opposes the decrease intrapulmonary pressure generated during diaphragm contraction preventing paradoxical or inward movement of upper chest wall during inspiration.
3. *Scalene muscles:* Primary muscle of quiet ventilation. The scalene muscles attach on the transverse processes of C3 to C7 and descend to the upper borders of the first rib (scalenus anterior and scalenus medius) and second rib (scalenus posterior)
   - **Action:** Lifts sternum and 1st two ribs in the pump handle motion of upper rib cage.

- Along with parasternal muscles counteract the paradoxical movement of upper chest caused by the decrease in intrapulmonary pressure created by diaphragm contraction.

Accessory Muscles of Ventilation

- Muscles that attach the rib cage to the shoulder girdle, head, vertebral column, or pelvis.
- Assist in inspiration or expiration, in situation of stress, such as increased activity or disease.

1. *Sternocleidomastoid muscle*
   - **Origin:** Manubrium and superior medial aspect of clavicle
   - **Insertion:** Mastoid process of temporal bone
   - **Action:** Bilateral neck flexion
   - With help of trapezius muscle stabilizing head, sternocleidomastoid muscle moves rib cage superiorly, which expands the upper rib cage in pump-handle motion.
   - Occurs at end of maximal inspiration.
2. *Pectoralis minor:* Help elevate the 3rd, 4th and 5th ribs during a forced inspiration
3. *Subclavius:* A muscle between the clavicle and the first rib, can also assist in raising the upper chest for inspiration
4. *Pectoralis major:* It elevates upper rib cage it has a humeral and clavicular head when the arm is positioned beside the truck, humeral attachment of pectoralis major is below the level of the clavicle. The clavicular portion acts as an expiratory muscle, by pulling the manubrium and upper ribs down with the humeral attachment of pectoralis major above the level of the clavicle, such as when the arm is raised, the muscle becomes an inspiratory muscle, pulling the manubrium and upper ribs up and out
5. *Levator costarum:* Elevation of the upper ribs
6. *Abdominal muscles* (Transverse abdominis, internal and external oblique abdominis and rectus abdominis)

- Are expiratory muscles (forced exhalation)
- Assist in both inhalation and exhalation

- **Inhalation by:**
  - Increased intra-abdominal pressure
  - Pushes diaphragm cranially and exerts passive stretch on costal fibers of the diaphragm.
  - Increase intra-abdominal pressure created by lowering of diaphragm in inspiration must be countered by tension in abdominal muscles.

DEVELOPMENTAL ASPECTS OF STRUCTURE AND FUNCTION

Difference Associated with the Neonate

- Newborn has a cartilaginous and thus extremely compliant.
- Infant chest wall muscles act as stabilizers rather than mobilizers.
- Complete ossification of ribs occurs after several months.
- Ribs in adults slope downward and diaphragm is elliptically shaped. Infant shows a more horizontal alignment of ribs.
- Very little motion of ribs cage during tidal breathing of an infant.
- Only 20% of muscle fibers of diaphragm are fatigue-resisted fibers in healthy newborn, compared with 50% in adult.
- Accessory muscles of ventilation are at a disadvantage until infant can stabilize upper extremities, head, and spine.

Difference Associated with the Elderly

- Articulations of chest undergo fibrosis.
- Interchondral and costochondral joints fibrous and chondrosternal joints obliterated.
- Reduced mobility in chest wall articulations.
- Costal cartilages ossify.
- Reduction in diaphragm abdomen compliance.
- Airways narrow, alveolar duct diameter increase, shallow alveolar sac
- Decrease in elastic recoil and increase pulmonary compliance
- Decrease of elastic fibers
- Increase in functional residual capacity
- Decrease in inspiratory capacity
- Skeletal muscles of ventilation—loss of strength, fewer muscle fibers, a lower oxidative capacity, a decrease in number of size of fast twitch type two fibers and a lengthening time to peak tension.
- Diaphragm less domed, with decrease in abdomen tone in aging
- Early recruitment pattern for accessory muscles.

LUMBAR SEGMENT

TYPES OF VERTEBRA AND ITS STRUCTURE

The lumbar segment is the truncal part between the thorax and sacrum consisting of 5 lumbar vertebrae. It is numbered from above to below with L1 communicating with T12 and L5 communicating with S1 (**Fig. 12.10**). The lumbarvertebrae are much stronger than any other vertebrae as it has to take the load of the whole of the trunk and balance it including the weight of the head and upper extremities (**Figs. 12.11A to C**).

The vertebra parts broadly are:
- Vertebral body
- Neural arch

Neural arch (broadly) consists of:
- Pedicle
- Lamina
- Superior articular pillar
- Inferior articular pillar
- Spinous process
- Transverse process

Single vertebral segment consists of 2 vertebrae and 1 intervertebral (IV) disc in-between.

Intervertebral Disc

The intervertebral disc is a fibroelastic structure present between the two vertebral bodies. The intervertebral disc has three parts:
1. Annulus fibrosis
2. Nucleus pulposis
3. Vertebral end plate

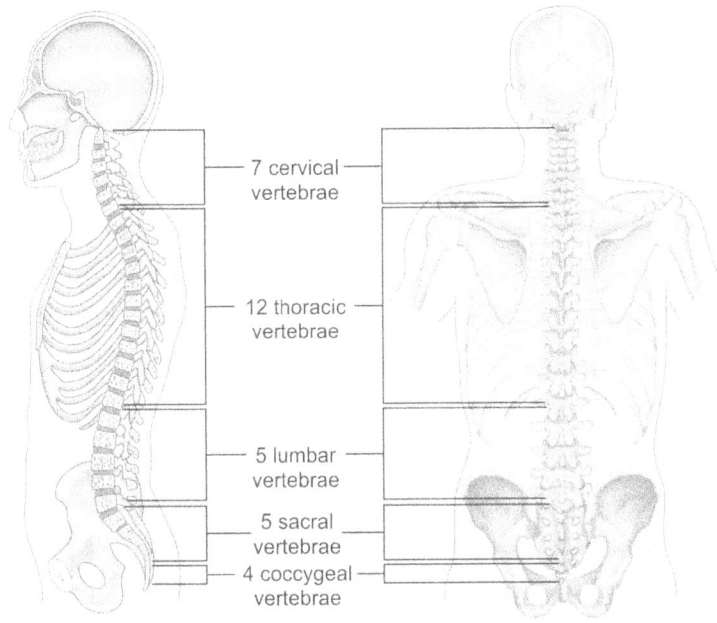

Fig. 12.10: Five distinct regions of the vertebral column

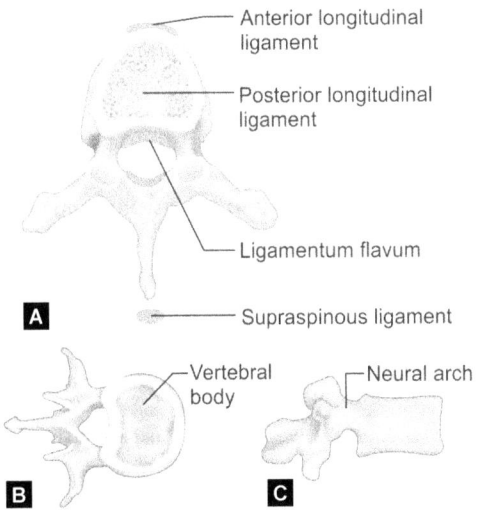

Figs. 12.11A to C: (A) Structure of typical lumbar vertebra; (B) Lumbar vertebrae Axial (overhead) view; (C) Lateral view

Functions of intervertebral disc:
- Shock absorbing mechanism
- Distribute the weight load
- Provide movement between the segments
- Provide nutrition to the vertebra
- It guides the direction of motion.

- It helps in the formation of primary and secondary curves.
- It gives up to 20% of the height of the spinal segment.

Because of the intervertebral discs property of water retention and drainage, there is variation of a person's height in a day. The disc is similar to a sponge which absorbs the water and swells and on loadings the water drains out. Thus in the morning a person is taller by 1 cm to 1.5 cm as the spine is resting throughout the night and the disc absorbs the water and swells. Though if each disc is seen separately the quantity is less (about 0.7 mm water retention) adding up the 23 discs in the spine brings about 1-1.5 cm. As the day goes the loading happens and at the end of the day the person is less short. This system is very important as this is how the nutrients are transported into the discs. This osmotic system loses its efficiency as the person ages.

- **Nucleus pulposus (Fig. 12.12):** It is a gelatinous structure present in the center of annulus fibrosus. It contains 70-90% of water, 65% of glycosaminoglycans, and 15-20% of collagen fibers.

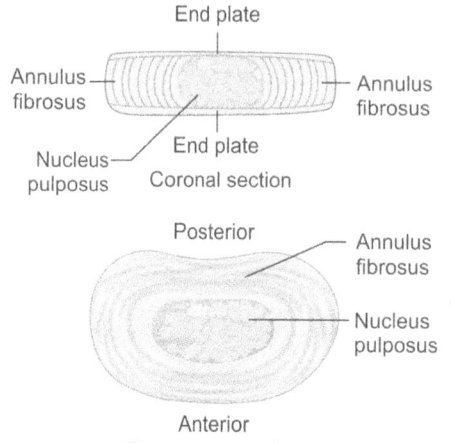

Fig. 12.12: A schematic representation of a lumbar intervertebral disc showing the nucleus pulposus, the annulus fibrosus, and the vertebral end plate

- **Annulus fibrosis (Fig. 12.12):** It is a layered fibrous structure surrounding the nucleus pulposus. It is tougher than nucleus pulposis and has up to 15–25 concentric layers. Its main function is to hold the water content in the nucleus pulposus. The design of the fibers is annular in nature.
- **Vertebral end plates (Fig. 12.12):** These are thin cartilaginous layers above and below the discs. This vertebral end plate communicates the vertebral body to the disc.
- **Hydrodynamics in the intervertebral discs:** 80% of the overall load is taken by the intervertebral discs and 20% is by the facet joints thus the disc plays a predominant role in dissipating the pressure.

The intervertebral disc dynamics can be discussed under the following points:
- **Hydrostatic pressure:** The pressure exerted in the disc (nucleus pulposus).
- **Hoop stress:** The exerted pressure getting transmitted into circumferential pressure causing the disc to stretch outward thus reducing the vertical load on the lower vertebra.
- **Pascal's law:** It states that when pressure exerted onto the water, the force distribution is of equal magnitude, at all the points in the water.
- **Radial expansion:** Because of the Pascal's law and the hoop stress, there is an equal distribution on the disc radially resulting in the radial expansion of the disc.
  - **Compression:** Consider nucleus pulposus as a round ball in the middle of the annulus fibrosus. Under compressive loading, the hydrostatic pressure is exerted in all directions as nucleus pulposus tries to expand. Tension in the anulus fibrosus rises as a result of nuclear pressure. A force equal in magnitude but opposite in direction is exerted by anulus fibrosus on the nucleus pulposus, which limits radial expansion of nucleus pulposus and establishes equilibrium. The nuclear pressure is transmitted by anulus fibrosus to the end plates. This works under fluid dynamic mechanism (or hydrodynamic mechanism).
  - **Bending:** The behavior of IV disc during bending motions occurs with the activities of daily life. Nucleus pulposus deforms in the direction opposite to the motion during sagittal or frontal plane motions, so that during lumbar extension, the nucleus pulposus displaces anteriorly and vice versa. Hence, nucleus pulposus functions as a ball bearing during spinal motions.
  - **Rotation:** The oblique arrangement of fibers present in the annulus fibrosis helps the disc to withstand torsional forces while eliciting trunk rotation.

THE JOINTS IN THE LUMBAR SEGMENT

In each lumbar segment, there are two zygapophyseal joints and one interbody joint. Thus both the joints kinematics and kinetics will be discussed simultaneously.
- **Zygapophyseal joint/facet joints:** It is also called as facet joints. These are plain synovial joints. The joints have a synovial capsule.
- **Interbody joint:** The interbody joint is a symphysis joint of amphiarthrosis variety.

Articulating structures:
- **Facet joints:** Superior articulating surface of the below vertebra articulates with the inferior articulating surface of the vertebra above.
- **Interbody:** The superior surface of the lower vertebral body and the inferior surface of the upper vertebral body join together with the help of intervertebral disc.

Degrees of freedom: 3

STABILITY OF THE LUMBAR SPINE
- **Intervertebral disc:**
  - As a rubber ferrule
    - Hydrodynamic mechanism
- **Ligaments:**
  - Anterior longitudinal ligament
  - Posterior longitudinal ligament
  - Ligamentum flavum
  - Interspinous ligament
  - Supraspinous ligament
  - Intertransverse ligament
  - Iliolumbar ligament
- Capsule of the facet joint
- Orientation of the facet joint
- Three points segment
- Thoracolumbar fascia
- Vertebral curvature

Intervertebral Disc as Stabilizer

It acts as a rubber ferrule as seen with the rubber tip at the end of tables and chairs. It is not a great stabilizer but gives a good grip from vertebra to the vertebra. Another way the disc helps in stability is by the hydrodynamic mechanism. As discussed earlier because of the disc sharing the load (radial expansion mechanism), the load sharing helps in the stability of the spine.
- **Capsule of the facet joint:** The capsule and the meniscoids hold the facet joints in place and check the micro movements.
- **Orientation of the facet joint:** The facets are oriented medially and posteriorly (lower articular pillar) lying between the sagittal and frontal plane. This arrangement may allow flexion and extension but it allows very little rotation, thus helping in maintaining stability.
- **Three-point segment:** The vertebra to vertebra contact is on three-point distribution. Around 80% the weight is borne by the vertebral body point and 20% weight is taken by the facet point. Take the example of a two-wheeler and autorickshaw. The two-wheeler is always unstable and requires another point in the form of stand to be stable. Compare to it the autorickshaw, it is more stable, and obviously the car is the most stable with four-point contact.
- **Vertebral curvature:** The curvature itself acts like a spring mechanism, assume if the vertebrae is placed one above other vertically, there would be no spring-like mechanism.

Ligaments (Fig. 12.13)

Anterior Longitudinal Ligament
- The anterior longitudinal ligament is a long band extending from C2 up to the sacrum. Above C2 it continues as anterior atlanto-occipital ligament (C0-C1 joint) and anterior atlanto-axial ligament (C1-C2 joint). It is twice the stronger to that of posterior longitudinal ligament.
- It is attached to the anterior aspect of vertebral body and anterior aspect of intervertebral disc extending all along from C2 to the sacrum.
- The ligament is band like almost covering the entire anterior side of the spine.
- **There are two types of fibers:** Superficial and deep. The superficial fibers run parallel and the deeper fibers run horizontally and attach to the anterior side of the intervertebral disc. This ligament becomes taut in extension and slack in flexion.
- This ligament helps in limiting lordosis.
- This ligament increases in thickness and width from thoracic to lumbar vertebrae.

Functions of anterior longitudinal ligament:
- It resists excessive extension.
- It resists extension torque at the lumbosacral junction.

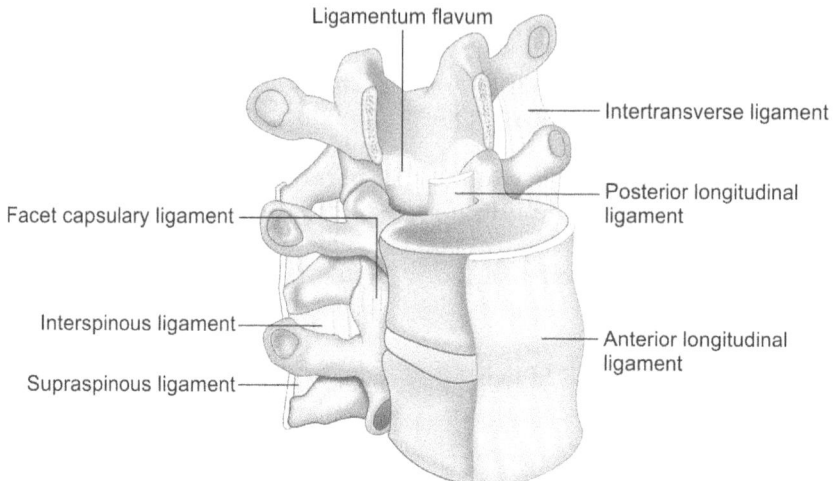

Fig. 12.13: Ligaments surrounding the lumbar vertebrae

- It resists excessive lordosis.
- It prevents (along with facet joint) anterior translation of vertebrae.
- It prevents (along with posterior long ligament) collapse of the stack of the vertebrae.
- In quadruped position, it holds up the vertebral column.
- It prevents anterior disc prolapse.

Posterior Longitudinal Ligament
- The posterior longitudinal ligament is a long band extending from C2 up to the sacrum. Above C2 it continues as tectorial membrane. It is half the strength of anterior longitudinal ligament.
- It is attached to the posterior aspect of vertebral body and posterior aspect of intervertebral disc extending all along from C2 to the sacrum.
- **There are two types of fibers:** Superficial and deep. The superficial fibers run parallel and the deeper fibers run horizontally and attach to the posterior side of the intervertebral disc. This ligament becomes taut in flexion and slack in extension.
- This ligament helps in limiting kyphosis.
- The ligament is band like but in the lumbar region the ligament narrows to a thin ribbon thus causing commonly posterolateral disc prolapse.

Functions of posterior longitudinal ligament:
- It resists excessive flexion.
- It resists excessive kyphosis.
- It holds up the vertebral column in standing.
- It prevents (along with facet joint) posterior translation of vertebrae.
- It prevents (along with anterior long ligament) collapse of the stack of the vertebrae.
- It resists posterior disc prolapse.

Ligamentum Flavum
- The word flavum means yellow. It is called so because the fibers are predominantly made up of elastin fibers which are yellow in color.
- 80% elastin and 20% collagen fibers. It is also known as yellow ligament.
- Ligamentum flavum attaches from lamina to lamina. To be specific it is attached from upper border of lamina of lower vertebra to the lower border of the lamina of the upper vertebra. This series of paired ligaments extends throughout the vertebral column present immediately posterior to the spinal cord extending from C2 to sacrum.
- The ligamentum flavum along with the lamina forms the posterior wall of the vertebral canal.
- The ligamentum flavum is a thick elastic ligament.

- Above C2 it continues as posterior atlanto-occipital ligament (C0-C1 joint) and posterior atlanto-axial ligament (C1-C2 joint).
- This is the only ligament in the human body to have a predominant contractile element.
- It is essential to have the contractile elements in this ligament otherwise the ligament would buckle during extension.
- The ligament is stretched in flexion position.
- Even in neutral position it is in tension because of the elastic property of the ligament. Thus, it continuously creates compressive forces on the disc and the ligament provides overall stability.

Functions of ligamentum flavum:
- Control flexion
- Assist extension (since it has contractile property)
- Spine stabilization even in neutral position
- Constant compressive force on the disc
- Dynamic stabilizer during the movements
- Prevent buckling onto itself during extension due to elastic property
- Prevent the capsule, menisci and other soft tissue going into the facet joint. The ligament is attached to the capsule which pulls back during extension.
- Maintain passive extension force

Interspinous Ligament
- The interspinous ligament connects from the shaft of spinous process above to the shaft of spinous process below.
- It prevents excessive flexion and becomes slack in extension.
- This is one of the first ligaments to get injured while sustaining flexion injuries and can be a source of low back pain.

Functions of interspinous ligament:
- It resists excessive flexion.
- Maintains extension
- Prevents separation of spinous process of two adjacent vertebrae

Supraspinous Ligament
- It is a cord-like ligament attaching from the tip of spinous process above to the tip of spinous process below.
- The ligament resists separation of the adjacent spinous process. This ligament becomes stretched during flexion and slack during extension.
- This is the first ligament to get injured during flexion injuries.
- This ligament is not very distinct in the lumbar region.
- In the cervical region, this ligament continues as ligamentum nuchae.

Functions of supraspinous ligament:
- It prevents flexion.
- Maintains extension
- Prevents separation of spinous process of two adjacent vertebrae
- It has mechanoreceptors thus can play a role in the recruitment of spinal stabilizers such as multifidus muscle.

Intertransverse Ligament
- The intertransverse ligament is attached from the transverse process above to the transverse process below.
- It is situated on both the sides.
- Not so well developed in the lumbar segment
- In side flexion, the ipsilateral ligament becomes slack and contralateral ligament becomes stretched.
- This ligament forms the part of thoraco-lumbar fascia.

Iliolumbar Ligament
- The iliolumbar ligament is a series of bands that run from the transverse process of L5 to the ilium.
- It acts to resist the movements at the lumbosacral joint.

KINEMATICS

Osteokinematics
The possible movements in the lumbar spine are:
- Flexion
- Extension

- Lateral flexion
- Rotation (minimal)

Planes and axis
- Flexion and extension occur in sagittal plane around frontal axis.
- Lateral flexion occurs in frontal plane around antero-posterior axis.
- Rotation occurs in transverse plane around vertical axis.

Range of motion
- On an average the lumbar spine is around 45° lordotic

Movement	Range of motion
Flexion (**Fig. 12.14**)	40–50°
Extension	15°
Lateral flexion	20°
Rotation	5°

The range of motion of each segment varies and generally, there is maximum flexion at L5-S1 and as we go up ROM reduces. About 13° happens in L5-S1, 11° happens at L4-L5 and keeps reducing as you go up. Overall flexion is 50°.

It is the opposite during side flexion. Maximum movement happens at the higher level and as we go down the ROM reduces. It is the stiffest at the L5-S1.

Factors resisting flexion
- Posterior longitudinal ligament, ligamentum flavum, supraspinous ligament, and interspinous ligament
- Thoracolumbar fascia
- Posterior spinal muscles

Factors resisting extension
- Facet joints
- Anterior longitudinal ligament
- Abdominal muscles

Factors resisting side flexion
- Quadratus lumborum
- Thoracolumbar fascia
- Intertransverse ligament

Factors resisting rotation
- Facet joint

Coupling

- In lumbar spine a movement in one plane is often associated with an automatic movement in another plane this is called as spinal coupling. That is for example the side flexion in neutral position is often associated with rotation in opposite direction. Thus, rotation and side flexion occur simultaneously (**Fig. 12.15**).
- **The common coupling patterns are:**
  - In flexion position—side flexion is often associated with same side rotation.
  - In extension position—side flexion is often associated with opposite side rotation.
  - This particular coupling patterns is because of the orientation of facet joints.

In a broader perspective any 2 movements happening together is called as combined

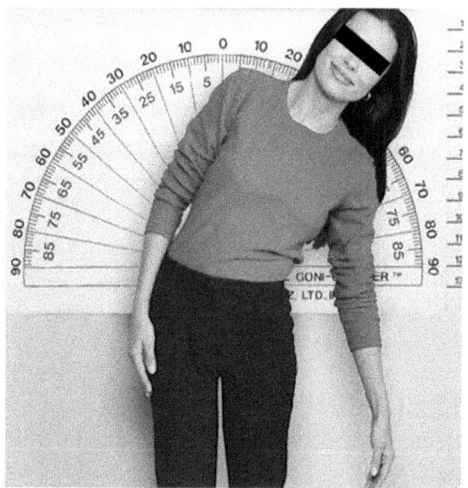

Fig. 12.14: Trunk lateral flexion

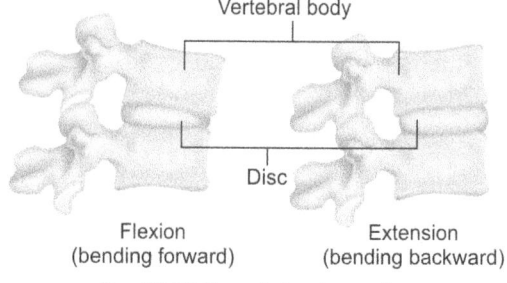

Fig. 12.15: Facet joints in motion

Chapter 12 | Vertebral Column

movements. Combined movements further divided into:
- Coupling movements
- Noncoupling combined movements

As discussed coupling movements are 2 movements happening together naturally due to the joint mechanics. For example, knee extension with lateral rotation of tibia is 2 natural movements which happen automatically.

Noncoupling combined movements are the 2 movements happening together in which one movement is induced by an external force or therapist. For example, knee extension along with induced tibial medial rotation by a therapist.

ARTHROKINEMATICS (TABLE 12.7)

Flexion

Facet joints:
- There is opening up of the facet joint.
- In facet joints the superior facets anteriorly tilting and glides superiorly

Interbody joint:
- There is anterior compression of the disc and posterior stretch.
- The posterior longitudinal ligament holds the excessive flexion.

Extension

Facet joints:
- There is closing up of the facet joint.
- In facet joints the superior facets posteriorly tilting and glides inferiorly

Interbody joint: There is posterior compression of the disc and anterior stretch.

Lateral Flexion

Facet joints:
- There is closing of ipsilateral facet and opening up of contralateral facet.

◢ **Table 12.7:** Arthrokinematic movement.

Osteokinematic movement	Zygapophyseal joint	Interbody joint	Ligaments
Flexion	Lower facet of upper vertebra glides **anterosuperiorly** and away from the upper facet of the lower vertebra	• Posterior side disc stretches • Anterior side disc shortens • Nucleus pulposus tends to move **anteriorly**	• Stretching of posterior longitudinal ligament, ligamentum flavum, interspinous and supraspinous ligament • Shortening of anterior longitudinal ligament
Extension	Lower facet of upper vertebra glides **posteroinferiorly** and toward the upper facet of the lower vertebra	• Anterior side disc stretches • Posterior side disc shortens • Nucleus pulposus tends to move **posteriorly**.	• Shortening of posterior longitudinal ligament, ligamentum flavum, interspinous and supraspinous ligament • Stretching of anterior longitudinal ligament
Lateral flexion	• Ipsilateral facet moves **downward** • Contralateral facet moves **upward**	• Contralateral side disc stretches • Ipsilateral side disc shortens • Nucleus pulposus tends to move **contralaterally**	• Stretching of contralateral intertransverse ligament • Shortening of ipsilateral intertransverse ligament
Rotation	• Contralateral facet moves **forward** toward the lower facet of upper vertebra • Ipsilateral facet moves **backward** away from the lower facet of upper vertebra	• Rotational • Torque	—

- Ipsilateral facet glides inferiorly and contralateral facet glides superiorly.

Interbody joint: There is compression of the disc ipsilaterally and contralateral side stretch.

Rotation

Facet joints:
- There is coupling movement happening, rotation is associated with side bending.
- Pure rotation is very minimal.
- Theoretically there is compression of ipsilateral side and opening up of contralateral side.

Interbody joint: The disc undergoes torsional force and the annulus fibrosis resists it.

KINETICS (FIG. 12.16)

Forces at the lumbar spine are:
- Axial compression
- Bending
- Shear
- Torsion

The forces are due to:
- Gravity
- Ground reaction
- Muscle generated
- Forces due to the structure and soft tissue

The compression force is generated by the gravity due to the body weight. 80% of the force is borne by the IV discs and 20% is borne by the facet joints. Not just gravity, fascia, ligaments, and muscles also induce axial compression passively. Best example being the ligamentum flavum. Shear force is due to the lordotic nature of the spine which makes upper spine shear away from the lower spine. But this is protected by the facet joints. Torsional force in the lumbar is very minimal and the spine is protected by facet joints. Bending forces are mainly guided and controlled by the lumbar musculature. The bending happens in four direction, flexion, extension, and lateral rotation on both sides.

Lumbar flexors:
- **Abdominal muscles:** Rectus abdominus, internal oblique, external oblique, transverse abdominus
- **Iliospoas**

Lumbar extensors:
- **Erector spinae:**
  - Iliocostalis
  - Longissimus
- **Multifidus**

Lumbar lateral flexors: Quadratus lumborum

Rotators:
- Rotatores
- Multifidus

Dynamic Stabilizers
- Multifidus
- Rotatores
- Interspinalis
- Intertransversarious
- Ligamentum flavum

LUMBOPELVIC RHYTHM

Lumbopelvic rhythm is the coordinated movement between the hip joint and the

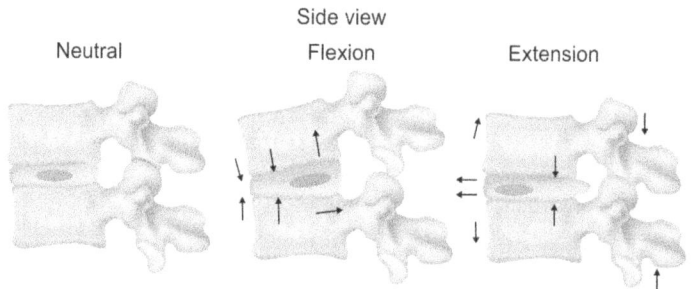

Fig. 12.16: Forces exerted on the disc during trunk flexion and extension

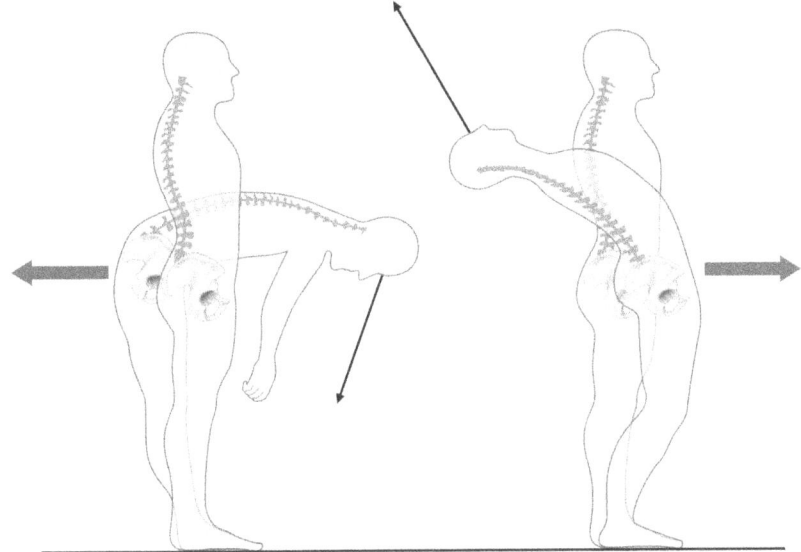

Fig. 12.17: Lumbopelvic rhythm

lumbar spine to bring about a larger range of motion. For example, bending down to touch the feet **(Fig. 12.17)**.

Take an example; the person is standing and he has to touch the ground with knee straight. The possible ROM of a lumbar segment is only 50. The ROM of the hip joint with knee straight is about 80. The ROM of thorax is 45. Thus working in isolation it is not possible to touch the ground. The required ROM to touch the ground is 180. Thus the joints have to share the ROM to complete the task.

Sequence of the Lumbopelvic Rhythm

Flexion: Open book phenomenon
- Flexion of lumbar, simultaneous posterior shift of pelvis
- Counternutation of sacrum, simultaneous open book of pelvis
- Anterior pelvic tilt
- Hip flexion
- End position

Extension: Closed book phenomenon
- Hip extension
- Posterior pelvic tilt
- Nutation of sacrum, simultaneous close book of pelvis
- Extension of lumbar, simultaneous anterior shift of pelvis
- Back to neutral position

Why the sequence is necessary?
As you see in the sequence the lumbar motion occurs only at the initial ranges. At the end ranges, the movement is taken over by the hip. This protects the spine from injury in the long run.

Note: Close book is nothing but the tendency of both ASIS to come toward each other like closing a book. Open book is the tendency of the ASIS to go away from each other like opening a book.

Any disruption in this sequence or failure of the segments fulfills their ROM results in altered lumbopelvic rhythm. Common causes of altered lumbopelvic rhythm are:
- Stiff lumbar segment
- Excessive lumbar flexion
- Stiff hip joint
- Excessive hip flexion
- Muscular imbalance

Advantages
- Achieve larger ROM
- Stable and less compromised joints

Consequences if lumbopelvic rhythm is absent:
- Less ROM
- Stress on the joints
- Injury

THORACOLUMBAR FASCIA (FIGS. 12.18A AND B)

- Most superficial structure associated with several major muscle groups.
- It is a diamond-shaped structure presents posteriorly at the thoracolumbar area.

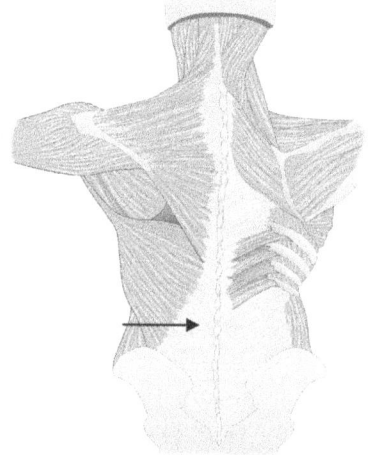

Fig. 12.18A: Thoracolumbar fascia (arrow)

- Tension on TL fascia will produce a force that exerts compression of the abdominal contents—external corset.
- Thoracolumbar fascia is a biological corset present in the lumbar region for the mechanical stability of the lower back and sacroiliac joint.
- The attachments are spinous process of thoracic, lumbar and sacrum at the midline, lower borders to the gluteus maximus, sacrum, iliac crest, upper side to the latissimus dorsi, and it goes anteriorly to attach with the anterior abdominal muscles.
- **It is organized into:**
  - The anterior layer is located anterior to the quadratus lumborum muscle and
  - Middle layer is located posterior to quadratus lumborum muscle. It starts from the transverse process. Both anterior and middle layers are anchored at the transverse process and inferiorly to the iliac crest.
  - The posterior layer of the thoracolumbar fascia starts at the spinous process covers the posterior surface of the erector spinae.

  All the three layers move laterally joins together and go on anteriorly to blend with the anterior abdominal muscles.

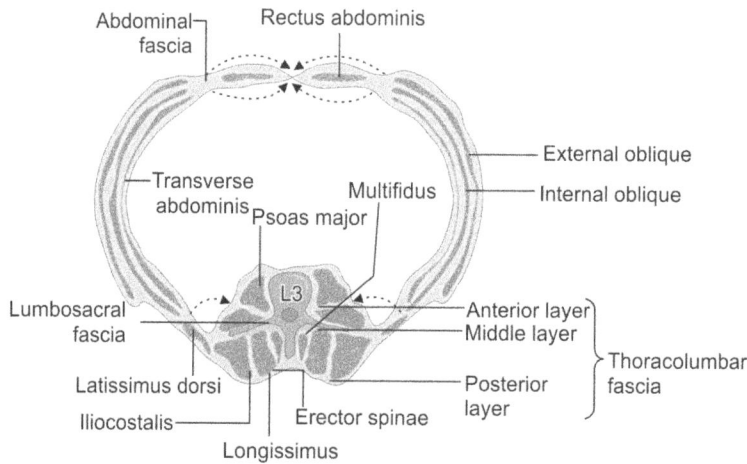

Fig. 12.18B: Thoracolumbar fascia

- It provides mechanical stability to the sacroiliac joint. Stability is enhanced by attachment of gluteus maximus and latissimus dorsi.
- The posterior and middle layers fuse at their lateral margins forming a lateral raphe. This blends with the fascia of the transverse abdominis and internal oblique.

Functions of the thoracolumbar fascia:
- Support the back in its position
- Support the back during motion, as it is connected to the anterior abdominal muscles. The more the spine flexion happens the more the fascia tightens the spine.
- It connects opposite side latissimus dorsi to the gluteus maximus. This forms the oblique chain to perform sporting activities, e.g., bowling.

LUMBOSACRAL JOINT

It is just a part of the lumbar spine L5 articulating with the S1 which is referred to as the lumbosacral joint.

Types
- Symphysis joint at interbody
- Synovial joint at the facets

Articulating structures:
- **Facet joints:** Inferior articulating surface of L5 articulates with superior articulating surface of S1
- **Interbody:** The superior surface of the lower vertebral body and the inferior surface of the upper vertebral body join together with the help of intervertebral disc.

Degrees of freedom: 3

Stability
- **Iliolumbar ligament:** Iliolumbar ligament attaches from the transverse process of L5 to the iliac crest on both the sides. It stabilizes lateral flexion and flexion.
- **Lumbosacral ligament:**
  - Dorsal
  - Ventral

Kinematics

Osteokinematics

Movement	Range of motion
Flexion	12–13°
Extension	3–4°
Lateral flexion	Negligible
Rotation	0°

Lumbosacral Angle (Fig. 12.19)
- The angle formed between the horizontal lines to the lower border of the L5 vertebral.
- Lumbosacral angle is formed by the fifth lumbar vertebra and first sacral segment. It is also called as Ferguson's angle. Lumbosacral angle can be defined as the first sacral segment, which is inclined slightly anteriorly and inferiorly forms an angle with the horizontal.
- **Normal angle is 30°**
  - Excessive angle may be predisposing to cause spondylolisthesis.
  - Fewer angles may be a predisposing factor causing disc prolapse.

PATHOMECHANICS
- Intervertebral disc prolapse
- Spinal canal stenosis
- Lumbar spondylosis/facet joint syndrome
- Lumbar radiculopathy
- Lumbar spondylolisthesis

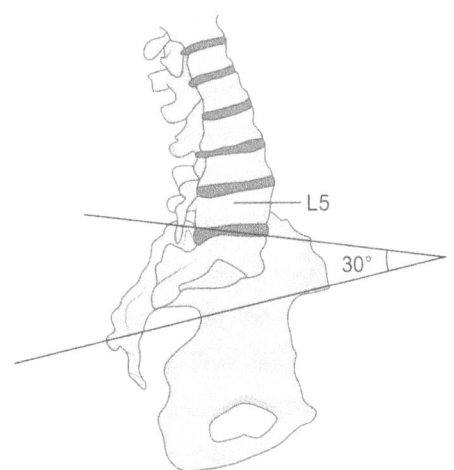

Fig. 12.19: Lumbosacral angle

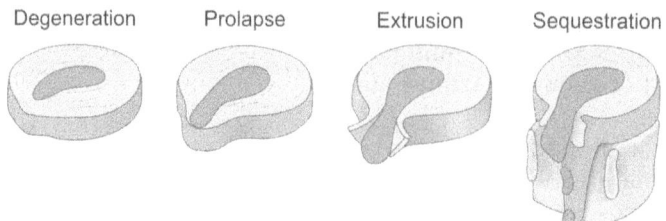

Fig. 12.20: Four stages to a disc herniation

Intervertebral Disc Prolapse

The stages of disc prolapsed are (**Fig. 12.20**):
- **Disc bulging:** Extension of the disc margin beyond the margins of the adjacent vertebral end plates.
- **Disc protrusion:** The posterior longitudinal ligament remains intact but the nucleus pulposus impinges on the annulus fibrosus.
- **Disc extrusion:** The nuclear material emerges through the annular fibers but the posterior longitudinal ligament remains intact.
- **Disc sequestration:** The nuclear material emerges through the annular fibers and posterior longitudinal ligament is disrupted. A portion of nucleus pulposus has protruded into the epidural space.

Disc herniation is a condition, in which a tear in the annulus fibrosus of an intervertebral disc allows the soft nucleus pulposus to bulge out.

Most herniations involve posterior lateral or posterior migration of nucleus pulposus.

L5-S1 segment is most common.

Two mechanisms of disc herniation: Sudden and gradual
- Very large, sudden compressive force delivered on a flexed and axially rotated spine, e.g., fall or lifting large load.
- Series of multiple, low magnitude compression forces over a flexed spine, e.g., repetitive lifting or bending with flexed back.

Spinal Canal Stenosis

Spinal stenosis occurs when the space around the spinal cord narrows. This puts pressure on the spinal cord and the spinal nerve roots, and may cause pain, numbness, or weakness in the legs.

Extension of the lumbar spine narrows the spinal canal. It is insidious in onset. Pain increases on standing and decreases while sitting and bending forward.

Lumbar Spondylosis

It is the age-related degenerative process occurring at the lumbar spine. In this
- Reduced water content in the disc
- Narrowed joint space
- Osteophyte formation
- Articular cartilage damage
- Joint erosion

Lumbar Spondylolisthesis

- Spondylolisthesis describes the anterior displacement of a vertebra above in relation to the vertebrae below.
- Stress fracture of the pars interarticularis is occurring bilaterally results in spondylolisthesis.
- Increased lumbosacral angle which increases the stress on pars interarticularis is a predisposing factor for spondylolisthesis.
- Frequently occurs at L5/S1 segment
- **Types**
  - Grade I: 25% slippage
  - Grade II: 50% slippage
  - Grade III: 75% slippage
  - Grade IV: 100% slippage

Lumbar Radiculopathy

The disc prolapse impinging on the nerves or the spinal canal stenosis squeezing the nerves results in the pain and tingling sensation of

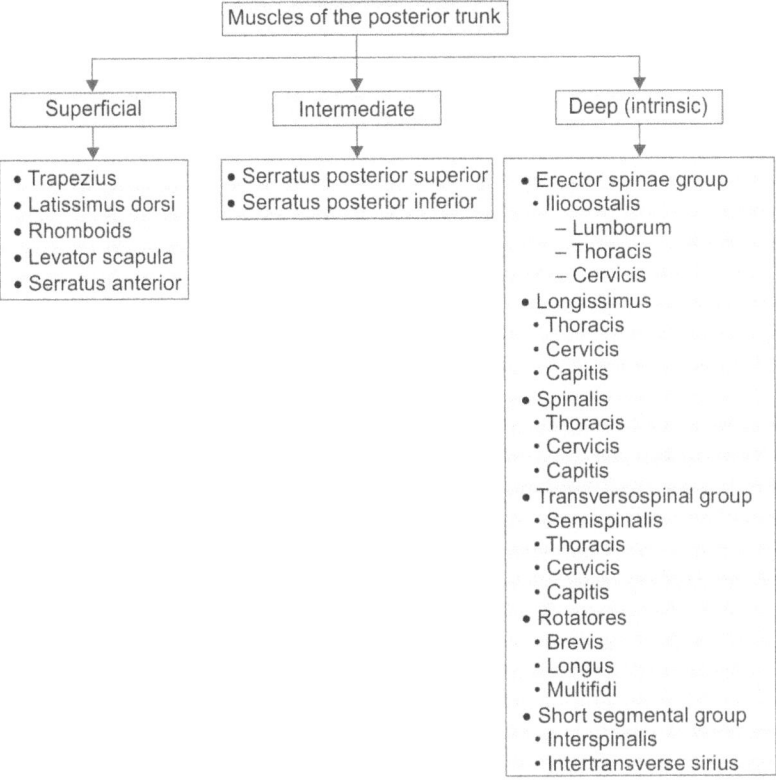

Flowchart 12.1: Muscles of the vertebral trunk

the particular nerve. In the long run it will also lead to loss of sensory and motor functions of the nerve.

MUSCLES OF TRUNK REGION

Set 1: Muscles of Anterior-lateral Craniocervical Region

- **Sternocleidomastoid**
- **Scalene:**
  - Anterior
  - Posterior
  - Medius
- **Longus colli**
- **Longus capitus**
- **Rectus capitus anterior**
- **Rectus capitus lateralis**

Set 2: Muscles of Posterior Craniocervical Region

- **Splenius:**
  - Cervicis
  - Capitus
- **Suboccipital muscles:**
  - Rectus capitus posterior major
  - Rectus capitus posterior minor
  - Obliqus capitis superior
  - Obliqus capitis inferior

All the posterior trunk muscle are shown in **Flowchart 12.1**.

SACROILIAC JOINT

INTRODUCTION

The sacroiliac joints mark the transition between the caudal end of the axial skeleton and the lower appendicular skeleton.

The joint is formed by the sacrum and innominate. The word "sacrum" refers to being "sacred," probably named as this is the keystone of spine, the place of child birth, seat

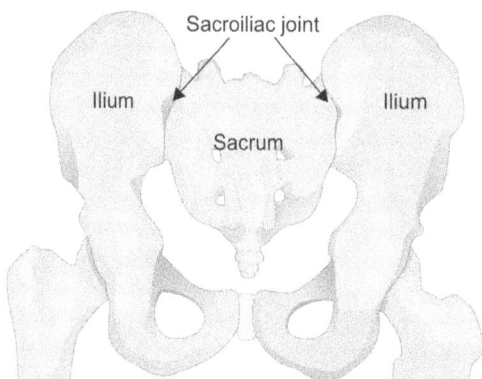

Fig. 12.21: Pelvic girdle

of various emotions, and key feature of human evolution. Many in the medieval centuries worshipped this bone. The "word innominate" literally means "without a name." Probably, it was of less significant than sacrum to the people in the old era **(Fig. 12.21)**.

Type: The joint has two parts:
1. Anterior part is a synovial joint.
2. Posterior part is a syndesmosis.

Articulating surfaces: Proximal—on either side of the posterior surface of the sacrum situated laterally to the sacral foramina from S1 to S3.

Distal: On the medial corner of anterior side of innominate.

The articulating surfaces are ear-shaped with uneven surface. This creates the stability for the joint. The surfaces are covered by hyaline cartilage with a thickness of 1–3 millimeter.

Age-related changes:
- 0–20 years: Smooth gliding planes
- 20–50 years: Interlocking irregularities
- >50 years: Hypomobility
- >80 years: Osteophytic, immobile

Functions of this joint:
- Stress relief within the pelvic ring
- Stable means of load transfer
- Accommodate aberrant motion during larger movements
- Triplanar shock absorber

Resting position: Neutral

Capsular pattern: Pain when joints are stressed

Close pack: Nutation
Loose pack: Counternutation

STABILITY

- Articulating surface
- Ligaments
- Joint structure

Articulating surface
The articulating surface is uneven. This fits into each other well like ridges fitting into depressions. This creates a very stable joint.

Ligaments
- **Primary:**
  - Anterior sacroiliac ligament
  - Interosseous ligament
  - Short and long dorsal sacroiliac ligaments
- **Secondary:**
  - Iliolumbar ligament
  - Sacrotuberous ligament
  - Sacrospinous ligament.
- The anterior sacroiliac ligaments are capsular ligaments as it gets connected to the capsule anteriorly.
- The short and long dorsal sacroiliac ligaments attach to the posterior superior iliac spine (PSIS) and ilium, sacrum posteriorly, thoracolumbar fascia, and aponeurosis of erector spinae.
- The interosseous ligament creates the syndesmosis in the joint and bond the joint.
- The sacrospinous ligament attaches to the ischial spine to lateral border of sacrum and coccyx.
- The sacrotuberous ligament attaches from ischial tuberosity to the posterior spine of ilium and lateral sacrum and coccyx.
- The iliolumbar ligament is a series of bands that run from the transverse process of L_5 to the ilium. It acts to resist the movements at the lumbosacral joint

JOINT STRUCTURE

Joint structure for stability can be discussed under the following **(Figs. 12.22 and 12.23)**:
- Form closure (passive stability)
- Force closure (active stability)

Chapter 12 | Vertebral Column

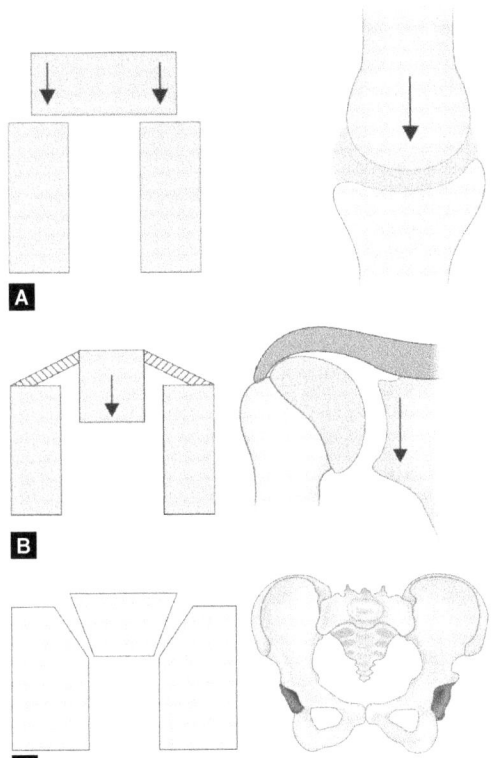

Form closure is the passive stability which is created by the bone-to-bone stability which is shown in the **Figure 12.22A**. Force closure is the active stability which is done by the musculature, fascia and ligaments. This is shown in the **Figure 12.22B**.

The sacroiliac joint is a combination of both the form closure and the force closure as shown in **Figure 12.22C**.

KINEMATICS

Osteokinematics (Figs. 12.24 and 12.25)

The movements in this joint have varied response from researchers from no movements possible to six movement patterns.

Overall all one could agree that about 1° to 3° or 1–3 mm movement of movement is seen in the joint.

Movements of sacrum
- Nutation
- Counternutation

Movements of innominate
- Anterior rotation/tilt
- Posterior rotation/tilt

Nutation is the anterior tilt of the sacrum. It is also called as flexion.

Figs. 12.22A to C: Sum of force closure and form closure resulting in holding power. (A) Example of form closure (stability through bone support); (B) Example of force closure (stability through muscles and ligaments); (C) Combination of form closure and force closure

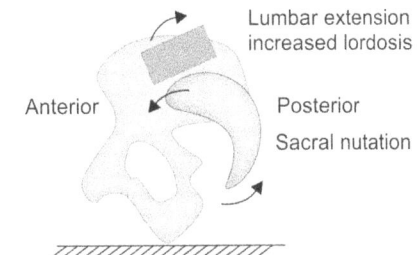

Fig. 12.24: Sacral motion: Closed kinematic chain

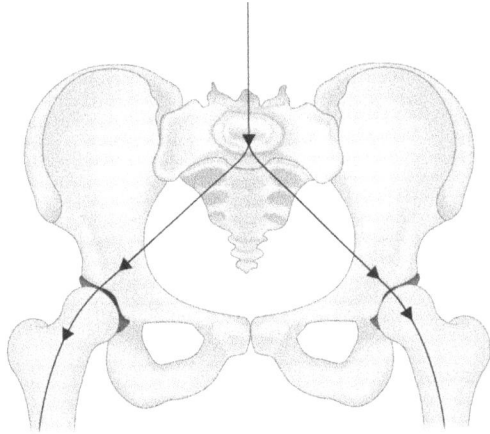

Fig. 12.23: Line of force along the lines of trabecular pattern of hip and pelvis

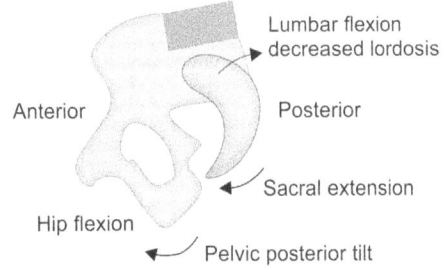

Fig. 12.25: Pelvic motion secondary to hip motion

Counternutation is the posterior tilt of the sacrum. It is also called as extension.

Base of the sacrum moves anteriorly and inferiorly while coccyx moves posteriorly.

Base of the sacrum moves posteriorly and superiorly while coccyx moves anteriorly.

Hip motion	Innominate motion (hypothetical and unproven)
Flexion	Posterior rotation
Extension	Anterior rotation
Internal rotation	In-flare
External rotation	Out-flare
Abduction	Superior shear
Adduction	Inferior shear

Lumbar motion	Innominate motion	Sacral motion
Flexion	Anterior rotation	Nutation followed by counternutation
Extension	Posterior rotation	Nutation
Rotation	**Ipsilateral:** Posterior rotation **Contralateral:** Anterior rotation	**Ipsilateral:** Nutation **Contralateral:** Nutation
Side bending	**Ipsilateral:** Anterior rotation **Contralateral:** Posterior rotation	Side bending

- Movements are feeble in magnitude and irregular in direction.
- All muscles that cross the joint are designed to act on hip or lumbar spine.
- During flexion of hip the ipsilateral ilium glides backward and downward across the sacrum and compresses against it, pivoting at the pubic symphysis.
- During extension ilium glides forward and flares away from the sacrum.

■ KINETICS

Not many forces influence the sacroiliac joint. As the stability is both by form closure and force closure, the forces gets negated. The gravity gets negated by the ground reaction force.

The one force worth looking at is the shear force. Especially during one leg standing. This influences the joint. However, under normal circumstances, the joint is capable of holding up this force. Pubic symphysis joint might be the affected joint by this shear force.

Muscles influencing the sacroiliac joint
- Iliopsoas
- Rectus femoris
- Hip abductors and adductors
- Sartorius
- External rotators (mainly piriformis)
- Gluteus maximus
- Hamstrings
- Quadratus lumborum
- Multifidi
- Tensor fascia lata

Key landmarks for palpation
- Iliac crest
- Anterior superior iliac spine (ASIS)
- PSIS
- Ischial tuberosity
- S2
- Inferior lateral angle
- Sacrotuberous ligament
- Pubic tubercle

■ PATHOMECHANICS

Sacroiliac Joint Dysfunction
- Inflammatory
- **Mechanical:**
  - Instability
  - Intra-articular derangement
  - Altered myokinetics
  - Positional fault
  - Other mechanical disturbances

■ SYMPHYSIS PUBIS

Type: Symphysis joint of amphiarthrosis

Articulating surfaces: The end of both pubic bones join together with a symphysis disc in between. The joint surfaces are covered by hyaline cartilage.

Ligaments
- Superior pubic ligament
- Inferior pubic ligament
- Posterior ligament

The superior pubic ligament is a thick band attaching to pubic crest and pubic tubercle. It reinforces the joint superiorly.

The inferior pubic ligament arches from the inferior rami of one side to the other. This ligament reinforces inferiorly.

The posterior ligament is a fibrous membrane holding the joint posteriorly.

Anteriorly, the joint is supported by expansions from transverse abdominus, rectus abdominus, internal oblique, and adductor longus.

SACROCOCCYGEAL JOINT

The coccyx is made up of four rudimentary coccygeal vertebrae.

The sacrococcygeal joint is a true joint. It has a joint capsule and ligaments. The joint consists of fibrocartilaginous intervertebral disc

Type: Symphysis type of joint.

Articulating surface:
- **Proximal:** Apex of the sacrum
- **Distal:** The base of the coccyx (upper border as the triangle is upside down).

Ligaments:
- Sacrococcygeal ligament
- Posterior intercoccygeal ligament

Movements:
- Up to the middle age, there is movement in this joint. The movements are flexion and extension. The coccyx moves posteriorly during defecation, child birth.
- Flexion is done by levator ani and sphincter ani externus. Extension is due to the relaxation of these muscles.
- As the person ages old, this joint gets fused and no more movement possible in this joint.

Muscles influencing the joint:
- **Gluteus maximus:** The coccygeal fibers of gluteus maximus get inserted into the posterolateral part of coccyx
- **Levator ani:** Ischiococcygeal fibers of levator ani get inserted into the ventral surface of the coccyx.

SECTION 3

Analytical Biomechanics

SECTION OUTLINE

- Posture
- Gait
- Movement Analysis in Activities of Daily Living
- Movement Analysis in Sporting Activities
- Goniometry
- Walking Aids
- Orthotics and Prosthetics
- Ergonomics
- Starting and Derived Positions for Exercise

CHAPTER 13

Posture

Chapter Outline

- Static and dynamic posture
- Postural control
- Kinematics and kinetics of posture
- Sagittal plane analysis
- Optimal posture
- Postural sway
- Deviations
- Analysis of sitting posture
- Measurements in posture
- Evaluation of posture
- Pathomechanics
- Posture in relation to hip joint
- Musculoskeletal changes during pregnancy

DEFINITION

Posture refers to the alignment of the body from head to toe in a certain fashion. The word "posture" is derived from a Latin "ponere," which means "to put or place."

"Posture is the attitude assumed by the body either with support during muscular inactivity or by means of the coordinated action of many muscles working to maintain stability or to form an essential basis which is being adapted constantly to the movement which is superimposed upon it **(Fig. 13.1)**."

STATIC AND DYNAMIC POSTURE

- Posture can either be static or dynamic.
- **Static posture:** The body and its segments are maintained and aligned in the state of rest or equilibrium without any movement, e.g., standing, sitting, lying, and kneeling **(Fig. 13.2)**.

Due to the interaction of group of muscles which work more or less to stabilize the joints and in opposition to gravity or other forces, a constant pattern of posture has been maintained. In an erect posture the state of equilibrium is preserved, e.g., standing.

- **Dynamic posture:** A posture in which the body or its segments are in movement, e.g., walking, running, jumping.
- This type of active posture is required to form a gross movement. The pattern of the posture is adjusted and modified constantly to meet the changing situations which arise due to a demand and result in a movement, e.g., walking, running **(Fig. 13.3)**.
- **Base of support (BoS):** An area bounded anteriorly by line joining the tips of toes and posteriorly by tips of heels **(Fig. 13.4B)**.
- Considered smaller in bipedal stance compared to quadrupedal BoS **(Fig. 13.4A)**.
- **Center of gravity (CoG):** A point at which all the body mass is concentrated. It is also known as center of mass (CoM).
- With different positions such as sitting, kneeling, there is an alteration in the position of CoM.
- In midsagittal plane, CoM is at second sacral segment when adult is standing.
- **Good posture:** It is the state of balanced musculoskeletal activity that protects the body structures from injury or progressive deformation, irrespective of their working or resting position **(Fig. 13.5)**.

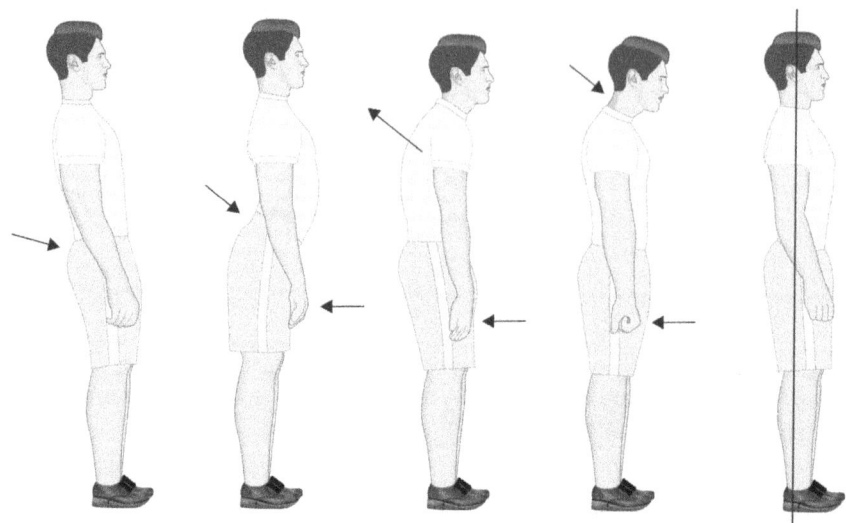

Fig. 13.1: Postural deviations

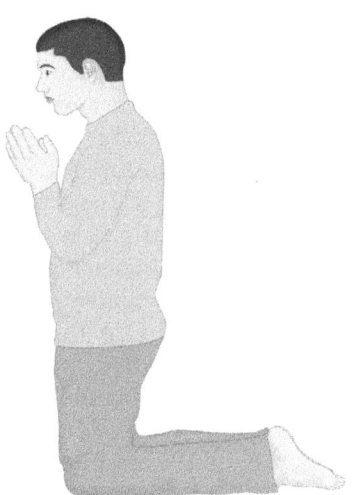

Fig. 13.2: Static posture

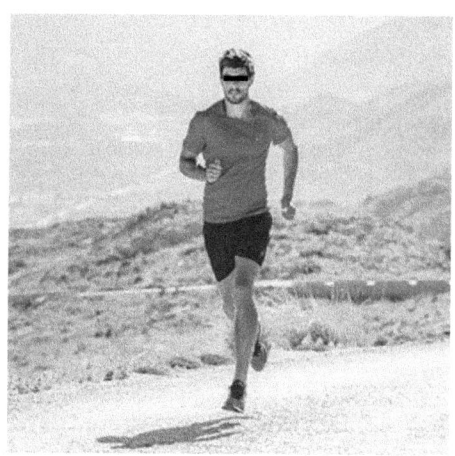

Fig. 13.3: Dynamic posture

- **Poor posture:** An altered body alignment which is inefficient in balancing body and increases strain on the structures **(Fig. 13.5)**.

Factors Affecting Good Posture

- **Developmental factors:**
  - It includes etiology of both congenital and acquired anomalies.
  - Congenitally, as the fetus grows in mother's womb it is prone to develop conditions such as congenital kyphosis, scoliosis.
  - As the child grows, bone growth occurs faster when compared to muscles in their body and at varying rates. This makes them prone for developing tightness of muscles, ligaments and fasciae, imbalance in muscular strength resulting in range of motion (ROM) limitation, and habitual postures.
- **Disease factors:**
  - Disabilities resulting due to amputation, neurological conditions or visual, skeletal, auditory impairments, and nutrition deficiency in an individual.

Chapter 13 | Posture

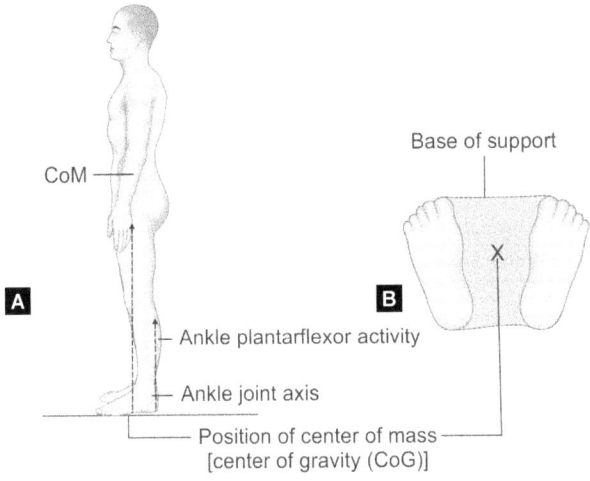

Figs. 13.4A and B: (A) Depicts CoM; (B) Base of support

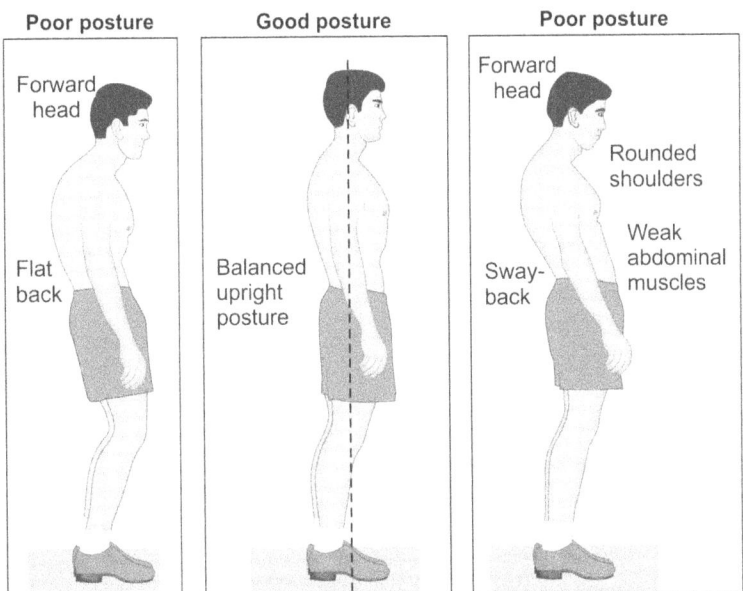

Fig. 13.5: Poor and good posture

- Muscular imbalance such as shortening or weakening of the muscle, any kind of pain.
- **Environmental factors:** Based on their home environment, environment at workplace, training centers which they are exposed to, and sports or hobbies an individual has, their posture can vary.
- **Psychological factors:** Emotional and mental status of an individual influence the posture.

ACTIVE POSTURE

The consolidated action of many muscles is requisite to maintain an active posture, which may be either static or dynamic.

INACTIVE POSTURE

These are the postures adapted for resting or sleeping which cause minimal demand on the muscles required for maintaining important body functions, such as respiration and

Flowchart 13.1: Theoretical model demonstrating systems contributing to postural control

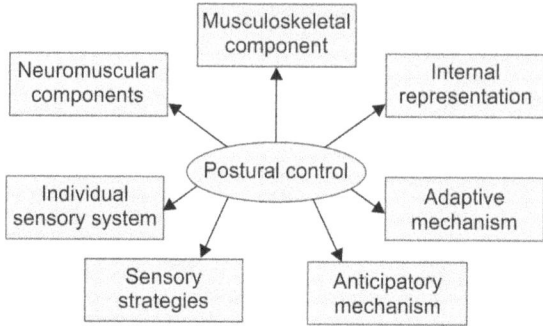

circulation. Such postures are used for training general relaxation.

Postural Stability and Control

Postural stability is defined as the ability of the body to maintain the CoG within the stability limits.

Stability limits is the area in which the body can sustain a posture without changing the BoS.

Postural Control and Stability Requirements

- **Sensory:** To assess the position and motion of body in space, the sensory information should be integrated.
- The capacity to generate forces for maintaining body position.

Neural components essential to postural encompasses (Fig. 13.6)

- **Motor system:** Neuromuscular response synergies
- **Sensory system:** Visual, vestibular, somatosensory systems
- Sensory strategies that organize these multiple inputs.
- Internal representation important for the mapping of sensation to action
- Higher level processes essential for adaptive and anticipatory aspects of postural control.

Postures are maintained as a result of neuromuscular coordination, the correct muscles being innervated by a complex reflex mechanism.

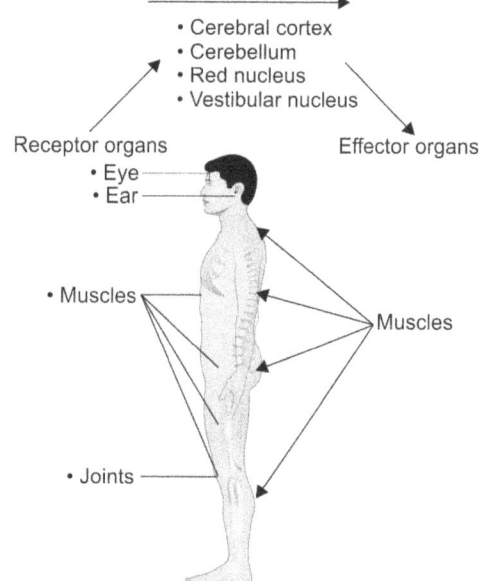

Fig. 13.6: Neural components essential for postural control

Postural reflexes
A reflex is a response to a stimulus. The afferent stimuli arise from the receptors situated all over the body, as the most of the receptors are situated in the muscles themselves, the ear, the eyes, and the joints. And the efferent response is a motor one, as antigravity muscles are the primary effectors organ.

POSTURAL CONTROL (FIG. 13.7)

- Can be either static or dynamic
- Refers to persons ability to maintain stability of the body and body segments in

Chapter 13 | Posture

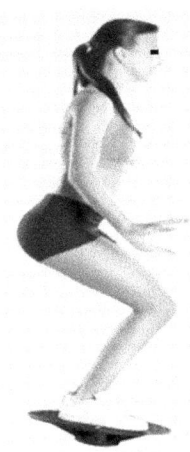

Fig. 13.7: Postural control

response to forces that threaten to disturb the body's equilibrium.
- Ability to maintain stability—multiple systems provide inputs which enable body to remain stable
- *Reactive (compensatory) responses*—occur as reactions to external forces that displace the body's CoM.
- *Proactive (anticipatory) responses* occur in anticipation of internally generated destabilizing forces such as raising arms to catch a ball or bending forward to tie shoes.

Major Goals and Basic Elements of Control
- Stabilizing the head with regard to vertical—primary goal
- Depends on integrity of CNS, visual system, vestibular system, and musculoskeletal system

None and Varied Inputs and Outputs
Alteration in inputs/absence of inputs can result in loss of stability or poor balance, e.g., ankle sprains lead to kinesthetic sense disturbance in ankle complex

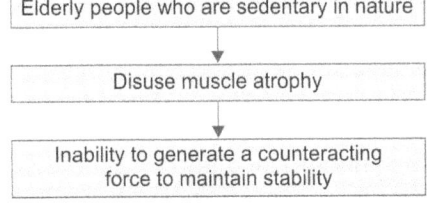

MUSCLE SYNERGIES
- Response of the body to any stimulus altering the balance, i.e., perturbation, is referred to as either synergies or strategies.
- "Perturbation is sudden change in conditions that displaces the body posture away from equilibrium".
- **Two types:** Sensory and mechanical
  1. *Sensory perturbation:* Changing visual input
  2. *Mechanical perturbations:* Movements of body segments or entire body displacing the CoM within the BoS of the body.
- "Synergies are centrally or organized patterns of muscle activity that occur in response to perturbations of standing postures".

Fixed-support Synergies
- These are patterns of muscle activity in which BoS remains fixed during perturbation and recovery of equilibrium.
- Stability is regained through movements of parts of the body, but feet remain fixed on BoS.
- Two examples of fixed support synergies (Fig. 13.8):
  1. **Ankle synergy:** It consists of bursts of muscle activity that occur in distal-to-proximal pattern on either anterior or posterior aspects of body in response to forward and backward motion of platform.

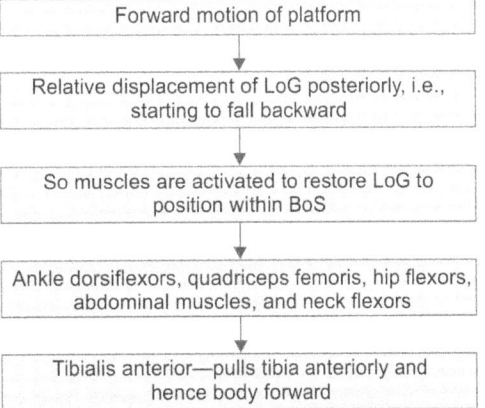

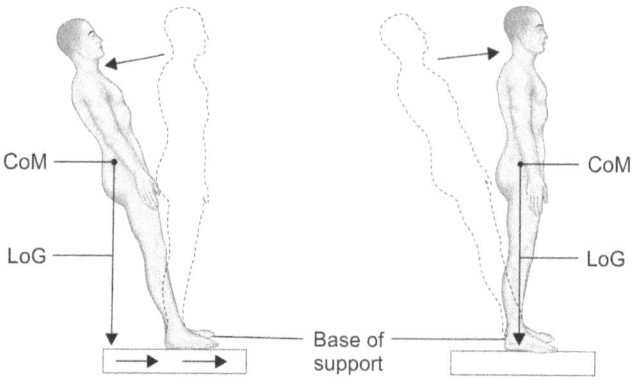

Fig. 13.8: Ankle and hip synergy when the surface is in motion
(CoM: center of mass ; LoG: line of gravity)

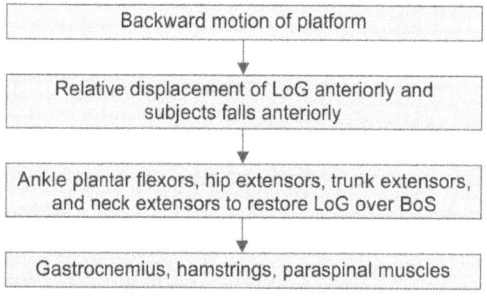

Change-in Support Strategies

- Includes stepping (forward, backward, and sideways) and grasping (using one's hands to grab a bar or fixed object).
- Are successful in maintaining stability during large perturbations.
- Younger subjects—take one step while elderly take multiple steps.

Head-stabilizing Strategies

- Used to maintain the head during dynamic tasks such as walking.
- To maintain the vertical stability of head, there are two strategies:
  1. Head stabilization in space (HSS) is a modification of head position in anticipation of displacements of body's CoG.
     - The anticipatory adjustments to head position are independent of trunk motion.
  2. Head stabilization on trunk (HST) is one in which head and trunk moves as single unit.

2. **Hip synergy:**
   - It consists of bursts of muscle activity in proximal to distal directions.
   - Fixed support hip strategy used primarily in situations in which change-in support strategies (stepping or grasping synergies) are not possible.

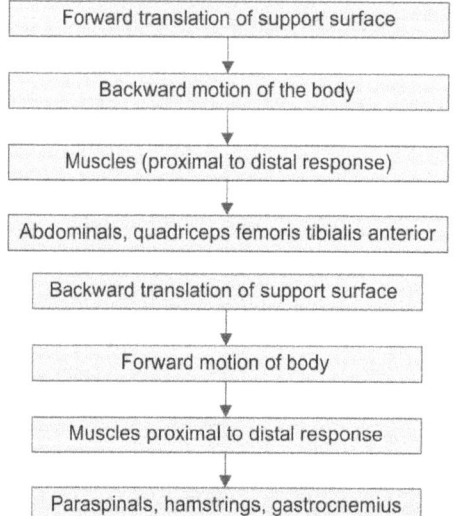

KINETICS AND KINEMATICS OF POSTURE

- External forces considered are: inertia, gravity, and ground reaction force.
- Internal forces—formed by muscle activity and passive tension in joint capsule, tendons, ligaments, and soft tissue structures.
- To maintain the body in a state of equilibrium, sum of all the forces and torque

acting on the body segments and full body must be zero.

Inertial and Gravitational Forces

- In standing position, there is nil or minimal body acceleration occurring. However, there is a constant swaying motion experienced by the body, which is referred to as postural sway or sway envelope.
- This sway is 12° sagittal and 16° in frontal plane for a normal individual.

Ground Reaction Forces

- Force acted upon body by ground, when body is in contact with the ground is ground reaction force (GRF), which is represented by a vector called ground reaction force vector (GRFV).
- **GRF has three components:**
  1. Vertical (along the y-axis)
  2. Two horizontal components:
     a. Medial lateral (along x axis)
     b. Anterior posterior (along z axis).
- The resultant GRFV is equal in magnitude but opposite in direction to the gravitational force in erect static standing posture.
- GRFV indicates the magnitude and direction of loading applied to the foot.
- Point of application of GRFV is at body's center of pressure (CoP), which is located in the foot in unilateral stance and between the feet in bilateral standing postures.
- GRFV and LoG have coincident action lines in static erect posture.

Sagittal Plane

Joints	Line of gravity
Atlanto-occipital	Anterior
Cervical	Posterior
Thoracic	Anterior
Lumbar	Posterior
Sacroiliac	Anterior
Hip	Posterior
Knee	Anterior
Ankle	Anterior

Standing (Coronal Plane–Anterior View)

Body segment	Line of gravity
Head/neck/shoulder	Passes through middle of the forehead, nose and chin
Chest	Passes through the middle of the xiphoid process
Abdomen/hips	Passes through the umbilicus
Hips/pelvis	Passes on a line equidistant from the right and left ASIS. Passes through the symphysis pubis
Knees	Passes between knees equidistant from the medial femoral condyles
Ankles/feet	Passes through ankle equidistant from the medial malleoli

Standing (Coronal Plane–Posterior View)

Body segment	Line of gravity
Head	Passes through middle of head
Arms	
Shoulders/spine	Passes along vertebral column in straight line, which should bisect the back into two symmetrical halves
Hips/pelvis	Passes through gluteal cleft of buttocks and should be equidistant from PSIS
Knees	Passes between the knees equidistant from medial joint aspects
Ankles/feet	Passes between ankles equidistant from the medial malleoli

OPTIMAL POSTURE

Ideal Plumb Line Alignment

Anterior View

See **Figures 13.9 and 13.10**.

Lateral View

See **Figures 13.11 and 13.12**.

Posterior View

See **Figure 13.13**.

Postural Sway (Fig. 13.14)

"The phenomenon of constant displacement and correction of the position of the CoG within the base of support" (Smith et al., 1996).

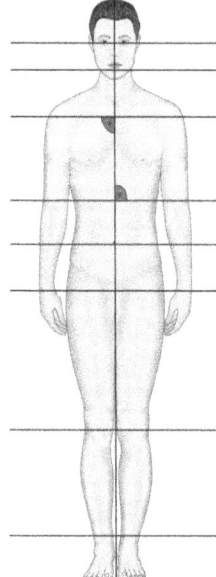

Fig. 13.9: Ideal plumb alignment: Anterior view

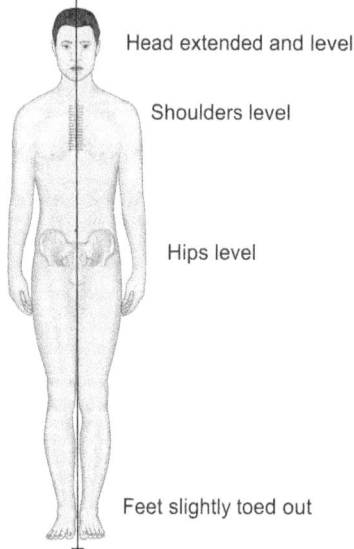

- Head extended and level
- Shoulders level
- Hips level
- Feet slightly toed out

Fig. 13.10: Line of gravity (anterior view)

Components	
Anteroposterior (AP) sway	5–7 mm at quiet stance in young adults
Mediolateral (ML) sway	3–4 mm at quiet stance in young adults

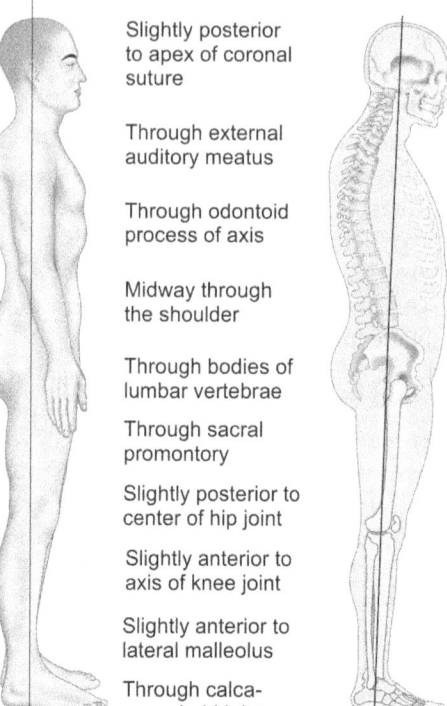

- Slightly posterior to apex of coronal suture
- Through external auditory meatus
- Through odontoid process of axis
- Midway through the shoulder
- Through bodies of lumbar vertebrae
- Through sacral promontory
- Slightly posterior to center of hip joint
- Slightly anterior to axis of knee joint
- Slightly anterior to lateral malleolus
- Through calcaneocuboid joint

Fig. 13.11: Ideal plumb line alignment: Lateral view

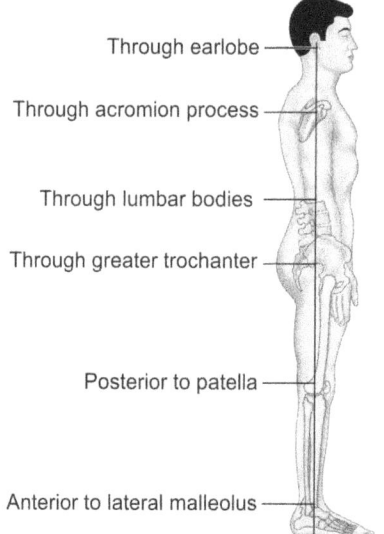

- Through earlobe
- Through acromion process
- Through lumbar bodies
- Through greater trochanter
- Posterior to patella
- Anterior to lateral malleolus

Fig. 13.12: Line of gravity (lateral view)

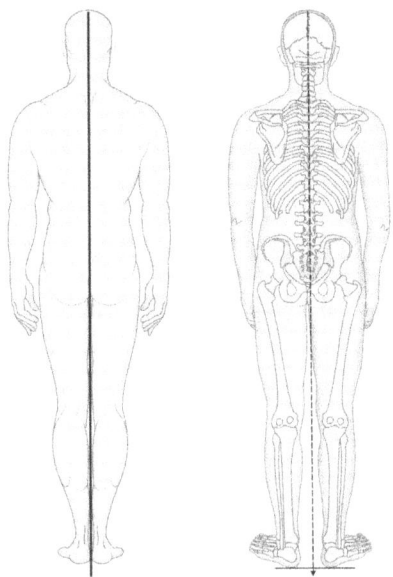

Fig. 13.13: Ideal plumb line alignment: Posterior view.

Mechanism:

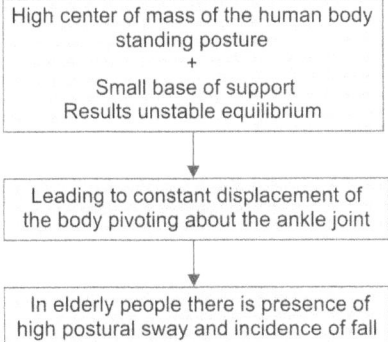

External and Internal Moments

- LoG passing through joint axis → No external gravitational torque created
- LoG passes away from joint axis → Results in external gravitational moment → Body segment rotation, if not opposed by counterbalancing internal moment (muscle contraction)
- LoG anterior to joint axis → External gravitational torque causes anterior movement of proximal body segment
- LoG posterior to joint axis → External gravitational torque causes posterior movement of proximal body segment

- These anterior and posterior movements are referred as flexion or extension moments.
- Note:

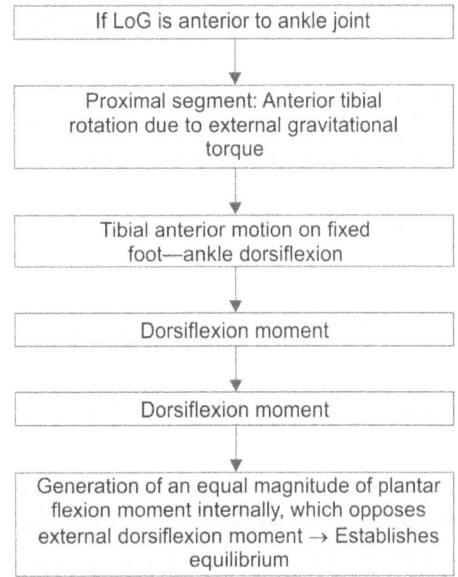

- Note:

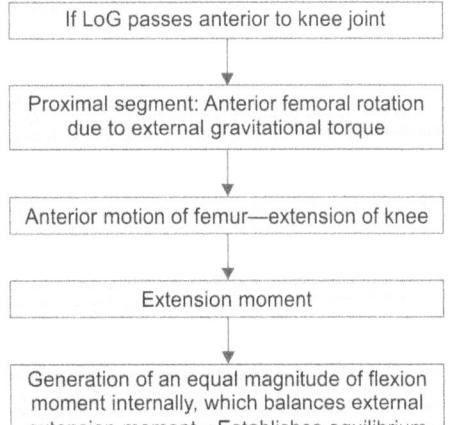

Optimal Posture or Ideal Posture

- Ideal posture—body segments aligned vertically and LoG passes through all joint axis.
- In ideal posture—small external gravitational moments; internal moments resulting from passive tension of capsule, ligaments and muscle and constant minimal muscle activity balance the external moment.

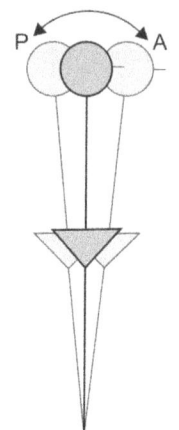

Fig. 13.14: Postural sway.

Analysis of Standing Posture: Viewed From Side

- A plumb line (a string with a weight tied at lower end) is used for observational posture analysis.
- Line released from ceiling and used to assess posture from either the lateral aspect or from anterior or posterior aspect.
- In anterior/posterior aspect—LoG should bisect body into two symmetrical halves.

Alignment and Analysis: Lateral View

1. Ankle

- In optimal posture—ankle joint is maintained in neutral, i.e., in between dorsi and plantar flexion.
- LoG is slightly anterior to lateral malleolus → anterior to ankle joint → external dorsiflexion moment is created, opposed by plantar flexion moment internally → preventing tibial forward motion.
- Soleus muscle contracts and posteriorly pulls the tibia—thus opposes dorsiflexion moment.
- Soleus—common function by acting to control anterior posterior sway between the legs.

2. Knee

- In an optimal posture—knee joint is in full extension.
- LoG is anterior to midline of knee and posterior to patella (**Figs. 13.15 and 13.16**).
- Thus creates external extension moment that keeps knee in extension.
- Opposing internal flexion moment is formed by passive posterior joint capsular and ligamentous tension → balances external gravitational moment and prevents hyperextension at knee.
- Minimal activity—in hamstrings

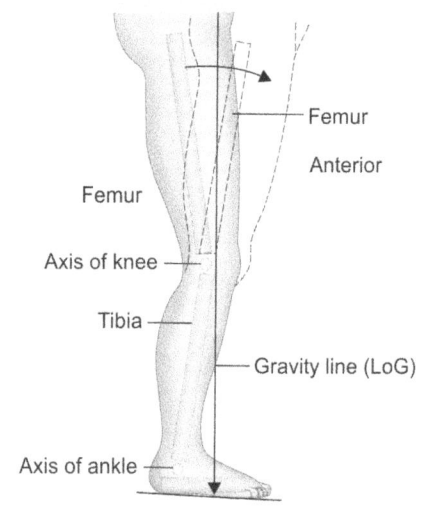

Fig. 13.15: Internal and external moment at knee joint

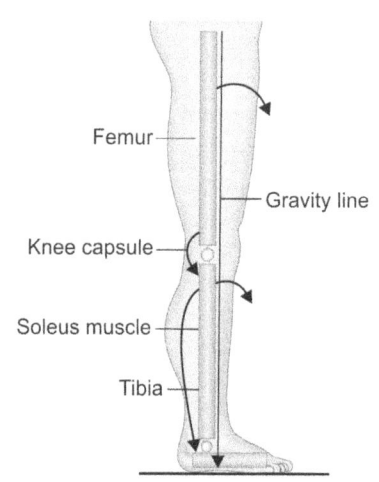

Fig. 13.16: During knee extension, LoG is located anterior to midline of knee and posterior to patella

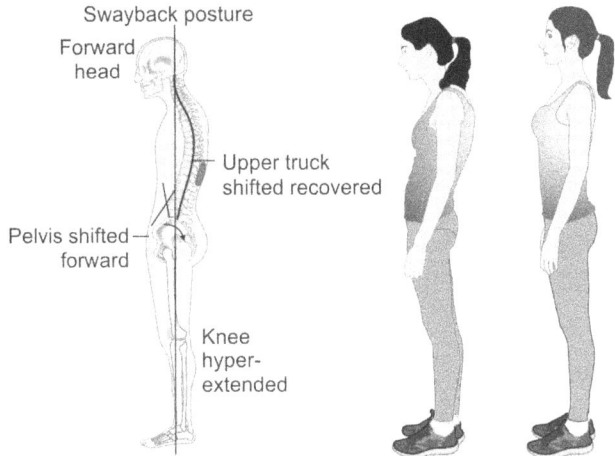

Fig. 13.17: Swayback posture

- Soleus exerts posterior pull on tibia.
- Gastrocnemius opposes the gravitational knee extension.

3. Hip and Pelvis

- Optimal posture—hips in neutral and pelvis at same level bilaterally, with neither anterior nor posterior tilt.
- LoG passes slightly posterior to axis of hip joint through the greater trochanter.
- Swayback posture **(Fig. 13.17)**

LoG drops behind the hip joint axes

• Forward head with extension of cervical spine • Trunk is displaced posteriorly with increased kyphosis • Lumbar spine flattened • Pelvis is rotated posteriorly • Hyperextended hips and knees

- Swayback posture causes excessive tension on anterior hip ligament. There is absence of muscular activity in subjects with swayback posture.
- Adaptive lengthening of anterior hip muscles—if posture becomes habitual
    ◆ Gluteus muscle—weakened by disuse atrophy
    ◆ Sway posture: There is increase in the magnitude of gravitational torque.

4. Lumbosacral and Sacroiliac Joints

- **Average lumbosacral angle:** 6–30°
- **Lumbosacral angle:** It is measured between bottom of L5 vertebra and top of sacrum S1 **(Fig. 13.18)**.
- Anterior tilting of sacrum—increases lumbosacral angle—increases shearing stress at lumbosacral joint—results is increase lumbar lordosis.
- **Optimal posture:** The LoG passes through the body of 5th lumbar vertebra and close to axis of rotation of lumbosacral joint.
- LoG passes anteriorly to sacroiliac joints, when sacrum is in optimal position.
- Anterior superior portion of sacrum is rotated anteriorly and inferiorly due to external gravitational moment.

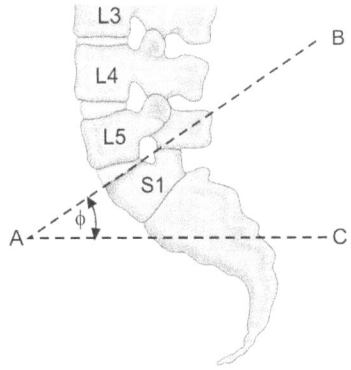

Fig. 13.18: Lumbosacral angle

- Internal moments are provided by passive tension in sacrospinous ligaments and sacrotuberous ligaments.

5. Vertebral Column
- Optimal position of the plumb line is through the midline of the trunk.
- Anterior to cervical and anterior to thorax and posterior to lumbar

6. Head
- LoG is anterior to vertebral body for flexion and extension, creating external flexion moment.
- External flexion moment → head tilts forward
- Opposed by tension in tectorial membrane, ligamentum nuchae, posterior part of zygapophyseal joint capsules and capital extensors
- In optimal posture, plumb line passes through the external auditory meatus of ear and head and passes over body's CoM at S2.

Deviations From Optimal Alignment Viewed From Side: Lateral View

Compensatory postures are those which are adapted for functional improvement or normalizing appearance.

1. Foot and Toes (Figs. 13.19A to C)
a. **Claw toes (Fig. 13.19B):** Is a deformity characterized by hyperextension of metatarsophalangeal joint, combined with flexion of DIP and PIP.
   - Abnormal weight distribution causes callus formation under metatarsal heads or distal phalanx.
   - Proximal phalanx might subluxate dorsally over metatarsal head.
   - In dorsal aspect of flexed phalanges, calluses grow due to constant rubbing on inside of shoes.
   - This deformity reduces BoS, increases postural sway.
   - *Causes:* Improper shoes, cavus foot, ineffective intrinsic foot muscles, and age

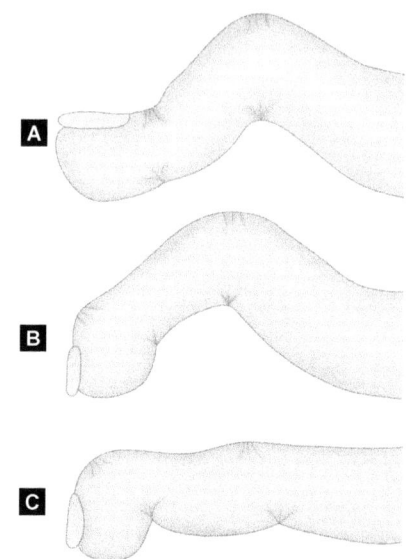

Figs. 13.19A to C: (A) Hammer toe; (B) Claw toe; (C) Mallet toe

   - Claw toes affect all toes (2nd through 5th), while hammer toes affect only one or two toes.

b. **Hammer toes (Fig. 13.19A):**
   - Deformity characterized by hyperextension of MTP joint, flexion of PIP, and hyperextension of DIP joint
   - Due to pressure from shoes, callosities might form on superior surfaces of PIP
   - Due to abnormal weight bearing, tip of DIP also shows callosities.
   - Over MTP joint, flexor muscles are stretched and extensor muscles are shortened.
   - At PIP joint, flexor muscles are shortened and extensor muscles are stretched.
   - *Note:* If paralysis of long and short toe extensors and lumbricals occurs, intrinsic and extrinsic toe flexor acts unopposed resulting in buckling of PIP and DIP joints→ hammer toe.

2. Knee
a. **Flexed knee posture (Fig. 13.20):**
   - In knee flexion contractures, LoG is posterior → results in external flexion

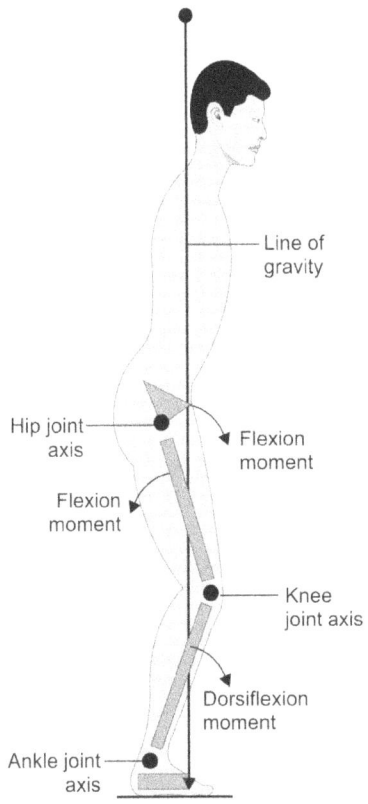

Fig. 13.20: Flexed knee posture

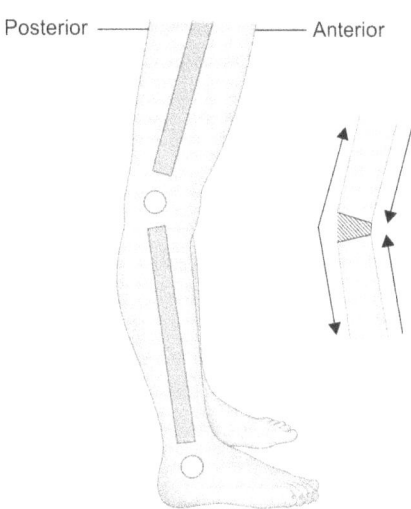

Fig. 13.21: Hyperextended knee posture (genu recurvatum).

→ quadriceps causes internal extension moment to balance external moment.
- Flexed knee posture - greater tibiofemoral and patellofemoral compressive stresses - leads to fatigue of quadriceps femoris.
- Flexed knee posture occurs along with flexion of hip and dorsiflexion of ankle.
- Thus, LoG is anterior at hip → external flexion moment→ hip extensors act to create internal extensor moment.
- At ankle—LoG falls anterior - creates external dorsiflexion moment - increases soleus activity to counteract internal plantarflexion moment.

b. **Hyperextended knee posture (genu recurvatum) (Fig. 13.21):**
- LoG passes anterior to knee joint → increases external extensor moment at knee → increases hyperextension and tension at posterior joint capsule.
- Adaptive lengthening at posterior capsule and cruciate ligaments
- *Knee hyperextension causes:* Limited ankle dorsiflexion or fixed plantar flexion position of foot and ankle called equinus.

3. Pelvis

a. **Excessive anterior pelvic tilt:** Leads the lower lumbar vertebrae to shift anteriorly, upper lumbar vertebrae move posteriorly → increasing lumbar lordosis
- Extension moment in lumbar spine is increased.
- Posterior convexity in thoracic
- Spine increases to balance lordotic lumbar curve and maintains head over the sacrum
- Anterior convexity of cervical spine increases to bring head back on the sacrum.
- In optimal posture, the lumbar disc are subjected to tension anteriorly and compression posteriorly, thus increases the anterior convexity of lumbar spine in turn increasing the compressive forces on posterior annuli and affect nutrition of posterior portion of intervertebral disc.

- Excessive compressive forces on the zygapophyseal joints.
b. **Excessive posterior pelvic tilt:** Posterior pelvic tilt causes straightening of lumbar spine and loss of flexibility.

4. Vertebral Column

a. **Kyphosis and lordosis:**
   - Kyphosis refers to normal posterior convexity in thoracic and sacral spine.
   - May develop as compensation for an increase in normal lumbar or poor postural habits or osteoporosis.
   - Two excessively kyphotic postures are Dowager's hump **(Fig. 13.22A)** and Gibbus deformity **(Fig. 13.22B)**—both lead to vertebral fractures.
   - Dowager's hump occurs often in postmenopausal women who have osteoporosis. Anterior aspect of bodies of vertebra collapse and increased compression stress on anterior portions of vertebral body.
     * Increase in posterior convexity and increase compression on anterior aspect of vertebral bodies and anterior annulus
     * Tensile stress increases on posterior aspect—affects posterior annulus and apophyseal joints.

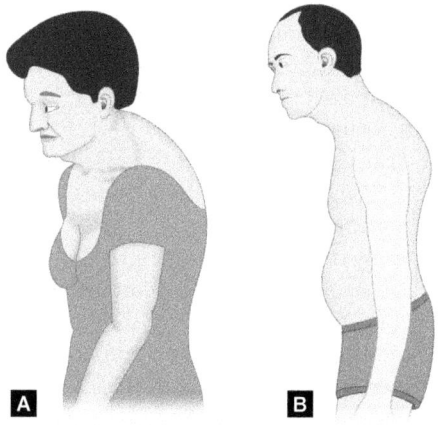

Figs. 13.22A and B: (A) Dowager's hump; (B) Gibbus deformity

* It comprises force generating capacity of back extensors.
* Causes limitations in chest expansion.
   - Lordosis—anterior convexity in cervical and lumbar region.
     * Abnormal increases in the curve
     * Compression on posterior part of vertebrae and posterior annulus and tensile forces increased on anterior aspect and anterior longitudinal ligaments.

5. Head

a. **Forward head posture:**
   - Head is positioned anterior.
   - The anterior cervical convexity is increased with apex of lordotic curve at distance from LoG in comparison with optimal posture
   - Large external flexion moment
   - Cervical extensors muscles become ischemic.
   - Posterior aspect of zygapophyseal joint capsules causes adaptive shortening and narrowed intervertebral foramen thus leading to nerve root compression
   - The following changes are seen namely-medial rotation of scapula, excessive thoracic kyphosis **(Figs. 13.23A and B)** leading to diminished thoracic cavity, reduced vital capacity and shortened body height.

Optimal Alignment and Analysis: Anterior and Posterior View

- LoG bisects body into symmetrical halves
- Head straight no tilting or rotation, face bisected equal halves
- Eyes, clavicle 7 shoulder are at level.
- Posterior view—inferior angle of scapula parallel and equidistant from LoG.
- Waist angles and gluteal folds should be equal.
- ASIS and PSIS should lie on a parallel to the ground.
- Joint axis of hip, knee, and ankle are equidistant from LoG.

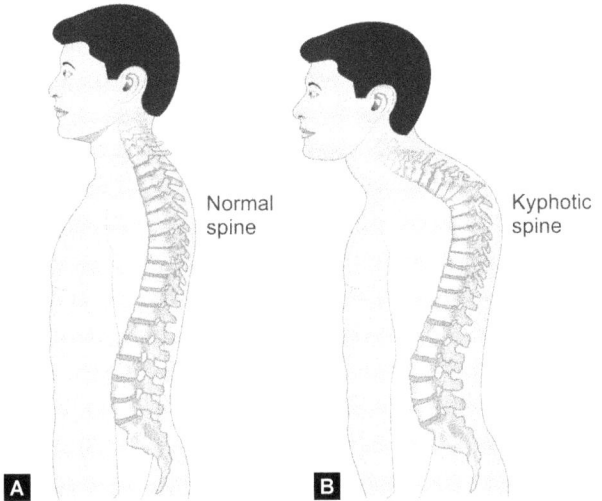

Figs. 13.23A and B: (A) Normal spine; (B) Excessive thoracic kyphosis

Deviations from Optimal Alignment

1. Foot and Toes

a. **Pes planus (flat foot) (Figs. 13.24 and 13.25)**
   - Pes planus or flat foot occurs when one malleolus is lower than the other and calcaneal eversion is present.
   - No calcaneal eversion should be present from 7 years of age.
   - Flat foot is characterized by reduced or absent medial arch.
   - It may be either rigid or flexible.
   - Rigid flat foot is a structural deformity that is hereditary, in which medial longitudinal arch is absent in nonweight bearing, toe standing, and normal weight bearing.
   - Flexible flat foot is a deformity in which arch is reduced during normal weight bearing, but reappears during toe standing or nonweight bearing.
   - In flat foot, the talar head is displaced anteriorly, medially, and inferiorly.
   - *Displacement of talus*
     - Causes depression of navicular bone
     - Tension in plantar calcaneonavicular (spring) ligament
     - Lengthening of tibialis posterior muscle
   - If the navicular bone is depressed, it will lie below the Feiss line.

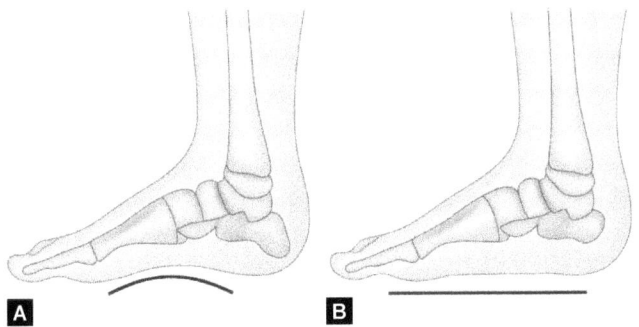

Figs. 13.24A and B: (A) Normal foot; (B) Flat foot or pes planus

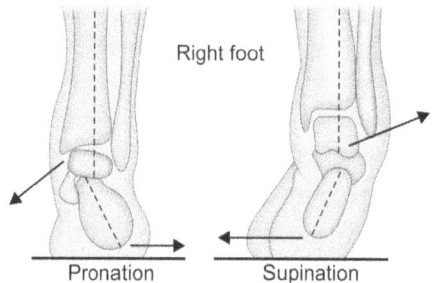

Fig. 13.25: Foot supination and pronation

- It require muscle contraction to support osteoligamentous arches during standing.
- In weight bearing pronation of foot causes medial rotation of tibia, affecting the knee joint function **(Fig. 13.26)**.

b. **Pes cavus (Fig. 13.27):**
   - The medial longitudinal arch is usually high.
   - Weight is borne on lateral borders of foot, lateral ligaments, and peroneus longus muscle is stretched.
   - It is unable to adapt to the supporting surface because subtalar and transverse tarsal joints tend to be near or at locked supinated position.
   - Cavus foot is not a good shock absorber.

2. Knees

a. **Genu valgum (knock knees):**
   - Valgus angulation at knees should be 5–7°.
   - Mechanical axes are displaced laterally.
   - Medial knee joint structures are subjected to abnormal stresses or distraction stress and lateral structures are subjected to abnormal compressive stress.
   - Patella is displaced laterally and is predisposed to subluxation.
   - Genu valgum produces pronation of foot, develops stress on medial longitudinal arch, and abnormal weight is distributed on posterior medial aspect of calcaneus.

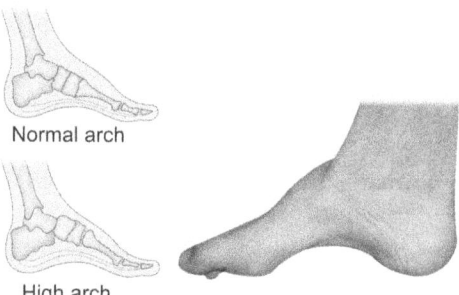

Fig. 13.27: Pes cavus

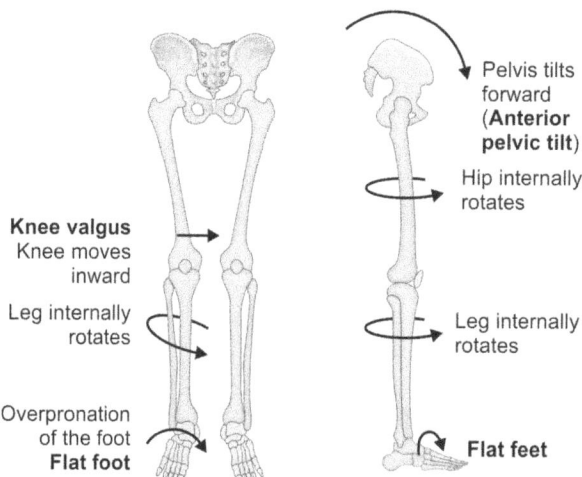

Fig. 13.26: Biomechanical alterations seen with flat foot

- Some added changes include flat foot, lateral tibial torsion, lateral patellar subluxation, and lumbar spine contralateral rotation.

b. **Genu varum (bow legs):**
- Knees are widely separated, when feet are together and malleoli are touching.
- There are compressive forces acting medially and patella is displaced in the same direction.
- The causes are vitamin D deficiency, renal rickets, osteochondritis, or epiphyseal injury.

3. Vertebral Column

a. **Scoliosis (Fig. 13.28):**
- It is a deformity in which there is presence of lateral deviation of spine in frontal plane.
- If one or more of medial or lateral structures fails to provide adequate support then the vertebral column tends to bend on one side.
- Lateral bending is accompanied by rotation of vertebrae because of lateral flexion and rotations are coupled motions below level of C2.
- *Two types:* Functional and structural

1. Functional/nonstructural curves are the types of curves that can be reversed if the cause of the curve is corrected, e.g., leg length discrepancy.
2. Structural curves involve changes in bone and soft tissue structures whereas idiopathic curves of unknown cause are categorized by age at onset: Infantile (0–3 years), juvenile (4–10 years), and adolescents (>10 years).
- The curves in scoliosis are named according to direction of convexity and location of curve.
- For example, curve convex to left in cervical area

Scoliosis can lead to pulmonary dysfunction, decreased vital capacity, impaired exercise capacity, and function of internal organs altered as well as cosmetically challenged appearance.

Home or school screening programs for identification **(Figs. 13.29A and B)**.
- Unequal waist angles
- Unequal shoulder levels or scapulae
- Rib hump
- Obvious lateral spinal curvature.

ANALYSIS OF SITTING POSTURES

Different sitting postures (Figs. 13.30A to C):
1. Active erect sitting posture is defined as unsupported posture in which person attempts to sit up as straight as possible.
   - LoG passes close to joint axes of head and spine.
   - Studies showed greater activity in superficial lumbar multifidus, thoracic erector spinae, and internal oblique abdominal muscles in erect sitting than in slumped sitting.
   - Flexion relaxation phenomenon explains to consist of flexion relaxation, sudden cessation of back extensors during trunk flexion than does active erect sitting posture, and passive tissues bear the load.

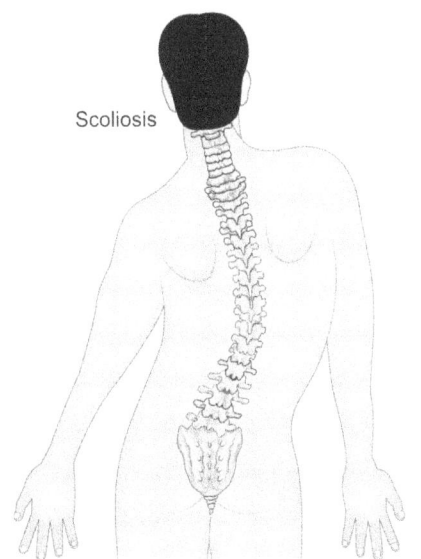

Fig. 13.28: Scoliosis

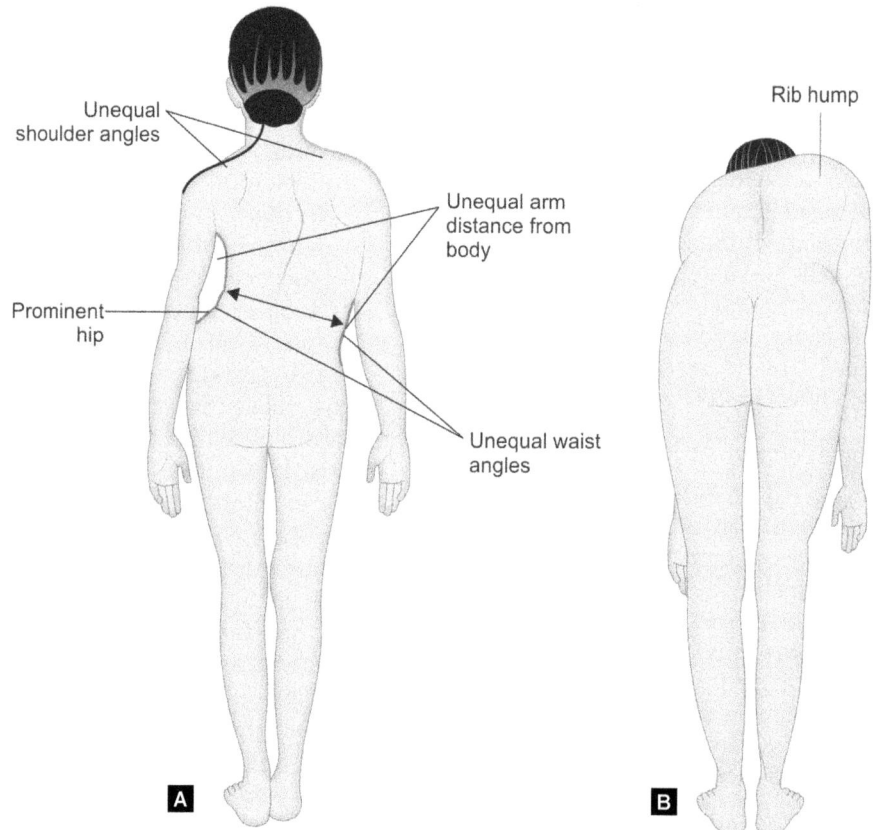

Figs. 13.29A and B: Alterations seen with scoliosis

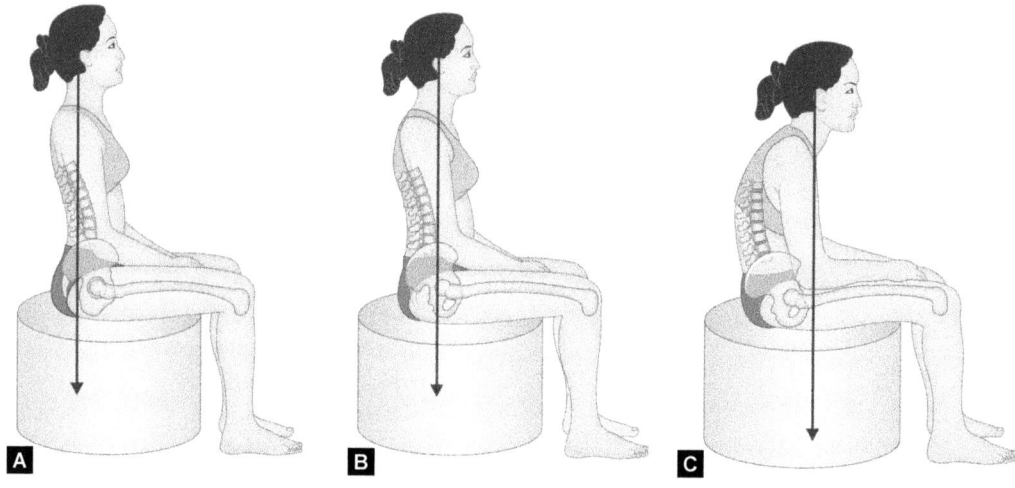

Figs. 13.30A to C: Different sitting postures: (A) Active erect sitting; (B) Relaxed erect sitting; (C) Slumped sitting

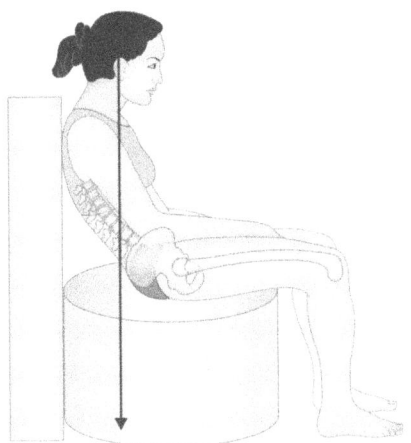

Fig. 13.31: Slouched posture

- Requires co-contractions of trunk extensors (erector spinae) and flexors (abdominal muscles) which cause higher pressures in disc between L4 and L5 than slumped sitting.

2. **Slumped posture:**
   - LoG is more anterior to joint axes of cervical, thoracic, lumbar spines.
   - Additional muscle activity is required to maintain a slumped posture.
   - In relaxed erect sitting, the LoG is slightly anterior to its position.
     ◆ In slouched posture (**Fig. 13.31**), the LoG is posterior to spine and hips, but the body weight is supported by back of chair and thus, less muscle activity is required.
     ◆ Sustained slouched posture increases the interdiscal pressure due to increase in compressive stress and load on anterior annulus and increase tensile forces on posterior annulus.
     ◆ Due to sustenance of load, creep increases in posterior annulus leading to stretching and thinning thus resulting in disc degeneration.

Muscle Activity in Sitting versus Standing

- Increase in muscle activity leads to increase in interdiscal pressure and vice versa.
- During sitting, pelvis is in posterior pelvic tilt position causing reduction in lumbar lordosis, thus upper and lower erector spinae activity is increased.
- Thus sitting > standing

Interdiscal Pressures and Compressive Loads on Spine

Interdiscal pressure is measured via insertion of pressure over sensitive sensors or transducers into one or more intervertebral disc.

Kyphosis developed during sitting postures

↓

- Increases intervertebral disk shear force
- Posterior annulus tensile forces
- Anterior annulus load hydrostatic pressure in nucleus
- Loading of posterior ligamentous structures

Seat Interface Pressures

- Pressure is defined as force per unit area.
- Pressure caused by contact forces between person's body and seat is termed as seat interface pressure.
- Paraplegia has significantly higher seat interface pressures due to continuous contact with the seat.

Note: Pressure sores (pressure ulcers)/ decubitus ulcers (**Fig. 13.32**).

1. Superficial pressure sores affect the layers of skin near epidermal tissue and progress downward into the subdermal layers.
2. Deep pressure sores cause deep tissue injury affecting subdermal tissue and muscle underlying the bony prominence

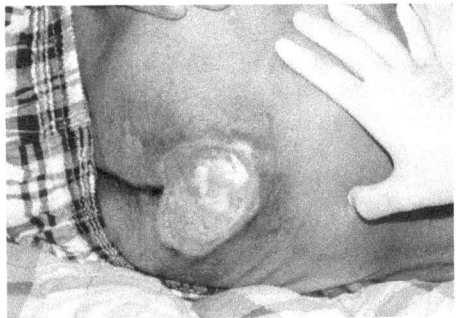

Fig. 13.32: Pressure sore

that progress upward through the epidermal tissue.

- *Deep tissue injury*
  ↓
  Compressive stress
  Inhibits blood flow
  Local tissue ischemia
  Failure of healthy capillaries → Tissue necrosis

Sustained increase in pressure leads to reduced lymphatic and venous circulation.

In supine lying → the risk areas are back of heels and head, scapulae, lower vertebral spine, and sacrum.

In side lying → shoulder, medial aspect of knees, lateral malleoli, greater trochanter of femur, and head of fibula.

Analysis of Lying Posture

- Interdiscal pressure is less in lying than in standing and sitting.
- Uniform pressure must be concentrated, e.g., for reducing mattress surfaces are foam, air, and water.

DIFFERENT TECHNIQUE/ INSTRUMENTS USED FOR MEASUREMENT OF POSTURE

A Plumb Line is a string with a weight on the end that may be hung next to a standing patient. It allows the evaluation of his/her posture in relation to the line. For a frontal plane view, the patient stands with the line midway between the heels; for a sagittal plane view, the patient stands with the line anterior to the lateral malleolus.

A Grid is a framework of evenly placed horizontal and vertical lines in front of which the patient stands. With a grid, the patient's posture can be evaluated in relation to ideal posture.

For Anterior Photograph

Client faces the camera (**Fig. 13.33**). The bold center, vertical line should line up with the vertical alignment line goes from the nose, chin, center of the chest, navel, and between the medial malleolus. Horizontal alignment

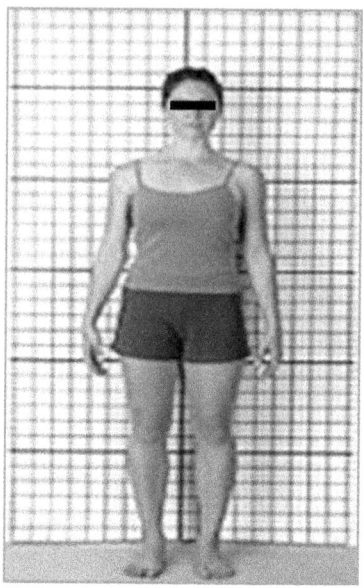

Fig. 13.33: Anterior photograph

lines provide reference for the level of the eyes, ears, shoulders, hands, pelvis, and knees.

For Lateral Photograph

Client faces sideways. Photograph right and left view. Bold center grid line directly behind and slightly anterior of the lateral malleolus. Look for line extending from ear to acromial process through greater trochanter of femur, slightly behind patella and one inch anterior to lateral malleolus. Bisecting vertically through these areas.

For Posterior Photograph

Client faces grid (**Fig. 13.34**). The bold center, vertical line should line up with the center of the body. Vertical alignment line bisects head, through neck, vertebrae, buttocks, and medial malleoli. Horizontal alignment lines provide reference for the level of the ears, shoulders, hands, pelvis, and ankles.

- **Posture boards (Figs. 13.35A to C)** are boards on which footprint has been drawn. Footprint may be painted on the floor of the examining room, but the posture board has the advantage of being portable.
- **Folding ruler with spirit level (Fig. 13.36)** is used to measure the difference in level

Chapter 13 | Posture

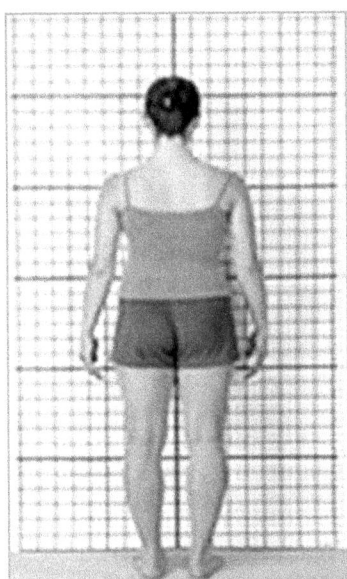

Fig. 13.34: Posterior photograph

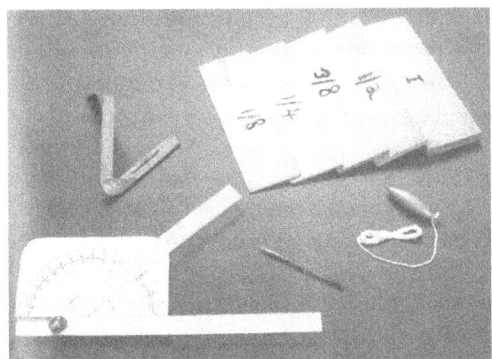

Fig. 13.36: The equipment consists of (left to right) protactor and caliper, folding ruler with spirit level, set of blocks, plumb line and marking pencil

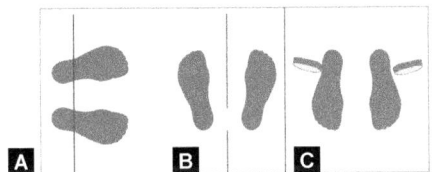

Figs. 13.35A to C: The posture boards with foot prints on which the subject stands for alignment tests. (A) Side view; (B) Back view; (C) Front view

of the PSIS. It also may be detected any difference in shoulder level. A background with a square is a more practical aid in detecting difference in shoulder level.
- **Set of six blocks (Fig. 13.36)** measure 4 inches by 10 inches and are of the following thickness: ⅛, ¼, ⅜, ½, ¾, and 1 inch. They are used for determining the amount of lift needed to level the pelvis laterally.
- **Marking pencil (Fig. 13.36)** is used for making the spinous processes to observe the position of the spine in case of lateral deviation.
- **Tape measure (Fig. 13.36)** is used for measuring leg length and forward bending in reaching the fingertips toward or beyond the toes.

APPROPRIATE CLOTHING

Clothing such as a two-piece bathing suit for girls or swim trunks for boys should be worn by subject for a postural examination. In hospital, gowns or other suitable garb should be provided.

Method and apparatus for diagnosing posture abnormalities includes a video camera, a video display terminal, and a subject platform positioned between the camera and the terminal so that the subject can view the terminal. A computer is employed to freeze a video image of the subject on said terminal so that an operator can obtain data regarding the relative positions of landmarks on said image using a light pen. The computer analyzes the landmark position data and generates a diagnosis of postural abnormalities of the subject. The method and apparatus may also employ a weight scale on the subject platform for transmitting data to the computer regarding the weight distribution on the feet of the subject.

EVALUATION OF POSTURE

Evaluating and treating postural problems require an understanding of basic principles related to alignment, joints, and muscles.
- Faulty alignment results in undue stress and strain on bones, joints, ligaments, and muscles.

- An assessment of joint position indicates which muscles are in an elongated and which are in a shortened position.
- A correlation exits between alignment and muscle test finding if posture is habitual.
- Muscle weakness allows separation of the parts to which the muscles is attached.
- Muscle shortness holds the parts to which the muscle is attached closer together.
- Stretch weakness can occur in one joint muscle that remains in an elongated position.
- Adaptive shortening can develop in muscles that remain in a shortened condition.

PATHOMECHANICS/FAULTY POSTURE

Kyphotic-Lordotic Posture

See **Figure 13.37**.

Head: Forward
Cervical spine: Hyperextended
Scapulae: Abducted
Thoracic spine: Increased flexion
Lumbar spine: Hyperextended
Pelvis: Anterior tilt
Hip: Flexed
Knee: Slightly hyperextended
Ankle: Slight plantar flexion because of backward inclination of the leg.

Lordotic Posture

See **Figure 13.38**.

Head: Neutral
Cervical spine: Normal curve
Thoracic spine: Normal curve
Lumbar spine: Hyperextended
Pelvis: Anterior tilt
Knee: Slightly hyperextended
Ankle: Slightly plantar flexed

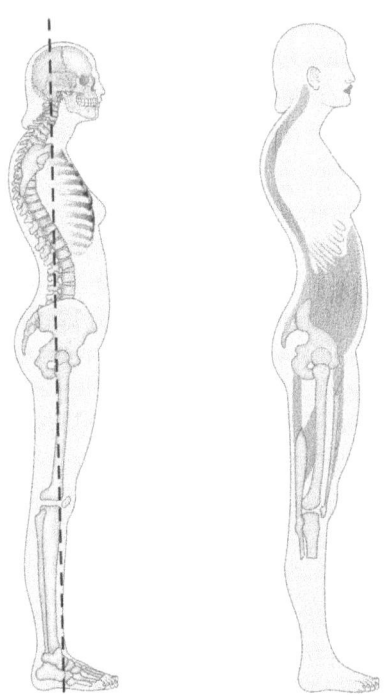

Fig. 13.37: Kyphotic-Lordotic posture

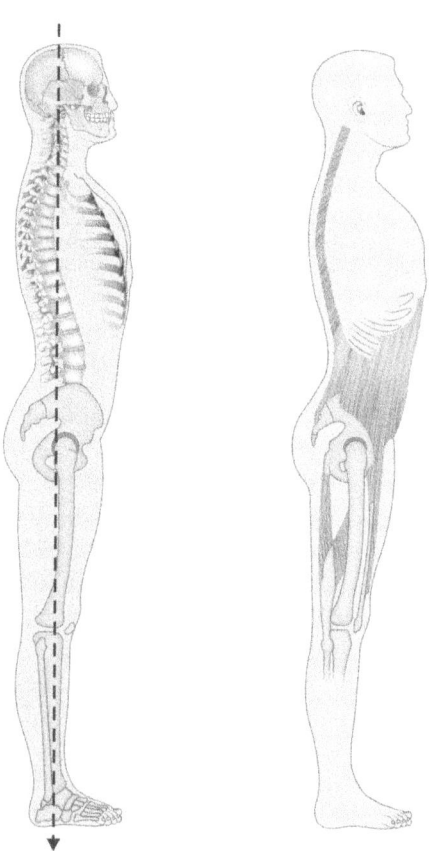

Fig. 13.38: Lordotic posture

Flat Back Posture

See **Figure 13.39**.

Head: Forward

Cervical spine: Slight extended

Thoracic spine: Upper part increased flexion, lower part straight

Lumbar spine: Flexed

Pelvis: Posterior tilt

Hip: Extended

Knee: Extended

Ankle: Slightly plantar flexed

Swayback Posture

See **Figure 13.40**.

Head: Forward

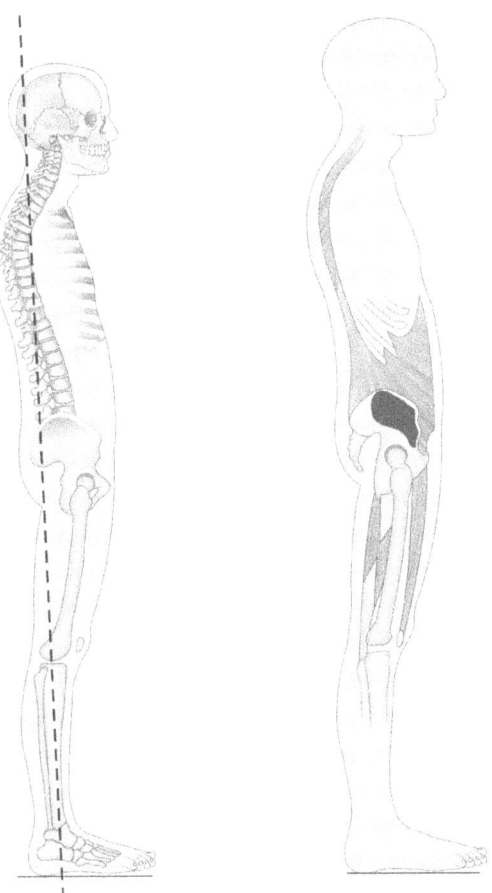

Fig. 13.40: Swayback posture

Cervical spine: Slight extended

Thoracic spine: Increased flexion with posterior displacement of the upper trunk

Lumbar spine: Flexion of the lower lumbar area

Pelvis: Posterior tilt

Hip: Hyperextended with anterior displacement of the pelvis

Knee: Hyperextended

Ankle: Neutral

Analysis of Standing Posture in Relation to Hip Joint

Sagittal Plane Alignment and Analysis

In optimal posture, the hip is in neutral position and the pelvis is at level and no

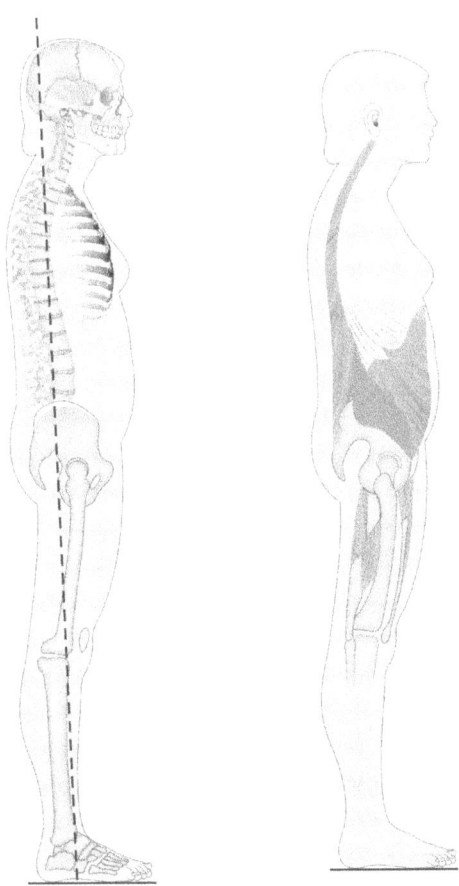

Fig. 13.39: Flat back posture

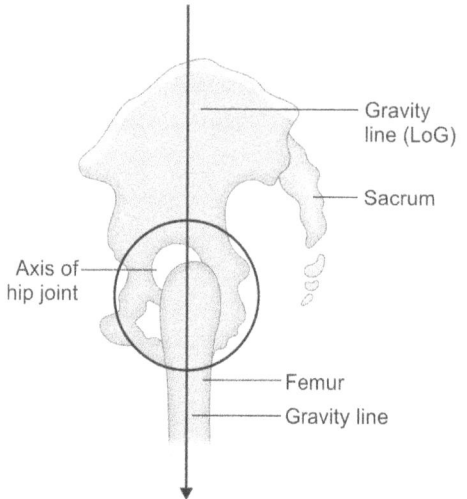

Fig. 13.41: LoG at hip joint

anterior or posterior tilt is observed. The LoG passes slightly posterior to the axis of the hip joint, and through the greater trochanter.

Thus, while postural sway, the LoG passes anterior to hip joint axis and the contraction of the hip to the exterior is required **(Fig. 13.41)**.

The location of gravitational force on the posterior side with respect to the hip joint axis produces an external torque causing extension moment at hip which tends to rotate the proximal segment of pelvis posteriorly on to the femoral heads.

When an EMG studies was taken, the iliopsoas muscle showed activity during standing, prevents hyperflexion via creating an internal flexion movement at the hip.

In swayback posture, the LoG drops farther behind the hip joint axes. Therefore, does not require any muscular activity at the hip therefore causing an increase in tension stress on anterior hip ligaments, which leads to adaptive lengthening of the same if posture tends to be habitual. Also, the gluteal muscles may be weakened by disuse atrophy due to reduced demand for hip extensor activity, if swayback posture is habituated. Different faults in posture are tabulated in **Table 13.1**.

MUSCULOSKELETAL CHANGES DURING PREGNANCY

Pregnancy is the period between conception to parturition, which lasts up to 40 weeks. It is calculated from the last menstrual period of a woman and is divided into three trimesters. During this phase of life, a woman's body

▲ Table 13.1: Types of postural fault

Postural fault	Anatomical position of joints	Muscles in shortened position	Muscles in lengthened position	Treatment
Forward head position	Cervical spine hyperextension	Cervical spine extensors, upper trapezius and levator	Cervical spine flexors	Stretch cervical spine extensors, strengthen cervical spine flexors, strengthen the thoracic spine extensors, deep breathing exe, stretch the pectoralis minor, shoulder adductor and internal rotators, strengthen middle and lower trapezius, stretch low back muscles, hip flexors, strengthen abdominals by posterior pelvic tilt, hip extensors
Kyphosis and depressed chest	Thoracic spine flexion, intercostals spaces diminished	Upper and lateral fibers of internal oblique, shoulder adductor, pectoralis minor, intercostals	Thoracic spine extensors, middle trapezius, lower trapezius	
Forward shoulders	Scapulae abducted and elevated	Serratus anterior, pectoralis minor, upper trapezius	Middle trapezius, lower trapezius	
Lordotic posture	Lumber spine hyperextension, pelvis anterior tilt, hip flexion	Lower back erector spinae, internal oblique, hip flexors	Abdominals especially external oblique, hip extensors	

Contd...

Contd...

Postural fault	Anatomical position of joints	Muscles in shortened position	Muscles in lengthened position	Treatment
Flat back posture	Lumbar spine flexion, pelvis posterior tilt, hip extension	Anterior abdominals, hip extensors	Lower back erector spinae, hip flexor	Strengthen lower back muscles, strengthen hip flexors to produce a normal anterior lumbar curve, stretch hamstrings
Swayback posture	Lumbar spine position depends on level of posterior displacement of upper trunk, pelvis posterior tilt, hip extension	Upper anterior abdominals, hip extensors	Lower anterior abdominals, hip flexor	Strengthen lower abdominals and hip flexors, wall standing exe, stretch hamstrings
Slight left C curve, thoracolumbar scoliosis	Thoracolumbar spine: lateral flexion, convex toward left	Right lateral trunk muscles	Left lateral trunk muscles	Stretch the right lateral trunk muscles, strengthen left lateral trunk muscles
Prominent or high right hip	Pelvis lateral tilt high on right, right hip adducted, left hip abducted	Right lateral trunk muscles, left hip abductor and tensor fascia lata, right hip adductor	Left lateral trunk muscles, right hip abductor, left hip adductor	Stretch the right lateral trunk muscles, strengthen the left lateral trunk muscles, stretch the left lateral thigh muscles and fascia, strengthen right gluteus medius
Hyperextended knee	Knee hyperextension, ankle plantar flexion	Quadriceps, soleus	Popliteus, hamstring	Overall posture correction, avoid hyperextension, short leg
Flexed knee	Knee flexion, ankle dorsiflexion	Popliteus, hamstrings	Quadriceps, soleus	Stretch knee flexor, stretch hip flexor is short
Medially rotated femur	Hip medial rotation	Hip medial rotator	Hip lateral rotator	Stretch the hip medial rotator strengthen the hip lateral rotator
Knock-knee	Hip adduction, knee abduction	Tensor fascia lata, lateral knee structure	Medial knee structures	Use inner wedge on heels if foot pronated, stretch tensor fascia lata
Bow legs	Hip medial rotation, knee hyperextension, foot pronation	Hip medial rotator, quadriceps, foot evertors	Hip lateral rotator, popliteus, tibialis posterior, long toe flexors	Perform exercises for overall correction of foot, knee and hip. Strengthen hip lateral rotators
Pronation	Foot eversion	Peroneals and toe extensors	Tibialis posterior, long toe flexor	Use inner wedge on heel, strengthen invertors
Supination	Foot inversion	Tibialis	Peroneals	Use outer wedge on heel, exercise to peroneals
Hammer toe and low metatarsals	MTP hyperextension, PIP flexion	Toe extensors	Lumbricals	Stretch MTP by flexion, stretch IP by extension, strengthen lumbricals by MTP flexion

undergoes multiple changes in various body systems, for accommodating and providing a suitable environment for the growing fetus.

The characteristic changes occurring are as follows:
- Increase in body weight
- Increase in circumference of breast and abdomen
- Remodeling of ligaments and other connective tissue
- Up to 2.5 cm descent of pelvic floor
- Stretching of abdominal muscles

We will now be discussing the anatomical, physical, musculoskeletal, and biomechanical changes occurring during pregnancy.

Anatomical and Physical Changes

- **Breast**
  - Enlarged
  - Tenderness—present
  - Nipples and areolas—darken
  - Glandular development
- **Uterus**
  - Expands in size, from 6.5 to 32 cm
  - Increase in weight, 20 times the original weight
  - Shape changes from oval to round
  - Placental development
  - Increase in vascular supply
  - Connective tissue surrounding it gets stretched
- **Abdomen**
  - Expands and drops due to fetus turning in downward position as trimesters pass
  - Hyperpigmentation of skin and linea alba
- Cervix is darkened and closed, during delivery dilates
- **Vagina**
  - Darkening of vagina and vulva
  - Softening of vaginal portion of cervix

Skeletal Changes

- Head position—more posterior as the pregnancy progresses from first to third trimester
- Protraction of shoulder girdle
- Increased thoracic kyphosis
- Increased lordotic curves at cervical and lumbar areas (by 5.9°) of vertebral column
- Exaggerated anterior pelvic tilt by 4°
- Hyperextension of knee
- Flattening of arches of foot

Muscular Changes

- Abdominal muscles get stretched, due to which its strength of contraction reduces, leading to mechanical disadvantage.
- Pelvic floor musculature descends down and gets stretched due to the growing weight of the fetus, increasing the risk of pelvic floor dysfunction.

Connective Tissue and Joint Changes

- Ligamentous tensile strength decreases with increase in relaxin and progesterone levels.
- Increase in contractile properties of thoracolumbar fascia resulting in decreased trunk stability
- Due to increase in laxity, joints and ligaments are predisposed to injury.

Biomechanical Changes

- **Location of CoG changes**
  - As the baby grows in size, the CoG shifts and the weight is distributed more anteriorly.
  - Forward pull of pelvis by gravity, due to increase in weight.
- **Wider BoS:** To compensate the positional changes and to maintain balance, the BoS increases.
- **Load:** The load on spine increases with increase in body weight.

Gait Alterations (Fig. 13.42)

- Waddling gait
- Increase in width of BoS while walking
- Decrease in step length and stride length
- Decreased single limb support time

- Increase in stance phase
- Increased cadence

Advantages

- To maintain balance
- To maintain CoM centered over BoS
- Protection and support
- Reduces strain during pregnancy

Clinical Applications

These body changes predispose a woman to developing the following conditions:
- Low back pain
- Neck pain
- Chest pain
- Leg pain/calf pain
- Pelvic girdle pain
- SI joint dysfunction
- Flat arches
- Nerve compression—sciatica and carpal tunnel syndrome

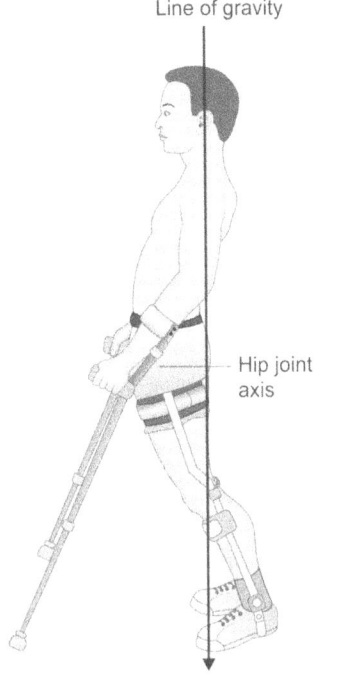

Fig. 13.42: LoG with crutch walking

CHAPTER 14

Gait

Chapter Outline

- Phases of gait cycle
- Parameters of gait
- Determinants of gait
- Kinematics of gait
- Kinetics of gait
- Gait analysis in relation to hip joint
- Pathological gait
- Treadmill gait
- Stair climbing gait
- Gait laboratory
- Gait analysis systems

INTRODUCTION

Gait

Gait is the human locomotion involving a series of rhythmical alternating movements of lower extremity resulting in forward propulsion of human body.

Gait Cycle

It is the cyclical pattern of gait, which constitutes from heel strike to the next heel strike of one foot. It is the unit of the gait.
- Continued repetition of this cycle results in gait.
- A typical gait cycle lasts for 1–2 seconds, depending on speed. The gait cycle is classified into (**Fig. 14.1**):
  - **Stance phase:** Heel strike
    - Foot flat
    - Midstance
    - Heel off
    - Toe off

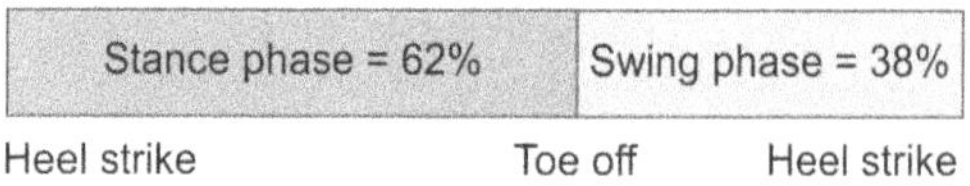

Stance phase = 62%	Swing phase = 38%
Heel strike Toe off	Heel strike

Fig. 14.1: Phases within a typical gait cycle

  - **Swing phase:** Acceleration
    - Mid-swing
    - Deceleration

Locomotion

The act or power of moving the body from place to place by means of one's own mechanisms or power. **Table 14.1** summarizes types of locomotion.

Table 14.1: Types of locomotion.

Types	Examples
On feet	• Walking (ambulation, level walking) • Race walking • Running • Ascending or descending ramp • Ascending or descending stairs • Jumping
On wheels	• Bicycling • Roller skating • Ice skating • Wheelchair propelling
On hands	• Walking on hands • Crutch walking • Stunts
On hands and knees	• Creeping • Crawling
On hands and feet	• Bear walking • Ropewalking
Rotary locomotion	• Cartwheels • Handsprings • Rolls

Ambulation

One type of locomotion which is characterized by moving the body on the level surface (**Fig. 14.2**).

STANCE PHASE

This is the support phase in which the limb under study is taking support from the ground (**Fig. 14.3**). This is further subclassified into five phases.

1. **Heel strike:** It is the first phase of the gait cycle where the gait is initiated by the heel of the foot touching the ground.
2. **Foot flat:** It is the phase of the gait cycle after the heel strike in which the foot is placed flat on the ground but without putting load on the limb.

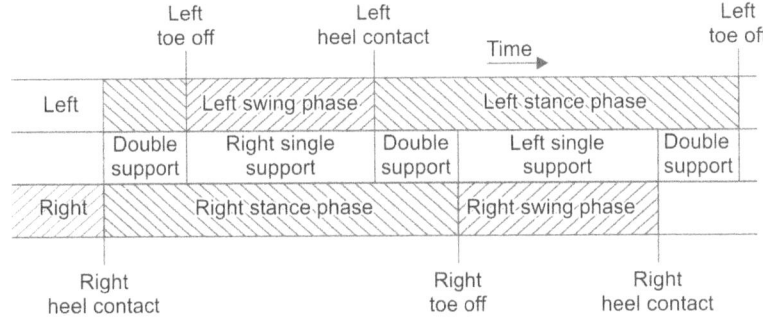

Fig. 14.2: Gait time duration

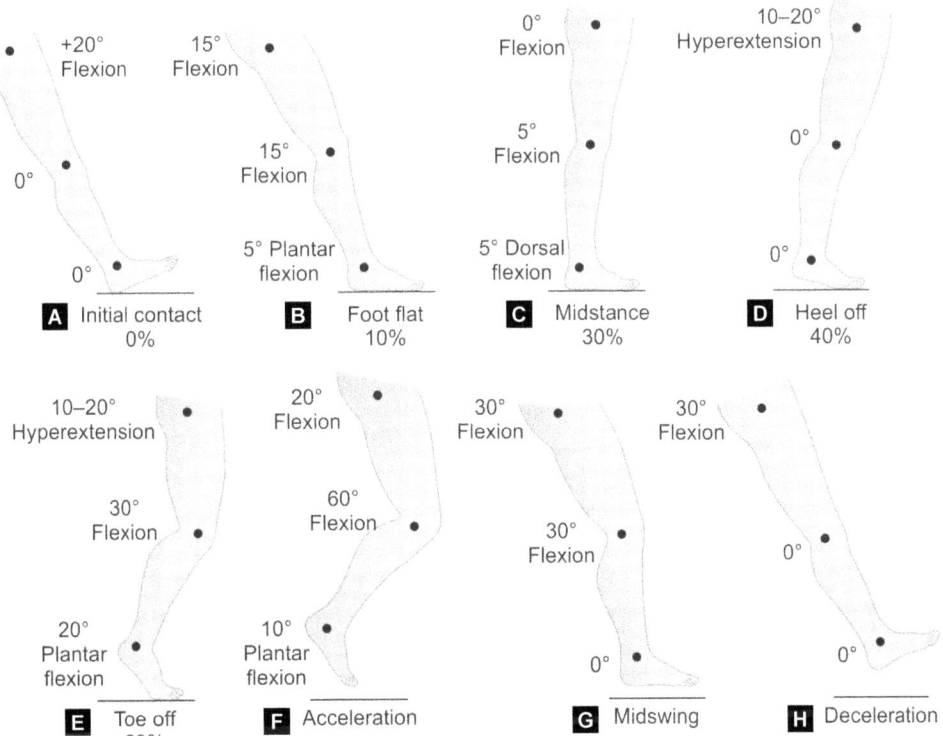

Fig. 14.3: Phases of gait

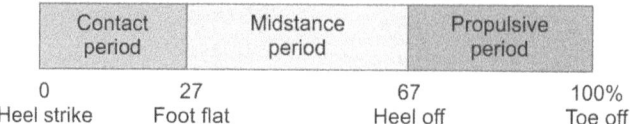

Fig. 14.4: Period within a typical stance phase

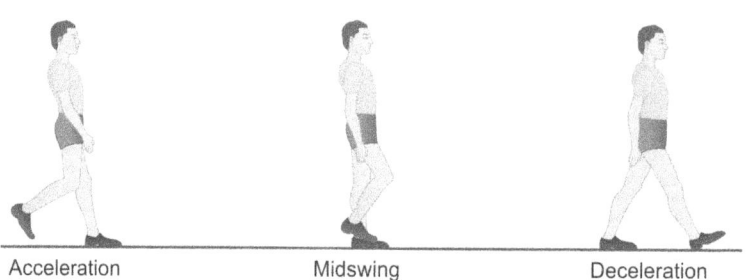

Fig. 14.5: Subdivisions of swing phase

3. **Midstance:** It is the phase of the gait cycle after foot flat in which the foot is placed flat on the ground and also loading the limb with body weight.
4. **Heel off:** It is the phase of the gait cycle after midstance in which the heel is taken off contact from the ground.
5. **Toe off:** It is the phase of the gait cycle after heel off in which the toe is taken off contact from the ground (**Fig. 14.3:A to E**).

Figure 14.4 shows period within a typical stance phase.

SWING PHASE

This is the recovery phase of the gait in which the limb under study is off the ground moving in the air getting ready for the next stance phase (**Fig. 14.3:F to H and Fig. 14.5**).
- **Acceleration:** This is also called as the early swing phase. It starts after the toe off phase in which the reference foot is in the air and accelerates forward toward mid-swing.
- **Mid-swing:** It is the phase after acceleration at the point where the reference leg is directly below the body and aligns with opposite side which is at midstance. The mid-swing leg is slightly flexed to clear the ground.
- **Deceleration:** It is also called as terminal swing phase. It is the phase after mid-swing in which the reference leg slows down to get ready to place the foot on the ground for heel strike.

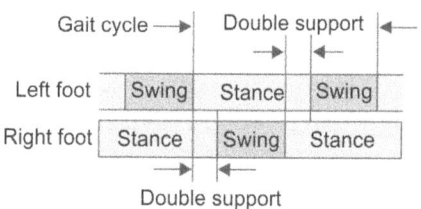

Fig. 14.6: Two double support phases within one gait cycle

Double Support Phase (Fig. 14.6)

It is the part of the stance phase which is characterized by both feet in contact with the ground simultaneously. Two double support periods during one gait cycle are seen.

About 22% of gait cycle constitutes double support.

Table 14.2 summarizes different terminology used to describe the gait cycle.

Table 14.2: Different terminology used to describe the gait cycle.

Phase	Traditional terminology	Rancho Los Amigos classification
Stance phase	Heel strike	Initial contact
	Foot flat	Loading response
	Midstance	Midstance
	Heel off	Terminal stance
	Toe off	Preswing
Swing phase	Acceleration	Initial swing
	Midswing	Midswing
	Deceleration	Terminal swing

PARAMETERS THAT DESCRIBE GAIT PATTERNS

Temporal (Time) Parameters

Parameter	SI unit	Definition	Significance
Stride time	Sec	The duration for the completion of a full gait cycle	Slightly > 1 sec
Step time	Sec	The duration for the completion of a right or left step	= the reciprocal of cadence for a symmetric gait
Stance time	Sec %	The duration when the foot is on the ground during one gait cycle	62% of one gait cycle
Single support time	Sec %	The duration when only one foot is on the ground during one gait cycle	
Double support time	Sec %	The duration when both feet are in contact with the ground simultaneously during one gait cycle	~22% of one gait cycle ↓ as walking speed ↑↑ in the elderly ↑ in patients with balanced disorders
Swing time	Sec %	The duration when the foot is in the air during one gait cycle	38% of one gait cycle ↓ as walking speed ↑

Spatial (Distance) Parameters

Parameter	SI unit	Definition	Significance
Stride length (Fig. 14.7)	cm	Distance between 2 successive heel contacts of the same foot	↓ in the elderly ↑ as ↑ walking speed
Step length (Fig. 14.7)	cm	Distance between 2 successive heel contacts of the opposite feet	
Step width/base	cm	Lateral distance between both heel centers of 2 consecutive foot contacts	7–9 cm in healthy adults
Foot angle (degree of toe-out)	Degree	Angle between the line of progression of the body and the longitudinal axis of the foot	7° in healthy adults

Speed Parameters (Fig. 14.8)

Parameter	SI unit	Definition	Significance
Cadence (step rate)	Number of steps	Number of steps per minute	Comfortable speed: 80–110 steps/min
			Slow speed: <70 steps/min
			Fast speed: >120 steps/min
Walking speed	m/s mph (m/h)	Distance per unit of time	↑ speed → ↓ in duration of all the component phases, especially double support phase
			↑ as cadence ↑, stride length ↑, or both
			↓ as angle of toe out ↓ or limb length ↑

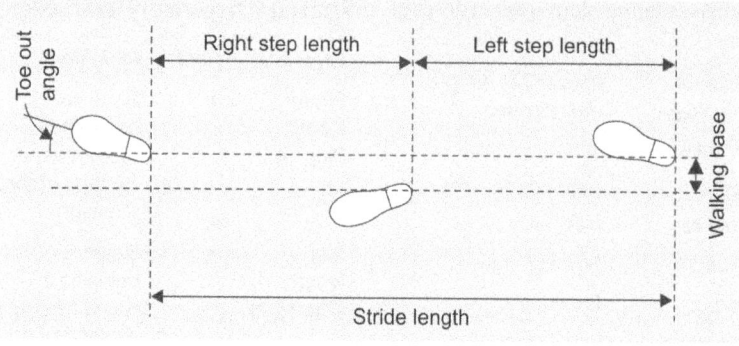

Fig. 14.7: Spatial parameters

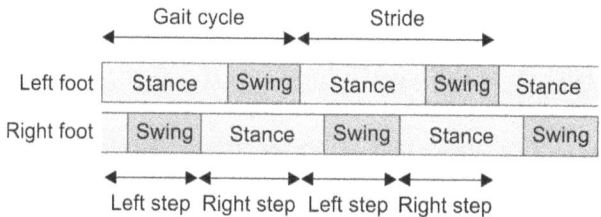

Fig. 14.8: Stride versus step. (1 stride = 1 gait cycle = 2 steps)

Average Values

	Male	Female	Total
Cadence (step/min)	105–125	100–120	113
Speed (m/min)	86	77	82
Speed (km/h)	5.2	4.6	4.9
Stride length (m)	1.46	1.28	1.41

Control of the Body COM

Walking and balance control

- **Walking** = a series of losses and recoveries of balance
  - Initially, the body leans forward to the limit of stability.
  - Momentary recovery of balance is achieved by placing one foot to a new position.
  - Forward progression is achieved by alternating relocation of the foot.
- **Requirement of walking balance**
  - *Efficiency:* Time consuming
  - *Effectiveness:* Minimum effort and minimum fatigue
  - *Safety:* Prevention from falls and associated injuries

Displacement of body COM during ambulation (Fig. 14.9)

- **COM:** The point in a body about which all the parts exactly balance each other
  - All the linear forces acting on the body are balanced, i.e., $\Sigma F = 0$
  - All the rotary forces acting on the body are balanced, i.e., $\Sigma M = 0$
- **Sinosoid pattern of movement in the sagittal plane:** 2 full sine waves
  - *Minimum height of COM:* At the midpoint of double support (5% and 55% of gait cycle)

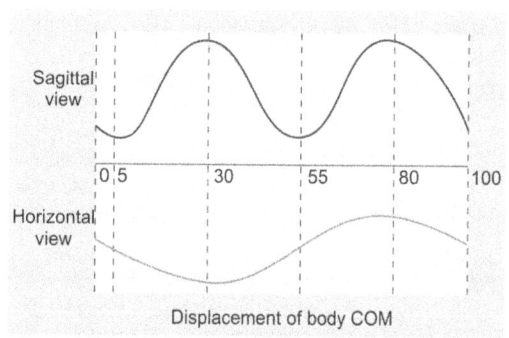

Fig. 14.9: Displacement of body COM during ambulation

- *Maximum height of COM:* At the midpoint of single-leg support (30% and 80% of gait cycle)
- *Total excursion:* 5 cm at the average walking speed
- Displacement depending on the stride length and speed of walking
- **Sinosoid pattern of movement in the transverse plane:** A single full sine wave
  - *Minimum right position of COM:* At the midpoint of stance phase of the right limb (30% of gait cycle as right foot initiates the gait)
  - *Maximum left position of COM:* At the midpoint of stance phase of the left limb (80% of gait cycle as the right foot initiates the gait)
  - *Total excursion:* 4 cm at the average walking speed
  - Displacement depending on the base of support of walking

DETERMINANTS OF GAIT CYCLE DURING AMBULATION

1. Lateral pelvic tilt
2. Pelvic rotation in transverse plane
3. Knee flexion in stance
4. Hip flexion
5. Interaction of knee, ankle and foot
6. Physiologic valgus at knee

The determinants are to accommodate:
- Vertical displacement of center of gravity (COG)
- Lateral displacement of COG

Lateral Pelvic Tilt in the Frontal Plane

Lateral tilt to the swing leg during the stance phase. This is to lower down the COG of the body in order to decrease energy expenditure. This stretches the hip abductors of the stance leg in order to facilitate their contraction and to increase their strength. It is controlled by hip abductors of the stance leg. The amount of pelvic tilt is about 8°.

Pelvic Rotation in Sagittal Plane (Fig. 14.10)

This is to minimize the motion of the COG. During normal walking the pelvis rotates toward the weight bearing side.
- **Pelvis:** 10–15°
- **Femur:** 14°
- **Tibia:** 20°
- **Foot:** 6–8° of pronation and 6–8° of supination

Knee Flexion in the Sagittal Plane (Fig. 14.11)

- 10–15° of knee flexion occurs during the first 15% of gait cycle in order to absorb the impact from ground reaction force (GRF). Maximum knee flexion of 60–70° occurs at the beginning of midswing (73% of gait cycle).
- Two times knee extension takes place during the stance phase. Knee extension at heel strikes. Knee extension again during the midstance period.

Hip Flexion in the Sagittal Plane (Fig. 14.12)

30° of hip flexion during initial contact period to lower the COG. Hip flexion again during swing phases, reaching maximum hip flexion prior to heel contact.

Interactions of the Knee, Ankle, and Foot (Fig. 14.13)

- During walking the ankle and foot acts as a rocker bottom along with knee. It acts like a chain with coordinated movement to accommodate COG.

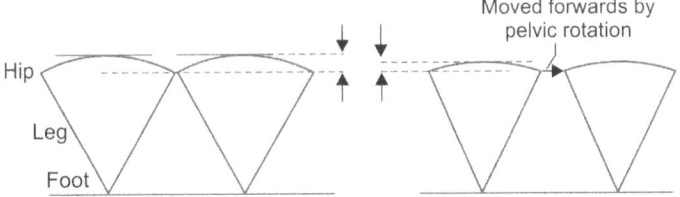

Fig. 14.10: Pelvic motion in saggital plane

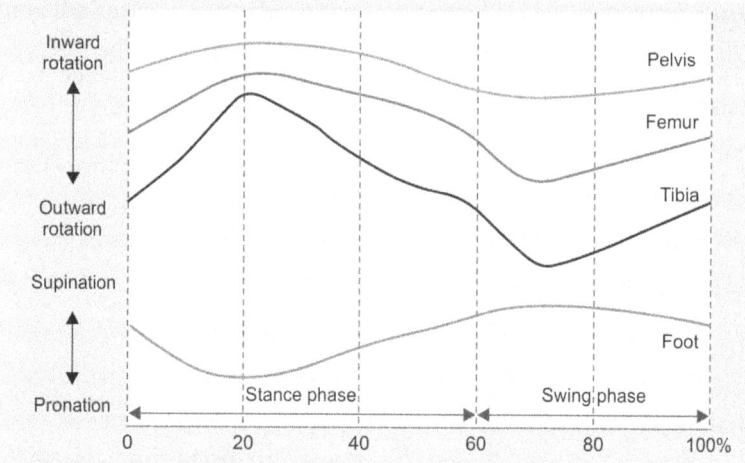

Fig. 14.11: Transverse rotation of lower extremity during one gait cycle

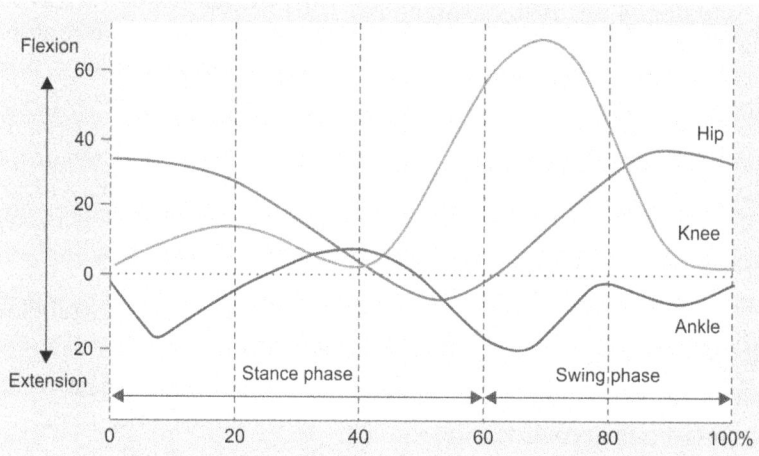

Fig. 14.12: Sagittal plane motion of lower extremity during one gait cycle

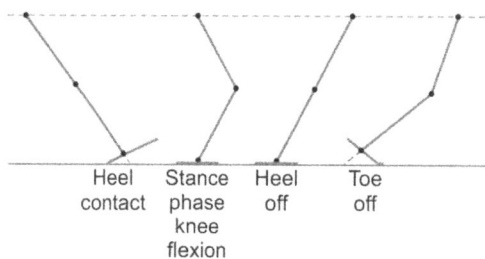

Fig. 14.13: Interactions of the knee, ankle and foot

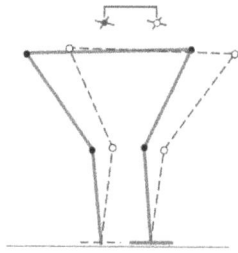

Fig. 14.14: Physiological valgus at the knee

- **Heel strike to foot flat:** Knee flexion, ankle plantarflexion, and foot pronation.
- **Midstance to toe off:** Knee extension, ankle plantarflexion, and foot supination.

Physiological Valgus of the Knee (Fig. 14.14)

In general, there is normal physiologic valgus at knee. This is to decrease the lateral motion of the COG.

KINEMATICS OF GAIT (FIG. 14.15)

Stance Phase

Kinematics of Heel Strike

Trunk	Neutral
Pelvis	5° rotation
Hip	30° flexion
Knee	Neutral
Ankle and foot	Neutral

Kinematics of Foot Flat

Trunk	Neutral
Pelvis	Neutral
Hip	20° flexion
Knee	20° flexion
Ankle and foot	15° plantarflexion

Kinematics of Midstance

Trunk	Neutral
Pelvis	5° pelvic tilt
Hip	Neutral
Knee	Slight flexion
Ankle and foot	10° dorsiflexion

Kinematics of Heel off

Trunk	Neutral
Pelvis	5° posterior rotation
Hip	10° extension
Knee	Neutral
Ankle	15° dorsiflexion
MTP	30° extension
IP	Neutral

Kinematics of Toe off

Trunk	Neutral
Pelvis	5° posterior rotation
Hip	15° extension
Knee	40° flexion
Ankle	20° plantarflexion
MTP	60° extension
IP	Neutral

Swing Phase

Kinematics of Acceleration

Trunk	Neutral
Pelvis	Neutral
Hip	20° flexion
Knee	60° flexion
Ankle and foot	Neutral

Kinematics of Mid-swing

Trunk	Neutral
Pelvis	5° pelvic tilt
Hip	30° flexion
Knee	30° flexion
Ankle and foot	Slight dorsiflexion

Kinematics of Deceleration

Trunk	Neutral
Pelvis	5° anterior rotation
Hip	30° flexion
Knee	Extension
Ankle and foot	Neutral

KINETICS OF GAIT

Stance Phase

Kinetics of Heel Strike

Hip	• GRF passes anterior to the joint • Eccentric contraction of gluteus maximus
Knee	• GRF passes anterior to joint axis • Eccentric contraction of quadriceps femoris
Ankle	• GRF passes slightly posterior to joint axis • Eccentric contraction of tibialis anterior, extensor halucis longus, extensor digitorum longus

Kinetics of Foot Flat

Hip	• GRF passes anterior to joint axis • Eccentric contraction of gluteus maximus
Knee	• GRF passes posterior to joint axis • Eccentric contraction of quadriceps femoris
Ankle	• GRF passes posterior to joint axis • Change up phase from eccentric contraction dorsiflexors to eccentric contraction of plantarflexors (gastrosoleus)

Kinetics of Midstance

Hip	• GRF passes posterior to the joint axis • Concentric contraction of gluteus maximus
Knee	• GRF passes anterior to the joint axis • Concentric contraction of quadriceps • Eccentric contraction of hamstrings
Ankle	• GRF passes anterior to the joint axis • Eccentric contraction of gastrosoleus

Kinetics of Heel off

Hip	• GRF passes posterior to the joint axis • Eccentric contraction of iliopsoas
Knee	• GRF passes anterior to the joint axis • Eccentric contraction of hamstrings
Ankle	• GRF passes anterior to the joint axis • Concentric contraction of gastrosoleus

Kinetics of Toe off

Hip	• GRF passes posterior to the joint axis • Change up phase from eccentric contraction of iliopsoas to concentric contraction of iliopsoas
Knee	• GRF passes posterior to the joint axis • Eccentric contraction of hamstrings
Ankle	• GRF passes anterior to the joint axis • Concentric contraction of gastrosoleus

Swing Phase

Kinetics of Acceleration

Hip	Concentric contraction of iliopsoas, sartorius, tensor fascia lata
Knee	Co-contraction of quadriceps and hamstrings
Ankle	Concentric contraction of dorsiflexors

Kinetics of Mid-swing

Hip	• Concentric contraction of iliopsoas • Eccentric contraction of hamstrings
Knee	• Concentric contraction of quadriceps • Eccentric contraction of hamstrings
Ankle	Isometric contraction of dorsifexors

Kinetics of Deceleration

Hip	Eccentric contraction of gluteus maximus
Knee	Eccentric contraction of hamstrings
Ankle	Isometric contraction of dorsiflexors

GAIT ANALYSIS IN RELATION TO HIP JOINT

Sagittal Plane Kinematics

At a typical walking speed, the hip is flexed approximately 30° at heel contact. Maximum hip extension of approximately 10° is achieved before toe off. Flexion of the hip is initiated during preswing phase, the hip further flexes to bring the lower extremity forward for the next foot placement. Maximal hip flexion (slightly more than 30°) is achieved just before heel contact.

Individuals with limited sagittal plane hip mobility, walk with movement at the pelvis, and lumbar spine without obvious gait deviation. Apparent hip extension can be achieved through anterior tilt, apparent hip flexion is achieved by posterior pelvic tilt.

Frontal Plane Kinematics

The pattern of elevation and depression of the iliac crests reflects the frontal plane motion of the hips. Excessive frontal plane movement is quite common, causing exaggerated medial-lateral shifts in the center of mass. It can be either in form of drop of contralateral iliac crest or hiking of the swing extremity.

Horizontal Plane Kinematics

Both femur and pelvis rotate simultaneously. At right heel contact, the right hip is in slight external rotation based on the relative posterior position of the contralateral ASIS (left). A net internal rotation movement of the right hip occurs during most stance on the right lower extremity, as contralateral ASIS brought forward.

Hip Muscle Activity During Gait

Hip Extensors (Fig. 14.16)

Activation of gluteus maximus begins at terminal swing. So at heel contact the gluteus maximus is already activated to extend the hip and prevent uncontrolled trunk flexion over the femur. It remains active from heel contact to midstance. During the

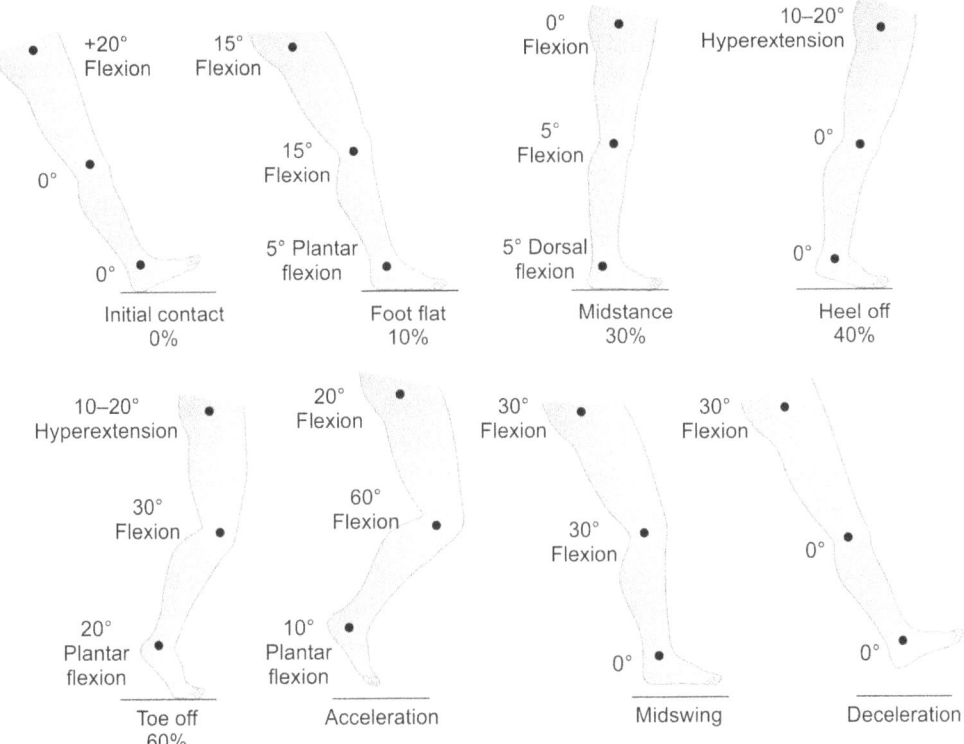

Fig. 14.15: Kinetic of gait cycle

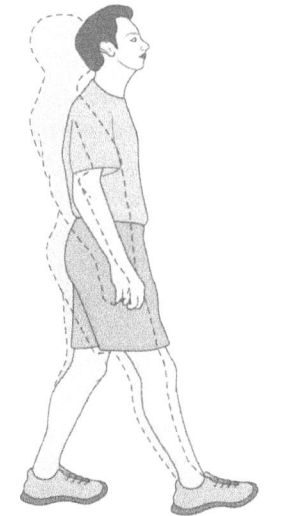

Fig. 14.16: Weakness of gluteus maximus

swing phase, the gluteus maximus is largely inactive until terminal swing, when a modest activation is needed to first decelerate the flexing hip and then initiates its extension. The hamstrings are active during the first 10% of the gait cycle.

Hip Flexors

The illipsoas becomes active well before toe off and remains so through initial swing. The activation at between 30% and 50% of the gait cycle is likely initially eccentric as the hip is extending at that time, followed by a concentric action to initiate hip flexion just before toe off. Despite the continued hip flexion into terminal swing, the hip flexors are active only in the first 50% of the swing phase. The second half of the swing phase is a result of the forward momentum that the thigh gains in initial swing.

Clinical relevance: In patient with weakness of hip flexors, the trunk will lean backward during swing phase of the affected limb, to propel the affected limb forward.

Hip Abductors

Hip abductors stabilize the pelvis in the frontal plane. The gluteus medius is active toward the very end of the swing phase in preparation for heel contact. The gluteus medius and minimus are most active during the first 40% of the gait, especially during single limb support. The hip abductors also control the alignment of the femur in the frontal plane. Inadequate muscular activation may result in excessive adduction of the femur, causing poor alignment of the lower extremity and excessive valgus torque at the knee during the stance phase.

Hip abductor weakness: Hip abductor weakness will not lead to any change of the alignment in bilateral stance.

Weakness of hip abductor manifests into the stance phase of the affected side, i.e., unilateral stance. As the single limb support begins and the abductors muscles are too weak to hold the pelvis level, the HAT-L weight tends to cause the pelvis to drop on the unsupported side. Because this is a very unstable phenomenon and puts subject at risk of falling, most subjects use a typical substitution. To avoid pelvic drop on the unsupported side, the subject leans the trunk the supporting side. This lean moves the center of mass of the HAT-L weight to the lateral aspect of the hip joint on the stance side. In this position weight of the HAT-L no longer tends to adduct the hip. In fact weight creates a slight abduction moment, thus eliminating the need for active abduction force. The resulting pattern of gait is known as gluteus medius limp.

Hip Adductors and Hip Rotators

The hip adductors show two bursts of activity during gait.

The first burst occurs at heel contact, which serves to stabilize the hip through coactivation with the hip extensors and hip adductors. The second occurs just after toe off, likely assists with initiating hip flexion.

Effect of weakness of adductors: Hip adductor weakness is not common but may result from an injury to obturator nerve. It leads to gait instability and abducted gait in which the affected limb contacts the ground with excessively abducted hip.

Effect of tightness of adductors: It is common. Extreme tightness of adductors leads to scissor gait. During swing, the limb with the tightness may have difficulty passing the stance limb. The limb with tightness also may land in front of the opposite limb at beginning of double limb support, again presenting a threat of tripping.

The hip internal rotators are active throughout much of the stance phase. They move the contralateral side of the pelvis forward in the horizontal plane.

The hip external rotators control pelvic rotation while lower limb is fixed to the ground, in conjunction with external rotators. Eccentric activation of the lower limb be especially important to control internal rotation of the lower limb in early stance.

PATHOLOGICAL GAIT

Common pathological gait:
1. **Antalgic gait (painful hip gait):** It is the gait assumed by the person when there is severe pain at one of the hip joint. It is also called as painful hip gait. It is characterized by longer stance phase of painless leg and shorter stance of painful leg. This is because since the leg is painful, the person tends to put least possible pressure and least possible time weight bearing on the painful leg.
2. **Stiff hip gait:** When one of the hip joints has become stiff due to various reasons, this type of gait is seen. In this the person is unable to flex the hip. Thus to clear the ground the person elevates the pelvis, abducts the hip, and propels forward to walk. It is nothing but the circumductory motion of the hip joint since. This gait is also called as circumduction gait.

3. **Trendelenburg gait:** When a person has weak or paralyzed gluteus medius, this type of gait is seen. In this gait, during stance phase there is pelvic drop on the opposite side. This is because the weak gluteus medius fails to hold the pelvis in its position when one leg is in the air and drops toward that side. This gait can be unilateral where there is only one side pelvic drop or bilateral where there is pelvic drop on both the sides alternatively as the gait progresses.
4. **Gluteus medius gait:** This is a Trendelenburg positive gait. In this also there is weakness or paralysis of gluteus medius. The difference is, to compensate for the weak gluteus medius which is unable to hold the pelvis, to maintain the COG, the person bends laterally opposite to that of the pelvic drop (same side of the stance leg).
5. **Waddling gait:** Bilateral weakness of the gluteus medius of results is bilateral lateral bending alternatively as the person walks. This gait looks like the walk of a duck. Thus it is also called as waddling gait or duck walking gait.
6. **Gluteus maximus gait:** This is seen when gluteus maximus is weak or paralyzed. A classical gait pattern resulting from gluteus maximus weakness is known as gluteus medius lurch. The lurch is a rapid hyperextension of the trunk prior to and continue through, heel contact on the side of the gluteus maximus weakness. Backward lurch moves the center of mass of the HAT weight to a position posterior to the hip joint, thus eliminating the need for the gluteus maximus to extend the hip. It is commonly seen in poliomyelitis cases.
7. **Quadriceps gait:** This gait is seen when quadriceps muscle is paralyzed. This is also seen in poliomyelitis cases. In this gait, since the quadriceps is not acting, the person pushes the knee into extension and locks with the help of the hand. He/she uses this position as a stabilizer and moves forward. It is also called as hand-on-knee gait.
8. **High stepping gait:** This gait is seen when there is foot drop deformity. In this since the dorsiflexors are not acting there is no heel strike. To place the foot on the ground the person lifts the leg high enough to clear the ground and slaps the foot onto the ground to move forward.
9. **Short leg gait:** When one leg is shorter than the other this type of gait is seen. This gait is only noticeable only when the difference in the leg length is more than 2 inches.
10. **Scissoring gait:** It is the common deformity seen in the cerebral palsy cases. It is characterized by bilateral hip adductor tightness. This results in excessive hip adduction each time the leg is taken forward. Bilateral movement of such pattern of crisscrossing looks like the action of a scissor. Thus it is also called as scissoring gait.
11. **Toe walking gait:** In this the person walks on the toes. This gait is commonly seen in diplegic cerebral palsy cases. In this the gastropsoleus is spastic and does not yield. The ankle is fixed in ankle dorsiflexion.
12. **Hemiplegic gait:** This gait is seen in hemiplegic cases. In hemiplegia due to the spasticity of hip flexors, adductors and knee flexors, the resultant gait pattern is that of the person is not totally erect, hips in flexion and adduction, ankles are everted, knee flexed. The person takes the steps as much range as is available.
13. **Parkinson's gait (Fig. 14.17):** This gait is seen in parkinsonism. This gait is characterized by short and quick steps. In this the person first the upper body and reluctant to move the legs. After moving the upper body to maintain the COG and avoid falling he takes a short step and again moves the upper body. These cyclical movements look like the person is hurrying up, but is actually afraid of falling and wants to cover the COG during the task of walking.

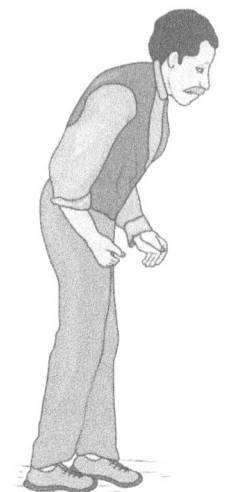

Fig. 14.17: Parkinson's gait

TREADMILL GAIT

Treadmill gait is similar to the normal over ground gait. The difference is the assistance provided from the treadmill to the person. Because of this assistance, the cadence is higher, the stride is longer. The person can put more effort in this gait. The treadmill also helps in reduced push off force from the person and also reduced GRF.

STAIR CLIMBING GAIT (FIGS. 14.18 AND 14.19)

It is the forward propulsion of human body with graded increase/decrease in height at every step.

The stair gait is the opposite to that of the treadmill gait. In this the person has to put more effort than the normal over ground gait. Broadly it is:
- Ascending stair gait
- Descending stair gait

Types of stair climbing
1. **Step over step**

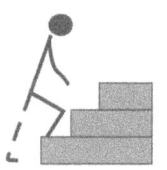 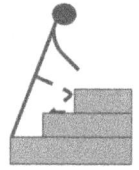 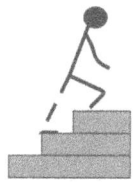

2. **Step by step**

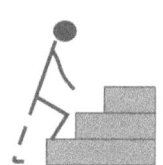 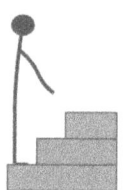 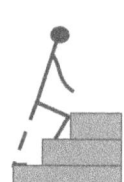

Irrespective whether it is ascending or descending, the gait is classified into the following phases:
- **Stance phase:**
  - **Weight acceptance (14%):** This is the first phase of stair climbing. In this the person puts the leg on the step higher or lower depending on whether it is the ascending stair or descending stair. After placing the leg on the step, the person may take the support of the railing by holding onto it.
  - **Pull up (14–32%):** In this phase the person pushes the step and pulls himself up (ascending stair) for forward continuance. In descending the person

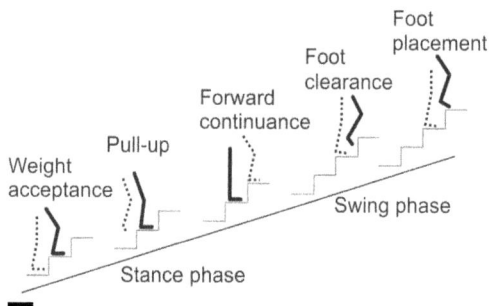

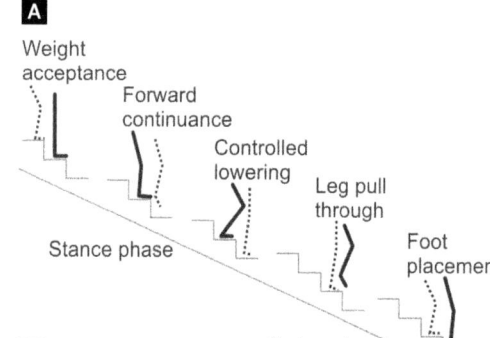

Figs. 14.18A and B: Phases during stair ascend and stair descend

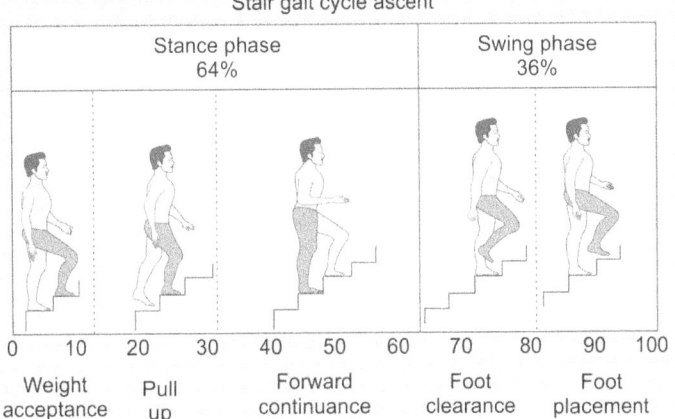

Fig. 14.19: Stair gait cycle

lets the eccentric contract of muscles control the forward propulsion of the body due to gravity.

- **Forward continuance (32–64%):** This is the end phase of the stance phase in which the body propels forward for the weight acceptance of the other leg.
- **Swing phase:**
  - **Foot clearance:** After the other leg has gone for weight acceptance, the reference leg clears the contact surface and is in the air.
  - **Foot placement:** This is the final phase of the stair gait cycle in which the reference leg gets ready for the next weight acceptance phase. During this phase the other leg is in forward continuance phase.
- **Types of stair climbing**

Kinematics and Kinetics

See **Tables 14.3 to 14.5**.

GAIT LABORATORY

Gait laboratories are the place wherein the individual gait examination is made with the help of complex computerized equipment.

As technological advances become more sophisticated and affordable, detailed biomechanical analyses of gait increasing can be performed in clinical setting.

Gait laboratories consist of a walkway which is 21.5 m long and 3 m in width.

The stride analyzer, which is one of the most recent advances in technology may occupy the latest gait laboratories to analyze the stride characteristics. There may be

◢ **Table 14.3:** Stance phase: Weight acceptance and through pull up.

Joint	Motion	Muscle	Contraction
Hip	Extension: 60 to 30 of flexion	• Gluteus maximus • Semitendinosus • Gluteus medius	Concentric
Knee	Extension: 80 to 35 of flexion	• Vastus lateralis • Rectus femoris	Concentric
Ankle	Dorsiflexion: 20 to 25 of DF	Tibialis anterior	Concentric
	Plantarflexion: 25 to 15 of DF	• Soleus • Gastrocnemius	Concentric

◢ **Table 14.4:** Stance phase: Pull up through forward continuance.

Joint	Motion	Muscle	Contraction
Hip	Extension: 30 to 5 of flexion	• Gluteus maximus • Semitendinosus • Gluteus medius	Concentric and isometric
	Flexion: 5 to 10–20 of flexion	• Gluteus maximus • Gluteus medius	Eccentric
Knee	Extension: 35 to 10 of flexion	• Vastus lateralis • Rectus femoris	Concentric
	Flexion: 5 to 10–20 flexion	• Vastus lateralis • Rectus femoris	Eccentric
Ankle	Plantarflexion: 15 of DF to 15 to 10 of PF	• Tibialis anterior	Eccentric
		• Soleus • Gastrocnemius	Concentric

◢ **Table 14.5:** Swing phase: Foot clearance through foot placement.

Joint	Motion	Muscle	Contraction
Hip	Flexion: 10–20 to 40–60 of flexion	Gluteus maximus	Concentric
	Extension: 40–60 flexion to 50 flexion		
Knee	Flexion: 10 of flexion to 90–100 of flexion	Semitendinosus	Concentric
	Extension: 90–100 of flexion to 85 of flexion	• Vastus lateralis • Rectus femoris	Concentric
Ankle	Dorsiflexion: 10 of PF to 20 DF		Concentric and isometric

electrogoniometers, dynamic EMG, and other equipment.

The walkway is surrounded by 6–8 cameras which gives the 3-D image of the subject.

There are infrared active markers which are attached to the subject's body at the specific landmark and then the subject is made to walk.

The subject is made to walk on force plate which senses the center of pressure and weight bearing points and the GRF.

GAIT ANALYSIS SYSTEMS

Gait analysis is the quantification and interpretation of human locomotion. The complexity of walking becomes very apparent as soon as one considers either referring a patient for objective analysis or establishing your own gait laboratory **(Figs. 14.20 and 14.21)**.

The gait may reflect compensations for underlying pathologies, or be responsible for causation of symptoms in itself. Aside from clinical applications, gait analysis is widely used in professional, sports training to optimize, and improve athletic performance.

Techniques Employed

- **Motion analysis system:** Defines the magnitude and timing of individual joint action.
- **Dynamic EMG:** Identifies the period and relative intensity of muscle function.
- **Force plate recordings:** Displays the functional demands being experienced during weight bearing.
- **GRF and vector analysis**
- **Stride characteristics:** To determine overall walking capability.
- **Energy cost measurement:** To determine the efficiency during walking.

Analysis of Systemic Gait

Systematic gait analysis involves mainly three steps:

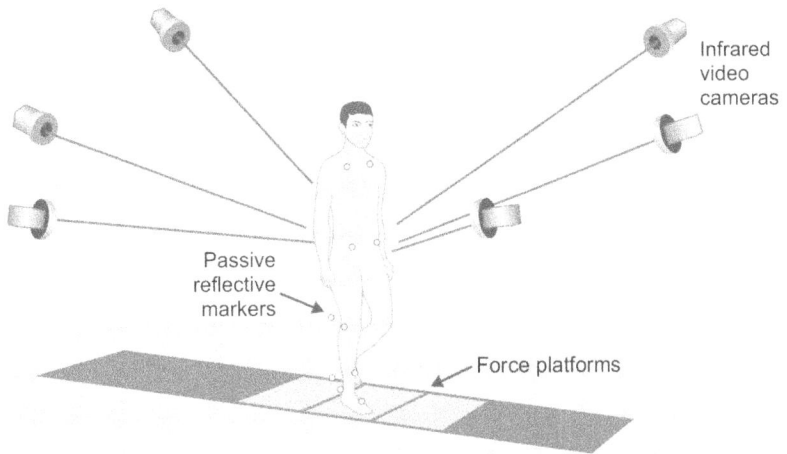

Fig. 14.20: Gait analysis using passive reflective markers, force platforms and infrared video cameras

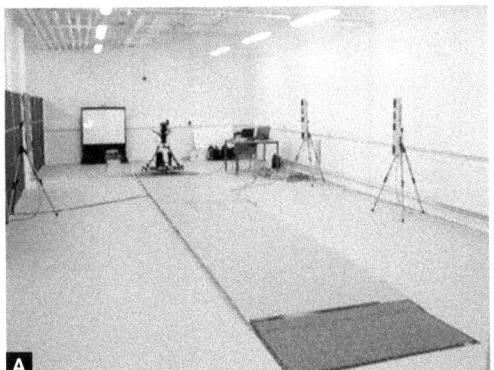
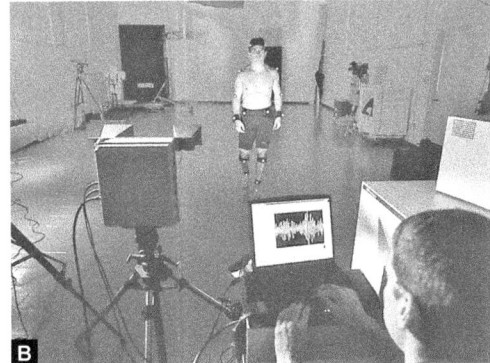

Figs. 14.21A and B: Gait laboratory

1. **Information organization:** Where the various information like age, height, weight, and BMI of the patient is collected.
2. **Data acquisition:** In which, first a gross review to sense the flow of action, and then the analysis should follow an anatomical sequence in order to sort the multiple events.
3. **Data interpretation:** Wherein the data formed on the computer is being interpreted and suspected conclusions made.

Motion Analysis System
(Figs. 14.22 and 14.23)

All motion quantification system depends on defining arcs and positions of individual joint numerically.

There are certain infrared markers which are placed on the joint axis of various joints that accurately represent the actions of the joints. And these markers are recorded by cameras and their locations translated into motion data by complex computer programs.

Dynamic EMG

With appropriate instrumentations, myoelectrical signals can be recorded and analyzed to determine the timing and relative intensity of the muscle effort. There are surface EMG electrodes available, which are connected to the computer via an infrared device.

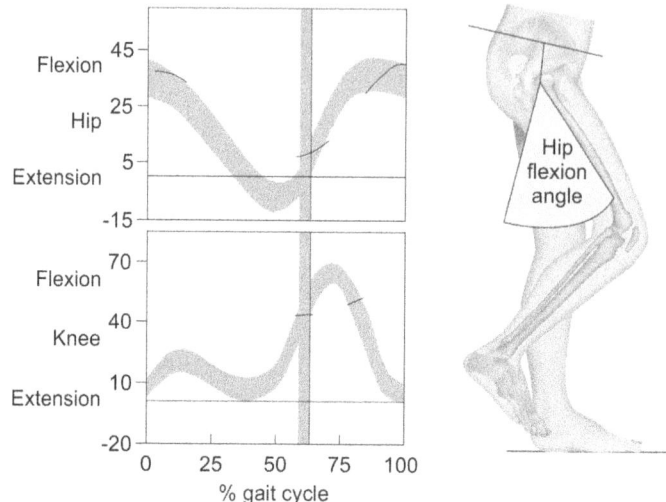

Fig. 14.22: Hip flexion range during gait analysis

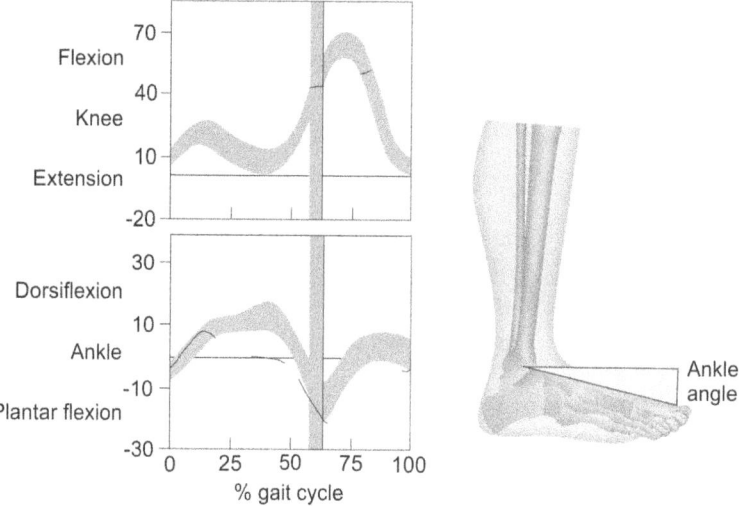

Fig. 14.23: Ankle range during gait analysis

The EMG recordings show the activity of the muscle during gait cycle, irrespective of the concentric or eccentric work done.
Muscle work is mainly done to:
- Provide a support moment through the stance phase, which is provided mainly by antigravity muscles.
- Generate energy to move.

There are two type of dynamic EMG recording, viz., surface EMG and wire EMG

Interval	Joint	Position	Muscle activity
Acceleration to heel strike	Hip	Flexed	Gluteus maximus hamstring, gluteus medius and minimus
	Knee	Flexed	Quadriceps femoris
	Ankle	Neutral	Anterior crural muscles

Contd...

Contd...

Interval	Joint	Position	Muscle activity
Heel strike to midstance	Hip	Neutral	Gluteus medius and minimus
	Knee	Extended	Quadriceps femoris
	Ankle	Dorsiflexed	Gastrocnemius; soleus
	Tarsal	Inverted	• Tibialis anterior • Tibialis posterior
Midstance to toe off	Hip	Extended	–
	Knee	Flexed	Gastrocnemius
	Ankle	Plantar	Gastrocnemius; soleus
	Tarsal	Everted	• Fibularis longus • Fibularis brevis

GRF and Vector Analysis

We all are aware about Newton's third law, i.e., for every action force there is an equal and opposite reaction force. The same applies here, when the foot strikes the ground, an equal and opposite force is applied by the ground onto the foot, this force is termed as ground reaction force (GRF).

GRF are described by using a coordinate system with forces expressed along vertical, anteroposterior, and mediolateral axes. The vector sum of the force components in each direction is a single expression of the GRF known as GRF vector (GRFV), which has typical pattern from initial contact to toe off.

GRFV combines both gravity effect on the body and the effects of the body's movement and acceleration in three planes of reference. This makes the GRFV especially suitable for the study of gait, during which the body's various masses undergo complex accelerations.

The point on the foot where GRF applies is known as Center of Pressure (CoP).

GRF cannot be viewed with the naked eyes, but nowadays with the technological advancement, there are certain cameras being invented which shows the GRFV on the computer screen with the help of force plate recordings.

Force plates are placed on the walkway on which the patients has to walk, so the information regarding the CoP and GRF can be obtained. Also it helps to get information regarding moments.

Moments

If a force is applied at a distance from the center of an axis of rotation or a joint center, this creates a moment that must be balanced by an equal and opposite moment at that joint. There are two moments:

1. **Internal moments:** Generated by the muscles, joint capsules, and ligaments to counteract the external forces acting on the body.
2. **External moments** which can be estimated from the product of the GRF and the perpendicular distance to a joint center.

Support moment: It is the algebraic sum of all the internal moments during stance phase.

Stride Characteristics

Various instruments are available to measure different parameters of stride or gait cycle. Stride analyzer is the latest available model which measures almost all of the temporal and spatial parameters of gait. Other stride measuring systems available are instrumented walkways, individual sensor system, insole footswitch systems, and stopwatch.

The patient is made to walk on a walkway, built in the gait laboratory. And the entire walk of the patient is being captured by 8 infrared cameras which are connected to the stride analyzer, and the values of different gait parameters are obtained on your computer screen.

Clinically, some of the gait parameters can be measured by use of a stopwatch and asking the patient to walk on the measured distance. But the reliability of the information depends of the experience of the therapist and other factors.

Time and distance are two basic parameters of motion and measurements of these variables provide a basic description of the gait.

Temporal variable includes step time, stride time, single and double limb support time, swing time cadence, and speed.

Distance variable includes stride length, step length, base width, and degree of toe out.

- **Base width:** Measuring the linear distance between the midpoint of the heel of one foot and the same point on the other foot.
  - Normally—5-10 cm (2-4 inch)
- **Step length:** Linear distance between successive points of contact of opposite extremity. Usually from one heel strike of one extremity to heel strike of another extremity.
  - Normally—35-41 cm (14-16 inch)
- **Stride length:** Linear distance between two successive events that are accomplished by the same lower extremity during gait, usually from heel strike to heel strike of the same extremity.
  - Normally—70-82 cm (27-32 inch)

Energy Cost Measurement

The main objective of the locomotion is to move the body through space with least expenditure of energy. Energy is the capacity to do work.

Muscles use metabolic energy to perform mechanical work by converting metabolic energy into mechanical energy. Metabolic cost is measured by assessing the body's oxygen consumption per unit of distance travelled (oxygen consumption for a person walking at normal speed of 4-5 km/h is 100 mL/kg body weight/min).

Muscle performs work on the parts of the body in order that they change their height or change their translational and/or rotational velocity.
- Concentric muscle work
- Eccentric muscle work

Analysis of work and energy in movement is usually done in two ways:
1. Kinematic approach
2. Mechanical power analysis

Kinematic Approach

- Total energy = Potential energy + Kinetic energy
- Kinetic energy = Translational energy + Rotational energy
- Potential energy = mgh (mass × gravitational constant × height)

In gait, during initial contact body has the lowest PE but is moving the fastest and as it moves into midstance, PE rises and is exchanged for KE. In this way, there are great energy savings, which is the sum of potential and kinetic components.

Mechanical Power Analysis

Power profiles across the hip, knee, and ankle are compared with joint angle and major muscle activity profile. Power is measured in joule/sec or N.m/sec.

CHAPTER 15

Movement Analysis in Activities of Daily Living

Chapter Outline

- Squatting
- Lifting
- Sit-to-stand
- Sitting
- Breathing

SQUATTING

Squatting is an active maneuver performed by co-contraction of quadriceps and hamstring muscles. The position of squatting is maintained with feet placed shoulder width apart. The squat has been described as the "King of Exercises" since it activates the largest, most powerful muscles in the body and is the greatest test of lower body strength. The major muscles that are activated are the ankle, knee and hip extensors, the spinal erectors and the abdominals. As a result, squatting is one of the most popular exercises for development of lower body strength and power. It constitutes one of the three competitive lifts in the sport of power lifting and the front squat variation is also a component of the "Clean" lift in weightlifting. Many athletes and fitness enthusiast today use the squat exercise when weight training. Since many years, it has been an affective training exercise in athletic conditioning, rehabilitation, and general fitness programs.

Squat Form Types

- **Parallel squat:** Where the squatter flexes the knee till the thighs are parallel to the floor.
- Deep squat or bottom squat: Where the squatter flexes the knee till the thighs move beyond a line parallel to the floor.
- Unilateral and bilateral squats
- Partial squats and full squats
- Squats with weights and without weights
- Squats on level surface and on wobble boards/foam
- Modified squatting: Wall squats, forward lean squats, and plyometric squats

Phases of Squat

- Phase of **descent**
- Phase of **ascent**

Technique of Squatting (Fig. 15.1)

If you bend the knees first, it limits the hip's freedom of movement. All the force is felt in the knees, and you will find yourself in a very awkward position on the balls of your feet. When performed properly the squat should start by gliding the hips backward before the

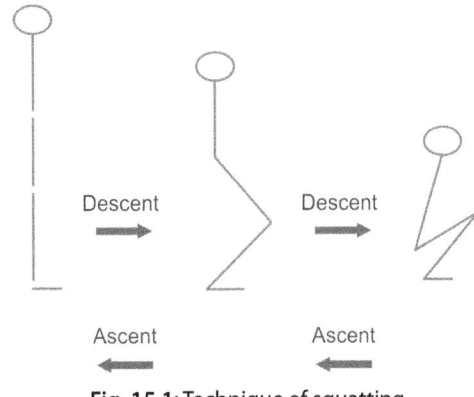

Fig. 15.1: Technique of squatting

knees break. This is done while keeping the torso upright and is not simply a lean forward (Chandler, Wilson and Stone, 1989). It should be similar to sitting in a chair, especially a low chair. This posterior movement actually helps you get the weight over the arch of your foot. Having the weight on the toes or heel of the foot will affect muscle function and balance. This weight positioning becomes even more crucial when you reach the bottom of the squat. As the top of the thigh reaches a parallel to the floor position or below, it is now time to come up. If the weight is forward on the toes, there is a tendency for the hips to rise up faster than the shoulders, leaving you in a potentially poor leverage position. This situation is when the squat becomes a good morning exercise. The opposite result of having the weight in the heel will leave you stuck at the bottom position or on your backside due to the balance problem.

Squatting is a movement, which involves the superoinferior shift, with a mild anteroposterior transition, of the center of gravity (COG). It is a closed kinetic chain activity and is functionally very significant and similar to sit-to-stand or stair-climbing in that it has two phases—ascent and descent.

The phase of ascent is movement up and against the gravity and thus it involves predominantly of concentric muscle activity whereas the phase of descent is just the opposite.

However co-contraction, proprioception, and stability are enhanced due to weight bearing.

Kinematics and Kinetics of Squatting: Review of Current Literature

Kinetics is the study of forces and **kinematics** is the study of movements.

Forces acting on the body are two—internal forces of muscle contraction, body weight and external forces of gravity, ground reaction forces.

Movements occurring in the body are movements of the bones (osteokinematics), joints (arthrokinematics), and of muscles (myokinematics).

The purpose of this material is to project the mechanics of squatting with respect to the kinetics and kinematics of the lower extremity joints and the spine only.

- **Descent:** This phase takes place in the direction of gravity, which is exactly opposite to that of the ascent and the muscle activity switches from concentric to eccentric predominant. Compared to that of ascent, the descent is always faster and more regular till the end of the squat down. In the ascent, the speed is slow and regular throughout.

- **Kinematics and kinetics:** A squat is considered a "full squat" or "deep squat" when the knees flex so that the proximal part of the thighs will pass the line parallel to the floor. At the deepest position of the parallel squat, Nisell and Ekholm (1986) found that the tibiofemoral shear force was of considerable magnitude. A shearing force causes the bones at the knee joint to slide across one another (i.e., the femur tending to slide anteriorly in relation to the tibia). The squat exercise is performed from the standing position, with feet placed shoulder width apart. An external rotation of approximately 10° is desired on the feet. The back is maintained in a flat position during the descent, with knees maintained over the toes. This alignment keeps the anterior shear forces across the tibiofemoral joint to a minimum (Panariello et al., 1994). Tendoachilles eccentrically controls the forward movement of tibia for ankle dorsiflexion and quadriceps for the knee whereas the hamstrings control the anterior tilt of the pelvis eccentrically during the descent. Care should be taken in maintaining a normal lordotic posture with the torso as close to vertical as possible during the ascend.

An approach that must be considered when examining biomechanics of the knee joint during a squat is the EMG activity of the hamstring and quadriceps muscle groups and the amount of co-contraction occurring during the exercise.

During the squat, an interesting phenomenon known as *Lombard's Paradox* occurs during contraction of the leg muscles (Holt, 1998). Eccentric contractions of the quadriceps and hamstring muscle groups occur during the descent, while concentric contractions of the same muscles occur during the ascent. This co-contraction is unique to the leg muscles and is not what is usually seen as the standard activity of opposing muscle groups, where the antagonist relaxes as the agonist contracts.

During extension of the knee, co-contraction of the hamstring muscle group reaches 20% of the maximum value, however, isometric contraction of the quadriceps with the knee between 10 and 20° of flexion produces only a 3% increase in hamstring muscle activity and a 90% increase in extension torque. This leads us to the conclusion that during squatting, the hamstring muscles produce a greater magnitude of contraction because they are required to stabilize the pelvis and trunk as well as the knee. The hamstrings being active neutralize the tendency for the quadriceps to cause anterior tibial translation.

- **Ascent:** The phase of squatting against the gravity is the ascent. This involves predominantly movement of the upper body relatively more than that of the lower body. The hips and knees move more than the feet.
- **Kinetics** of the ascent involves more of forces to counteract the effects of gravity and the body weight which comes from the concentric muscle activity of the spinal extensors, hip extensors, knee extensors, and ankle plantar flexors in a coordinated fashion. The anterior shear forces at the hip joint caused by the contraction of hamstrings causes posterior directed shear forces at the distal femur by the rotation of the shaft of the femur in the sagittal plane at an axis around its middle. This force shears tibia anteriorly thus helping knee extension which is associated with posterior shear at the distal tibia thus returning the ankle to neutral by a closed kinetic chain dorsiflexion.
- **Kinematics** of the ascent: The initial movement may involve a plantar flexion moment, followed by spinal extension with almost synchronized hip and knee extension happening together. The ankle moves from near maximum dorsiflexion to neutral position similar to the knee from full flexion to neutral extension. Hip flexion however is not full in the starting position and it returns also to neutral hip extension. Spinal extension occurs with an anterior pelvic tilt, which precedes the former. Thus the cycle of squatting is accomplished.

The point of minimal velocity during the ascent is often described as the "**sticking point.**" The sticking point is thought to result from the force-length properties of muscles and the torque produced by the load. The quadriceps' ability to produce tension decreases as they extend and hence so does their net extensor moment. At the sticking point, they are no longer able to produce sufficient force to continue extending the knees. Hip flexion at this point occurs to shorten the load's moment arm at the knee joints and enables the quadriceps to extend them (and also lengthen the hamstrings). The vasti muscles of the quadriceps group all show similar peak EMG activity during ascent and decent. The rectus femoris is the only biarticular muscle in the quadriceps group; it creates a hip flexor moment and shows ~30% greater activation during the descent yet still significantly less than the vasti. The vasti each has specific length tension relationships, and it may be a weakness in the lateralis that contributes to the sticking point since the medialis is the most active at the latter stages of knee extension.

The moment arm at the hip increases as it flexes at the sticking point but lengthening of the gluteal and hamstring muscles is advantageous for producing force since it improves their length tension relationships and hence increases net torque. The hamstrings are a biarticular muscle, crossing both knee and hip joints, during the ascent they shorten at the hip and lengthen at the knees. However, the shortening at the hip is disproportionate to the lengthening at the knee, and therefore their ability to produce tension is improved by hip flexion.

As the spine flexes, the spinal erector's length tension relationship moves closer to optimum but the net extensor torque decreases because there is a significant decrease in the angle the longissimus and iliocostalis muscle fibers make with the spine. This compromises their ability to support shear forces and hence, at full flexion, those forces are transferred to passive tissues, (i.e., ligaments and spinal discs) significantly increasing the risk of injury. Power lifters may allow their spine to flex to within 2 or 3° of full flexion hence preventing injury yet maximizing the ability to negotiate the "sticking region." Squatting typically stresses the spinal erectors isometrically in an extended position. Due to the specificity of this mode of training there is little cross over to the shorter muscle fiber lengths involved in spinal flexion. Therefore, if a lifter has not been conditioned to partially flex the spine, the muscles may not be able to maintain sufficient tension and it may "buckle."

Influence of Valsalva Maneuver in Squatting

When squatting lifters employ the Valsalva maneuver that is a voluntary increase in pressurization of the abdominal cavity achieved by closing the epiglottis and activating trunk and abdominal muscles. Increased intra-abdominal pressure improves the stability in the spine, however the mechanism is not fully understood. An early theory was that a hydrostatic force within the abdominal cavity induced an extensor moment by pushing down on the pelvic floor and up on the diaphragm. However, contraction of rectus abdominis and the internal/external oblique muscles causes a flexor moment that offsets the extensor moment caused by intra-abdominal pressure. It is now believed that increased coactivation of spinal flexor and extensor muscles increases spinal stiffness and hence spinal stability. This means that increased intra-abdominal pressure is simply a useful by-product that negates the flexor moment caused by the abdominal and oblique muscles as discussed above.

Influence of the Lower Extremity Kinetic Chain in Squatting: Pathomechanics

The act of squatting creates increased shear forces at the hip joint during the initial phase of ascent and torsional forces at the end of ascent. Hip flexion increases the moment arm of the load and therefore requires an increase in the isometric tension produced in the spinal erectors. At the beginning of the ascent some lifters (particularly in the front squat) hyperextend the spine to shorten the hip's moment arm and also to help keep the load-body center of gravity over the feet. Hyperextension of the lumbar spine places greater stress on the facet joints and may increase the risk of chronic lower back pain. Repeated training in this hyperextended position may cause an exaggeration of the lumbar curve—lordosis.

The knee however, is exposed to shear especially in the anterior direction at 60° flexion to 30° extension and this is clinically significant since this increases the strain on the ACL. The patellofemoral joint undergoes significant compression forces at around 90° to 45° knee flexion especially eccentrically loading on the quadriceps. The resultant of the two vectors, the forces of the quadriceps tendon and the patellar tendon at 60° increase the stress on the patellar articular cartilage. In the frontal plane, the Q angle is increased functionally by the increased adduction or internal rotation moment of the femur from coxa vara or anteverted hip respectively. Lateral shear forces on the patella or excessive compression of the lateral facets can occur at this phase.

The quadriceps muscles can contract more efficiently when the feet are pointing slightly outward. They should NEVER point straight ahead. If you squat with a very wide stance, your adductors tend to assist the quads. This can result in stress to the medial collateral ligament, abnormal cartilage loading, and improper patellar tracking. During the decent phase of any type of squat, do not allow the knees to extend beyond your feet. The further knees travel over feet, the greater the shearing forces on the patellar tendon and ligament. Make sure that knees point in the same direction as feet are pointing during the descent and ascent. Because of weak quads, many lifters inadvertently turn their knees inward during the ascent, placing great stress on the medial ligaments of the knee.

During squatting, range limitations at the ankle joint may cause restriction in the knee joint flexion or extension. A limitation in the ankle dorsiflexion (due to tight plantarflexors) may prevent the knee from being flexed; a limitation in ankle plantarflexion (due to tight dorsiflexion) may restrict the ability of the knee to fully extend. The rear foot varus with compensation of calcaneal eversion, which is a usual occurrence also functionally increases the external tibial torsion which in turn will again increase the Q angle. This occurs similar to pronated foot from either rear foot varus, pes planus secondary to forefoot varus, plantar flexed first ray, or hallux valgus.

Kinetic Chain Exercise Concept

Another area to be discussed is the concept of "open kinetic chain" (OKC) exercises versus "closed kinetic chain" (CKC) exercises. Closed kinetic chain exercise occurs when the terminal or distal segment of an appendage is fixed, such as during a squat, leg press, dead lift, power clean, or pull up. Conversely, open kinetic chain exercise occurs when the terminal or distal segment is free to move, such as during seated knee extension or flexion. The debate continues on whether to use OKC or CKC exercises within athletic training, rehabilitation and fitness programs. Discussed previously was one rational for using CKC exercises as opposed to OKC.

The rehabilitation communities in particular advocate the use of closed kinetic chain exercises because they stimulate and replicate many functional movements, such as squatting, stooping, and ascending or descending stairs (Wilk et al., 1996). Therapists also suggest that by performing specific close kinetic chain exercises, patients may be able to strengthen the quadriceps and hamstring muscles simultaneously while protecting a reconstructed ACL (Wilk et al., 1996). Furthermore, this group recommends that closed kinetic chain exercises are safer than open kinetic chain exercises because the CKC exercises minimize anteroposterior tibiofemoral shear forces and thus reduces stress on both the ACL and PCL. They also recommend closed kinetic chain exercises as the best form of exercise for the ACL-reconstructed knee.

Closed kinetic chain exercises allow for multijoint activities that simulate everyday as well as athletic movements. Performing a squat can aid in functional activity.

Comparison of Biomechanical Characteristics Between Few Common Lower Extremity Activities

Activity	Unilateral/ bilateral	Open/closed kinetic chain	Phases	Muscle activity
Gait	Combined	Combined	Stance, swing	Eccentric
Running	Unilateral	Combined	Stance, swing	Concentric
Stair climbing	Unilateral	Combined	Ascent, descent	Combined
Sit-to-stand	Bilateral	Closed	Ascent, descent	Combined
Squatting	Bilateral	Closed	Ascent, descent	Combined

■ MOVEMENT ANALYSIS OF LIFTING

Lifting

Lifting is the ability to raise or lower objects without assistive devices. It involves the movement of an object from one location to another location. Injuries due to lifting account for 15–65% of work related back pain.

Stages of Lifting
- Access
- Movement
- Placement

Classification

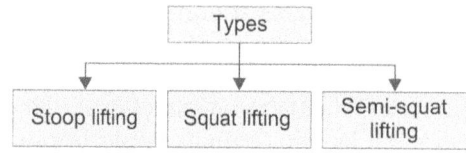

Other types of lifting are:
- Weightlifters lift
- Golfer's lift

Stoop Lifting
- Under stoop lifting, there is trunk flexion with no knee flexion.
- Trunk flexion, is achieved via, thoracolumbar flexion.
- There is disadvantage at extensor muscles of the trunk, due to shorter moment arm in this position.
- Intradiscal pressure is higher.
- Moderate use of thigh musculature

Position:
- Trunk → Flexion
- Thoracolumbar → Flexion
- Knee → Extension

Muscle work:
- Trunk flexion → Flexors of spine
- Concentric contraction of quadriceps at the beginning and at the end of lifting
- Hamstrings eccentric contraction at the middle of lifting
- High contraction of erector spinae

Squat Lifting
- This type of lifting is performed with spine being erect and by performing a squat to lift the object.
- The predominant movement is seen at the hip and knee
- Intradiscal pressure when compared to stoop lifting is lower
- Medium to high activity of thigh musculature

Position:
- Spine → Erect
- Trunk → Flexed
- Hip → Flexed
- Knee → Flexed
- Ankle → Dorsiflexed

Muscle work:
- Erector spinae works to maintain the stability
- Knee flexor acts at the beginning
- Knee extensors act the end
- High activity of vastus lateralis, and low activity of rectus femoris and biceps femoris

Biomechanical Criteria of Lifting
It is important to follow good practice of lifting to avoid musculoskeletal injuries.
- Keep the weight that is to be lifted close to the body as this reduces the stress on lumbar spine.
- Placement of a hand couple on weight, equalizes the weight while it is been lifted and thereby minimizes trunk instability.
- Face down, when lifting is in the uneven slope surface to negotiate the strain.
- Sagittal plane lifts are better.

Principles of safe lifting: Assess the area → Assess the load to be lifted → Lower the body, via bending the knees to the level of load → To ensure a broad, stable base, place the feet shoulder width apart → Keep the back straight → Use firm, palmar grip → Keep the arms close to trunk → Place the load close to the center of gravity and within the base of support → Pivot the feet in the direction of movement → Do not rotate the trunk while lifting → Lift using muscles in the legs → Avoid use of postural muscles in the trunk.
- Increase in intra-abdominal pressure
- Isometric back muscle strength
  When lifting is carried out one has to bend at waist and extend the upper body, this changes the back's alignment and the center of balance in the abdomen. Subsequently, the spine has to also support both the weight

of the upper body and the weight of the load being lifted.

The forces being transmitted through the low back can be estimated.

And is calculated by the moment and forces created by the weight of the load being lifted and the weight of the upper body

Moment = (Force) × (Distance)

Moment = (Weight of load) × (Distance from center of weight of load to a fulcrum)

NIOSH Lifting Equation

The National Institute of Occupational Safety and Health (NIOSH) issued a Work Practices Guide for Manual Lifting for establishing an **Action Limit (AL)** in the year 1981. When the action limit is exceeded, there is a requirement of implementation of job redesign. The Action Limit is the weight that one can safely lift. It is 75% for female and 99% for male population.

A **Maximum Permissible Limit** is three times the action limit.

The Maximum Permissible Load (MPL) = 3 (AL)

The 1981 NIOSH lifting equation is:

Action Limit (AL) = 90lbs. (6/H)(1−.01[V−30]) (.7+3/D)(1−F/Fmax)

where,

H = horizontal location of the load forward of the midpoint between the ankles at the origin of the lift (in inches)

V = vertical location of the load at the origin of the lift (in inches)

D = vertical travel distance between the origin and the destination (in inches)

F = average frequency of lifts (lifts/minute)

Fmax = maximum frequency of lifting which can be sustained (from a NIOSH table)

MOVEMENT ANALYSIS OF SIT-TO-STAND

Sit-to-stand is one of the most common movements of daily life. Rising from the seated

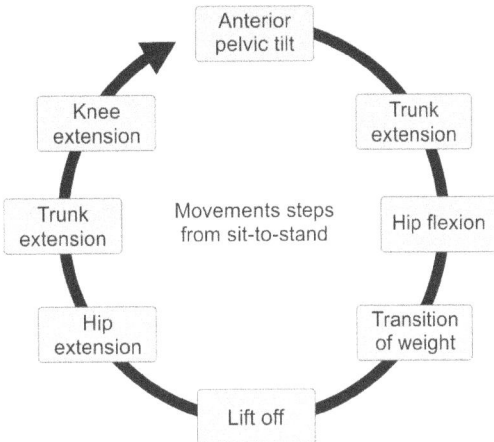

Fig. 15.2: Movement steps from sit-to-stand

position is a complex activity (**Fig. 15.2**). It requires adequate postural control during the motor transfer from a stable 3-points base, the sitting position, to a 2-points base, the standing position.

Phase 1: Flexion Momentum (Fig. 15.3)

This is used to start the initial momentum for rising; ends just before the gluteus are lifted from the seat of the chair.

Phase 2: Rising (Fig. 15.3)

Initiated just after there is maximum ankle dorsiflexion and ends when the hips first ease to extend, the hamstrings, gluteus allows the body to rise in a standing position. Hamstrings flex the knee and extend the thigh. Gluteus straighten out the hips while standing.

Phase 3: Standing (Fig. 15.3)

Gastrocnemius, soleus, plantaris calf muscles stabilize leg while standing, and aid in flexion while sitting.

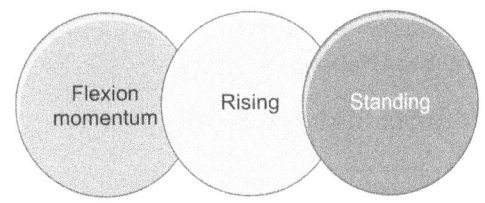

Fig. 15.3: Sit-to-stand concept

It requires the ability to move the body mass forward over a large BOS (thighs and feet) to a small BOS (feet) and to extend the lower limb joints to raise the body mass over the feet. This activity requires co-ordination, balance, adequate mobility, and strength. From a mechanical point of view STS provides an active stretch to calf muscles.

Sitting

The action of sitting down (on a seat of average height but without backrest) involves both knee flexion and trunk flexion on the thighs (of about 90° in both cases). Hip joint flexion is only about 60°, beyond which passive tension in the hamstring muscles increases quite rapidly. The sitting action is complete by a backward rotation of pelvis of >= 30°. The weight is taken on the ischial tuberosity, and on top of sacrum. If the overall line of trunk is to remain vertical, there must be a compensatory lumbar flattening or flexion equal to the backward pelvic rotation. Sitting up straight requires action of iliopsoas.

Standing

The fact that a symmetrical upright stance is sometimes called "the normal standing posture" is based on a misconception. When "standing at ease" in a symmetrical posture, we sway slowly back and forward within our foot base. The line of weight of the superincumbent body parts probably passes in front of ankle joints and behind the hip joints for most of the time so soleus and iliopsoas activity is seen. Quadriceps or hamstring shows minimum activity as moments about the knee is negligible. The anterior tibial muscles are only active when sway approaches posterior limits of the footbase. Only ligaments of foot, sacroiliac joints, and possibly knee joints could be of importance.

Sit-to-Stand Maneuver (Fig. 15.4)

Three phases:
1. The initiation phase
2. The seat unloading phase

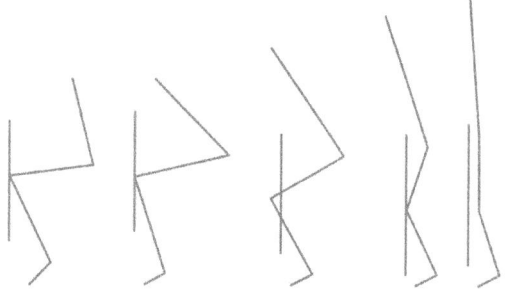

Fig. 15.4: Sit-to-stand phases

3. The lift or the ascending period
   - *Phase I:* Flexion momentum phase starts with initiation of movement and ends just before buttocks are lifted from seat of chair.
   - *Phase II:* Momentum transfer phase begins as the buttocks are lifted and ends when maximal dorsiflexion is achieved.
   - *Phase III:* Extension phase is initiated just after maximum DF and ends when the hips ceases to extend; including leg and trunk extension.
   - *Phase IV:* Stabilization phase starts after hip extension is reached.

Standing Up: Description of Action

- Pre-extension phase prepares for starting posture when feet are placed backward in such a way that LL extensor muscles get activated on the extension phase and backward horizontal component of GRF propels body mass forward.
- HAT is rotated forward at the hips.
- Velocity of trunk F, by reactive forces causes thighs to move forward.
- Since the feet are fixed, the shank rotates forward at the ankles, with movement taking place at the knee (flexion) and ankle (DF) **(Fig. 15.5)**.
- This movement of the thigh and shaft may augment the active dorsiflexion that together with the trunk rotation provide the horizontal momentum that moves the body.

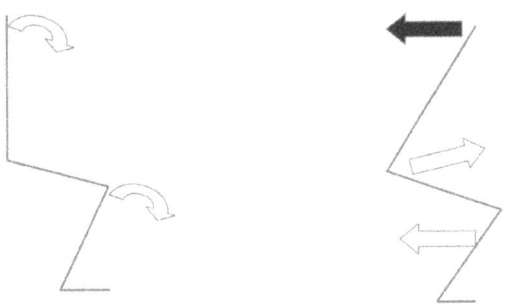

Fig. 15.5: ankle knee and trunk interaction during sit-to-stand

- Forward movement of the body by angular displacement at the hip and ankle in pre-extension phase can have a dynamic effect on the upcoming extension phase.

Kinematics

- Generation of *horizontal linear momentum* of body mass to move the body mass forward over the new BOS.
- Translation of horizontal momentum to *vertical momentum*, which propels body mass upward to the standing position.

Horizontal movement of the body mass is brought about principally by the clockwise rotation of the trunk at hips and of the shank segment of the ankle. Vertical movement of the body is brought about by the extension of hip, knee, and ankle [counter-clockwise rotation of the trunk and the shank segments and the clockwise rotation of thigh (at hip and knee)]. The later also extends the knee together with counter clockwise rotation of shank. The horizontal and the vertical movement of the body mass overlap, reflecting the overall sequence of the knee, hip, ankle, the knee starting to extend while the hip is still flexing.

Kinetics: Segmental rotations are brought about by muscle forces, along with gravitational, inertial, and interactive forces.

Major force generation occurs around the time the thighs are lifted off the seat in order to accelerate the body mass vertically into the standing position.

Decrease in force in one joint is compensated for by an increase in at the other joints to ensure the limb does not collapse.

Muscle Activity

- Tibialis anterior is the first muscle to be activated placing foot backward.
- Gluteus maximus, biceps femoris (hip extensors), and quadriceps tend to occur almost simultaneously. They show *peak activity* when thigh is lifted off the seat.
- Activity of iliopsoas in initiating trunk flexion is difficult to monitor as it is a deep muscle.
- The simultaneous onset of the biarticular rectus femoris and biceps femoris may be related to the contribution to the control of the hip flexion, with rectus femoris for the flexion and the biceps femoris exerting a breaking force at the hip and thus serving to slow down the hip flexion at the hip prior to the beginning of the lower limb extension.

Sitting Down

- Same action in reverse
- Angular displacement is same
- Control by extensor when flexion is increased
- Increase control at knee is required
- Takes longer time

Movement Impairment Syndrome of the Hip During Sit-to-stand

- **Femoral anterior glide syndrome:** It can occur with or without medial rotation. Most common is the one with medial rotation. This syndrome occurs because of inadequate posterior glide of the femoral head during hip flexion, the hip flexion is accompanied by medial rotation. Kinesiologic principles indicate that during flexion there will be posterior glide of the femur, but in this syndrome this posterior glide is insufficient. Similar is called shoulder impingement when there is anterior glide of humerus. In this the syndrome is often diagnosed to be iliopsoas tendonitis (pressure created by the femoral head against anterior joint structures, which occur when there is hyperextension of hip) this pressure combined with the diminished posterior glide of the femur during flexion causes femur to impinge on the anterior tissues of the joint capsule.

If pain is experienced during walking or during weight-bearing activities, the patient should be examined for it. Activities that emphasize on hip extension, such as running long distances or dancing, are often associated with femoral anterior glide syndrome. This is because the exaggerated extension of the hip joint is part of the movement pattern of running, similarly dancers.

- **Muscles and recruitment pattern impairment:** The action of TFL muscles is more dominant than the iliopsoas muscles. The TFL short on the affected side, despite standing alignment examination that shows a flat back, hip extension, and hyperextended knees, all of which are consistent with excessive length of iliopsoas.

  The action of the TFL is more dominant than the posterior gluteal medius (PGM) muscle. When the patient is in single limb stance, the hip rotates medially. During the PGM muscle test the hip rotates medially, which indicates that the TFL is dominant over PGM.

  The action of the medial hamstring is more dominant than the lateral hamstring. When patient is in sitting position and performs knee extension, hip rotates medially. When knee is slightly laterally rotated, the knee extension is limited or is performed more slowly, which is indicative of resistance from lateral hamstrings.

- **Common causes of mechanically induced hip pain**
  - Iliotibial tract irritation
  - Strain of muscle about the hip
  - Greater trochanter bursitis
  - Stress of femoral neck
  - Piriformis syndrome
  - Iliac crest
- Iliotibial tract irritation
- Downhill terrain
- Results due to constant need to control knee bend
- Along with this flexed knee position the lateral compartment of thigh attempts to stabilize the knee from buckling laterally.
- Examination of flexion of knee angulation in sagittal plane and the degree of varus and valgus in frontal plane is necessary.
- In this type, there is tightening of iliotibial tract (repeated contraction of the muscle). This tightness attenuates shock while running.
- Overactivity of the thigh muscle create overload to the muscle group or single muscle and may develop weakness of iliopsoas, rectus, sartorius, gluteus medius, and piriformis.
- Bursitis and stress
- As the muscular structure about the lateral compartment of the hip and thigh fatigue, an imbalance in musculature develops where one muscle group maintains the contracted position. Contacted muscle group becomes resilient to the firm structures rubbing beneath.
- Clicking of bursa can be felt with the leg flexed or rotated inward (pronated foot and the limb complex).
- The pronated foot cause inward rotation of the leg.
- **Hip flexor contracture on standing:** During normal standing line of force falls posterior to the hip joint and this creates an extension torque by gluteus muscle to extend the hip. Prevention of excessive hip extension is checked by iliofemoral ligament which is anterior to hip joint.

  With hip contracture, the line of force now is anterior to hip joint and this creates a flexion torque. To prevent flexion torque gluteus maximus acts to compensate. This standing interferes with the ability to optimally dissipate compressive loads normally on the articular cartilage. As a result articular cartilage is not able to protect the underlying bone from large forces produce due to activated muscles. This leads to arthritis, bursitis, and labral impingement, etc.

SITTING (FIG. 15.6)

Definition
"A body position in which the weight of the body is transferred to a supporting area, mainly by the ischial tuberosities of the pelvis and their surrounding tissues."
—*Schoberth, 1962*

- **Body weight transferring through:**
  - The ischial tuberosity to the seat and then to the floor
  - The foot directly to the floor
  - The forearm to the armrest and then to the floor
  - The back and pelvis to backrest and then to the floor
- **Comparisons of sitting posture with standing posture:**
  - Sitting posture provides stability required on tasks with high visual and motor control.
  - Sitting posture is less energy consuming than standing posture.
  - Sitting posture places less stresses on lower extremities than standing posture.
  - Sitting posture lowers hydrostatic pressure on lower extremity circulation.
  - The pelvis rotates backward and the lumbar spine flattens when standing to sitting.

Types of Sitting Posture (Fig. 15.7)
Middle sitting
- COM of the upper body directly above ischial tuberosity
- Floor support ~25%
- **Subtypes:**
  - Relaxed middle sitting with the lumbar spine straight or slight kyphosis
  - *Supported middle sitting:* With the lumbar spine straight or slight lordosis

Forward sitting (forward leaning sitting)
- COM of the upper body in front of ischial tuberosity
- Floor support >25%
- **Subtypes:**
  - Forward rotation of the pelvis with the lumbar spine straight or slight kyphosis
  - Little rotation of the pelvis but with large kyphosis of the lumbar spine
  - *Sitting on a chair with a forward sloping seat:* With the lumbar spine slight lordosis

Backward sitting (backward leaning sitting)
- COM of the upper body behind ischial tuberosity
- Floor support <25%
- **Subtypes:**
  - *Backward sitting without lumbar support:* Backward rotation of the pelvis and kyphosis of the lumbar spine
  - *Backward sitting with a lumbar roll support:* Backward rotation of the pelvis and lordosis of the lumbar spine

Standard Sitting Posture (Fig. 15.8)
- Chin-in
- Neck flexion 5–10°
- Keep lumbar lordosis
- **Hip:** 85–100°
- **Tibia:** Perpendicular to the floor
- Foot flat on the floor **(Fig. 15.9)**

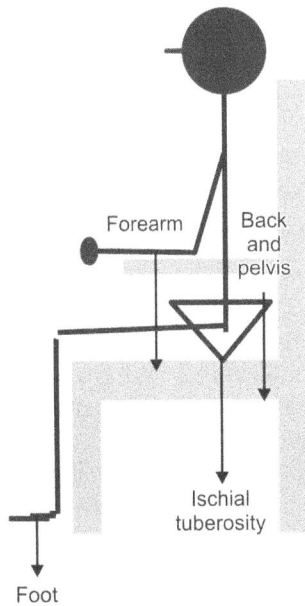

Fig. 15.6: Ideal sitting posture

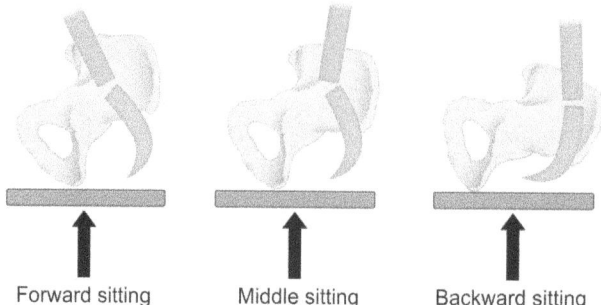

Fig. 15.7: Types of sitting posture

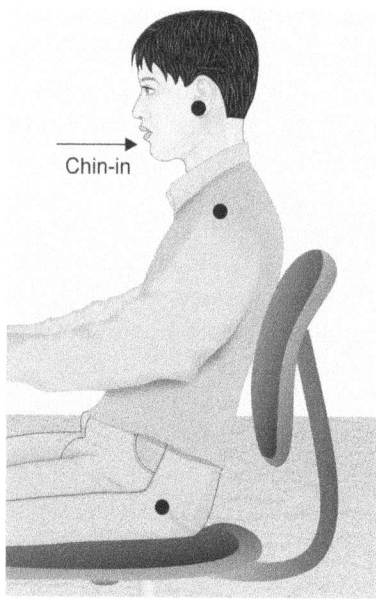

Fig. 15.8: Standard sitting posture

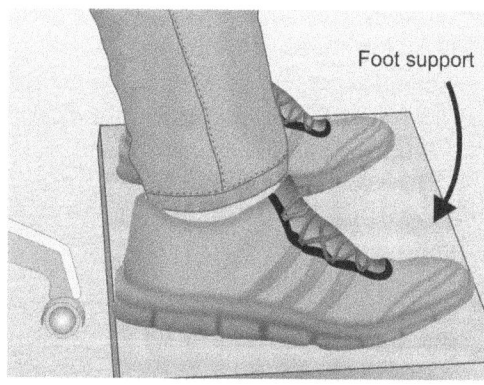

Fig. 15.9: Foot resting on foot stool

Sitting on a High Chair (Figs. 15.10A and B)
- Should have a foot support
- Without foot support, the weight of leg will form a moment at the hip joint to create anterior tilt of the pelvis, and then increase lumbar lordosis that might result in low back pain.

Semi-sitting Posture (Fig. 15.11)
- Good for "active" worker, e.g., grocery check-out person
- To encourage mobility
- To allow rapid changes between sitting and standing
- To preserve lumbar lordosis
- Inclination of the seat starts just in front of the ischial tuberosity to have full support of the trunk and the thigh.

Anthropometric Dimensions of Seated Workers

Vertical Anthropometric Measurements (Fig. 15.12)

All of the anthropometric measurements are based on the position when an individual sits with the popliteal fold 3–5 cm above the seat, with knee flexion of 90°, and with the foot flat on the floor.
- **Sitting height:** The vertical distance from the floor to the posterior aspect of the midpoint of the thigh.
- **Shoulder height:** The vertical distance from the sitting height to the superior aspect of the acromion.

Chapter 15 | Movement Analysis in Activities of Daily Living

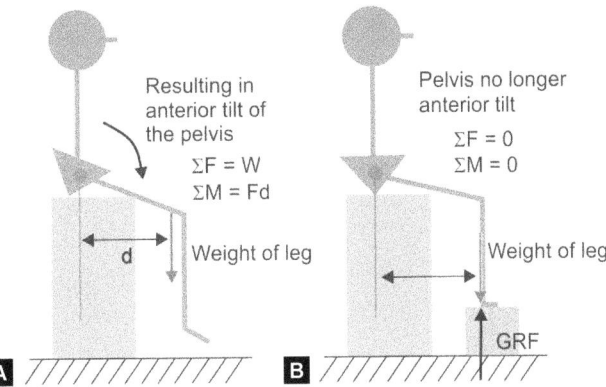

Figs. 15.10A and B: Sitting on a high chair. (A) Without foot support; (B) With foot support

- **Elbow height:** The vertical distance from the sitting height to the tip of the olecranon with the elbow being flexed to 90° and the upper arm being vertical.

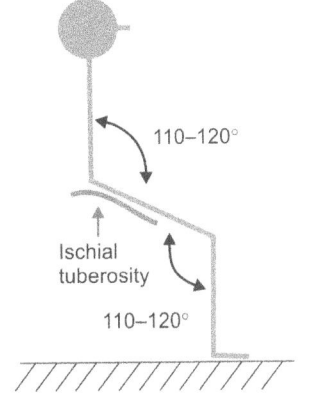

Fig. 15.11: Semi-sitting posture

- **Thigh height:** The vertical distance from the floor to the highest point of the thigh.
- **Patellar height:** The vertical distance from the floor to the superior aspect of the patella.
- **Orbital height:** The vertical distance from the floor to the orbit.

Sagittal Anthropometric Measurements (Fig. 15.13)

- **Abdominal depth:** The sagittal distance from the posterior aspect of the buttocks to the anterior aspect of the abdomen.
- **External sitting depth:** The sagittal distance from the posterior aspect of the buttocks to anterior aspect of the patella.
- **Internal sitting depth:** The sagittal distance from the posterior aspect of the buttocks to the posterior aspect of the popliteal fold.

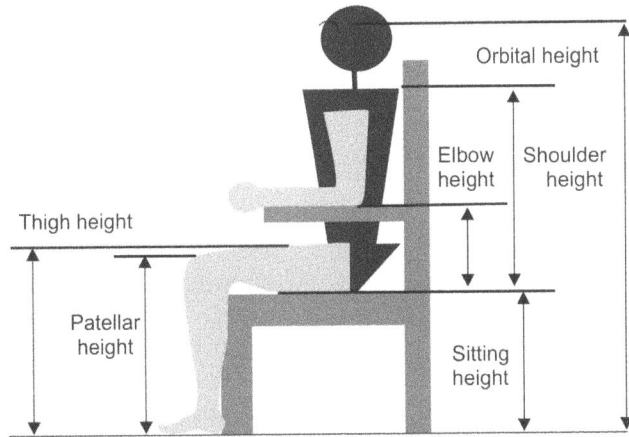

Fig. 15.12: Vertical anthropometric measurement (lateral view)

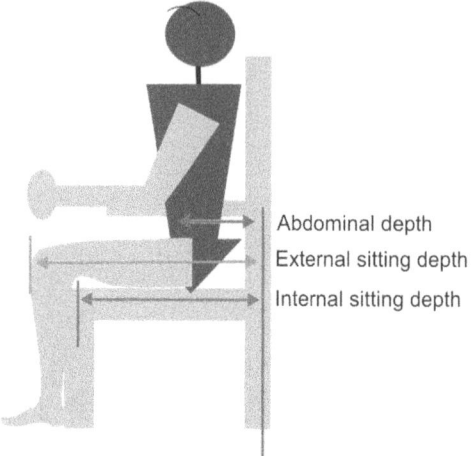

Fig. 15.13: Sagittal anthropometric measurement (lateral view)

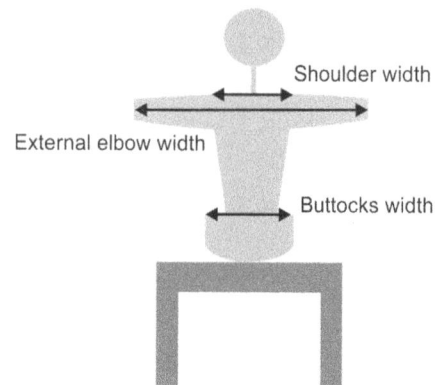

Fig. 15.14: Transverse anthropometric measurement posterior view

Transverse Anthropometric Measurements (Fig. 15.14)

- **Shoulder width:** The transverse distance between the tips of both acromion processes.
- **Buttocks width:** The maximum transverse distance at the buttocks.
- **External elbow width:** The transverse distance between the tips of both olecranon when the arms are placed at shoulder abduction of 90°.

Seated Work Place and Layout

Dimensions of the Seat (Figs. 15.15 and 15.16)

- Seat height = **Sitting height**
  - 3–5 cm below the knee fold when the low leg is vertical; otherwise it will cause compression of the posterior aspect of the thighs.
  - 3–5 cm above popliteal level if the chair is tiltable or the seat slope is forward (Bendix, 1987)
- **Seat width**
- **Seat depth (length):** 10 cm less than the **internal sitting depth** in order to facilitate rising from the chair.
- **Seat slope:**
  - Backward slope of 5°
  - *Adjustable seat slope:* Better used in the office
  - Forward slope of 20°

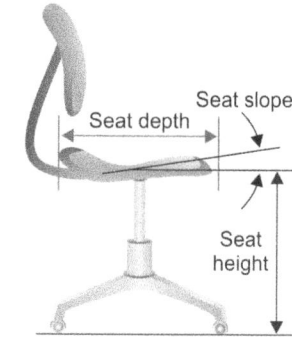

Fig. 15.15: Dimensions of the seat (lateral view)

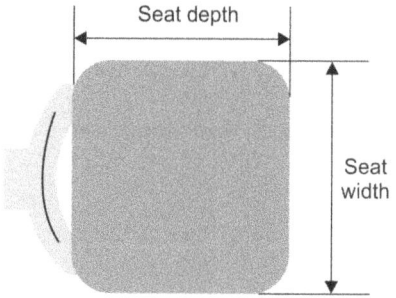

Fig. 15.16: Dimension of the seat (superior view)

- **Shape of the seat:** Front part of seat should be contoured so that the edges of the seat should not be detectable during seated work.
- Friction properties
- **Softness:** Pressure should be avoided on the posterior aspect of lower thigh.
- Adjustability
- Climatic comfort

Dimension of the Backrest (Fig. 15.17)

- Either with backrest or with lumbar support will decrease the pressure under the ischial tuberosity.
- Backrest should not restrict trunk or arm movements.
- Backrest top height = backrest bottom height + backrest height
- Backrest bottom height
- Backrest center height
- Backrest height
- Backrest width
- **Backrest horizontal radius:** Concave from side-to-side to conform the body contour
- **Backrest vertical radius (Fig 15.18):** Convex from the top to the bottom to conform to the lumbar lordosis
- Backrest-seat angle
- Pivoting and recline possibility
- Softness
- **Adjustability:** Adjustable in the vertical and/or horizontal planes
- Climatic comfort

Dimension of the Armrest (Figs. 15.19 and 15.20)

- Armrest can reduce the loading on the spine and facilitate the rising from the chair
- Armrest length
- Armrest width
- Armrest height = **Elbow height**
  - Shoulders shrug if the armrests are too high
  - Trunk slumps or leans to one side if the armrests are too low
- Armrest-to-armrest width
- Distance from armrest front to seat front

Dimension of the Chair Base

- Number of feet
- Base diameter
- Use of caster or wheel

Dimension of the Workbench

- Not necessarily the same for all types of work

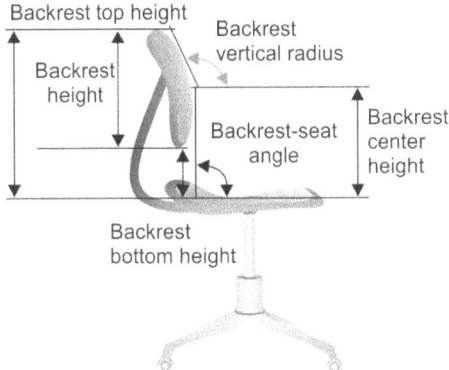

Fig. 15.17: Backseat dimension (lateral view)

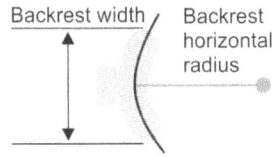

Fig. 15.18: Superior view of backrest

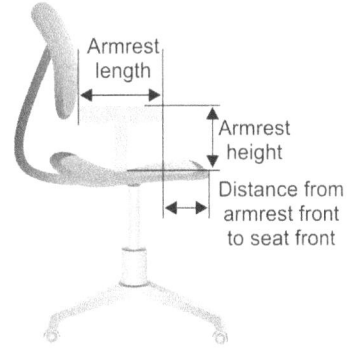

Fig. 15.19: Dimension of armrest (lateral view)

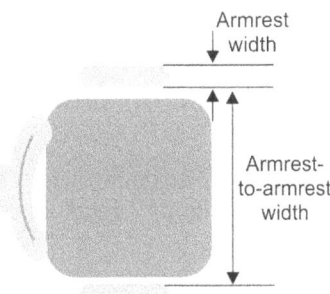

Fig. 15.20: Dimension of armrest (superior view)

- **Factors affecting workbench dimensions**
  - Size of the workpiece
  - Motions required by the task performer
  - Overall work layout
- **Workbench top height:**
  - 3–4 cm above the elbow level (Bendix, 1987)
  - Keyboard height = workbench top height if the computer is used
- **Workbench bottom height:** Greater than the thigh height in order to ensure sufficient space for the thigh
- **Workbench surface:**
  - Size large enough to accommodate work objects but not too far to reach
  - Friction high enough to prevent sliding of work
- **Inclination of workbench surface:**
  - The influence on lumbar posture from inclined table surfaces was actually greater than the influence of the seat slope (Bendix, 1987)
  - *For reading:* A slope of 45°
  - *For writing:* A flat desk
- **Field of vision**
- **VDT must be placed to prevent forward head or trunk flexion of the user**
- **Focal distance:** 20–40 cm

Video Display Terminal Users

Definition

- Maintaining the same posture >2 hours
- For one specific computer work
- Repeated using the same key(s) or mouse

Note: In most developed countries, approximately ¾ of labors is sedentary workers (Reinecke et al. 1992).

Cumulative Traumatic Syndromes in VDT Users

- Hultgren and Knave 1st, 1974: First reported about soft tissue problems among VDT users
- Muscle fatigue, soreness, stiffness, cramps, numbness, and/or pain were frequently found in VDT users.
- Associated with the frequency of key strikes
- More than half of computer users have reported local pain (1991 US statistics).
- **Location of pain:**
  - Neck and shoulder pain: 67%
  - Low back pain: 40%
  - Wrist pain: 29%
- **Resulting in:**
  - Increase in medical expenditure
  - Increase in work compensation
  - Decrease in productivity
- **Possible causes:**
  - *Physiological factors*
    - Endurance time decreases significantly when the posture required more than 30% of the strength of back muscles (Jorgensen, 1970) **(Fig. 15.21)**
    - Intradiscal pressure changes during various sitting postures **(Fig. 15.22)**
  - If the trunk leans forward, the moment loaded on the lumbar disc increased as the sine of α. For example, if the trunk leans forward at an angle of 30°, then the moment is Wd (sine 30°), i.e., 0.5 Wd **(Fig. 15.23)**.
  - Flexion of the neck depends on the visual demand and the height of work surface.
  - *Environmental or task factors:*
    - Malposture or maintaining the same posture for a long period of time
    - Improper workplace
    - Repetitive motions

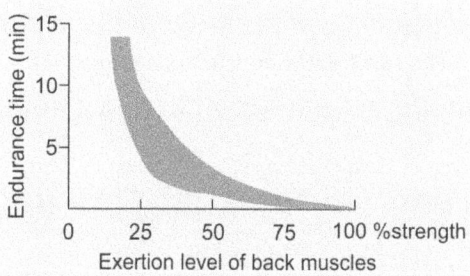

Fig. 15.21: Endurance time versus back exertion level

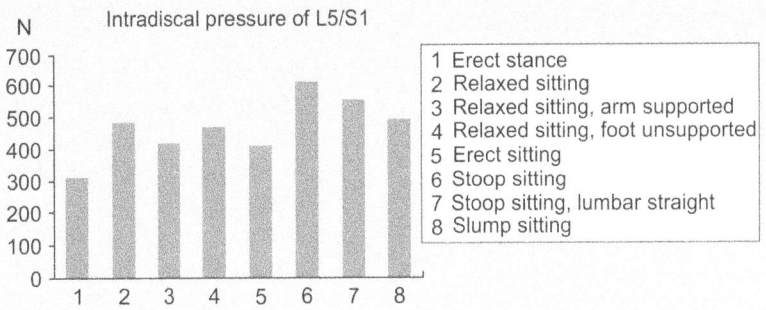

Fig. 15.22: Intradiscal pressure of l5/S1

- *Psychological factor*
  - Work stress
  - Time stress
- Social factors

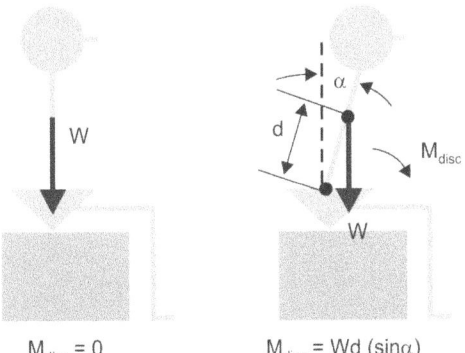

Fig. 15.23: Moment at the lumbar discs increases as the trunk leans forward

- Prevention of cumulative traumatic syndromes
  - To decrease the sustained duration
  - Muscle cannot sustain contractions over ~15–20% of their maximum strength without fatigue
  - To decrease the frequency
  - To increase muscle strength in the posture where the task requires

Biomechanical Considerations in VDT Workplace Design (Figs. 15.24 to 15.27)

- **Chair:** Chair with armrest
- **Seat slope**
- **Chair base**
  - Better to have 5-foot support
  - Radius = 30–35 cm
  - Use of casters or wheels

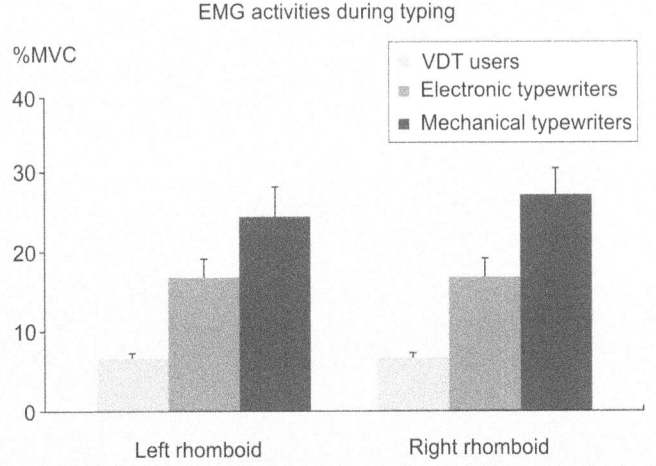

Fig. 15.24: EMG activities during typing

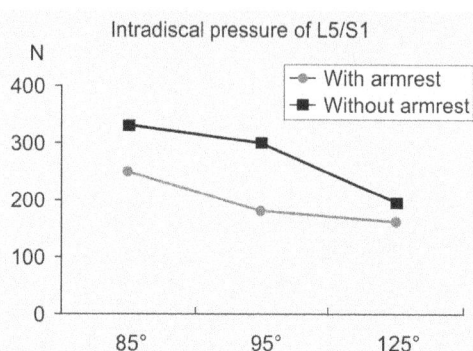

Fig. 15.25: Backrest-seat angle

- **Computer desk**
  - To provide sufficient space for the legs, i.e., work bench bottom height ≥ thigh height
  - If the desk is too low, an individual tends to lean forward and lower and protract the shoulder joints.
  - If the desk is too high, an individual tends to elevate and shrug the shoulder joint which is susceptible to muscle fatigue.
- **Keyboard**
  - *Keyboard height (from middle row to floor):* 70–85 cm
  - *Keyboard distance (from middle row to table edge):* 10–26 cm
  - In the position to have minimum wrist extension, flexion, and ulnar deviation
- **Screen**
  - *Screen height (from center of screen to floor):* 90–115 cm
  - *Screen inclination:* 88–105°
  - *Screen distance (screen to table edge):* 50–75 cm
- **Body posture**
  - *Visual distance (from eyes to center of screen)*
  - *Viewing angle (from eyes to center of screen):* <20°
  - *Trunk-seat angle:* Most people use the backward leaning posture that causes in a decrease in lumbar lordosis and is susceptible to herniation of the intervertebral disc.
  - *Elbow angle:* ~90°
  - *Shoulder flexion angle:* As small as possible.

MOVEMENT ANALYSIS OF BREATHING

Breathing includes the phases of inspiration and expiration together termed as respiration. Biomechanically the movement analysis of breathing can be known with the knowledge of movement of ribs and muscles responsible.

Rib Movements

Movement of rib cage depends upon:
- Type of articulating angle
- The movement of manubrium sterni
- The elasticity of costal cartilage
- Rib movement generated by intercostal muscles in a single interspace

Orientation of Axes

- Costovertebral and costotransverse joints are mechanically linked

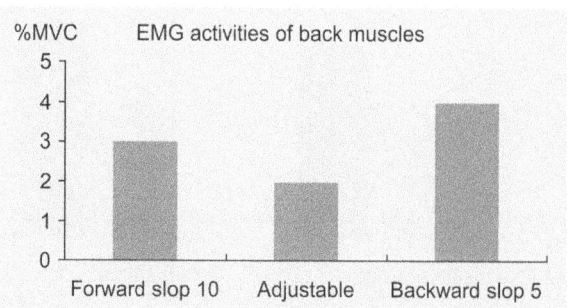

Fig. 15.26: Angle of seat slope

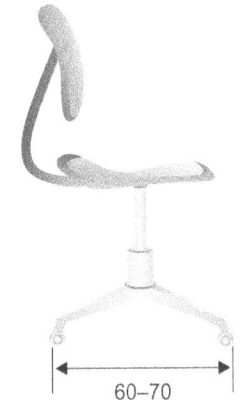

Fig. 15.27: Dimension of chair base

- For each rib length, shape and downward angle are different
- Axis of rotation in turn changes
- For upper ribs, the axis lies close to frontal plane
- For lower ribs, the axis lies to sagittal plane and movement occurs in frontal plane
- For floating ribs, the axis passes through costovertebral joints

The external and internal interosseous intercostal muscles in the interspace between rib 5 and 6 were activated, whereas the intercostal muscles could rotate the sternum and ribs.

Movements

First rib—attaches to manubrium → less mobile → elevates during inspiration

11th and 12th rib → only have postarticulations → do not participate in any movements

Pump Handle Movement

In this, the ribs that result in a change in the anteroposterior diameter, movement at costovertebral joints 2–6 about a side-to-side axis results in raising and lowering the sternal end of the rib. This occurs mostly in the vertebrosternal ribs.

2nd to 7th rib - attaches to the body of sternum → length and mobility is more → costocartilages rotate upward and become horizontal → sternum moves anteriorly, forward, upward → increases anteroposterior diameter of thoracic cage → movement occurs in sagittal plane → termed as pump handle movement.

Bucket Handle Movement

The bucket handle movement of ribs is a transverse increase in diameter of the chest due to movement of ribs during respiration. It expands and increases the volume of the chest to inhale air during inhalation.

8th to 9th ribs—indirectly attached to sternum → more angled → more mobile at lateral aspect of the rib cage → moves laterally, outward, upward → increases transverse diameter of rib cage → movement occurs in frontal plane → termed as bucket handle movement.

Muscles of Ventilation

These are the muscles attached to the rib cage, responsible for respiration, thus known as ventilatory muscles.

Features

- Increase fatigue resistance
- Greater oxidative capacity
- Contract rhythmically
- Have involuntary and voluntary effect

Primary Muscles of Ventilation

- Diaphragm
- Intercostal muscles
  - External intercostal
  - Internal intercostal
- Scalene muscles

Accessory Muscles

- Sternocleidomastoid muscle
- Pectoralis major and minor
- Subclavius
- Levators
- Abdominal muscles
- Transverse thoracic

Diaphragm

- A dome-shaped muscle
- It contributes to 70–80% of activity during respiration.

- The ventral segment of the muscle contributes to costal fibers.
- The dorsal segment of the muscle contributes to crural fibers.
- During inspiration → contraction of diaphragm → descends downward → increases in vertical diameter of rib cage → piston movement.

CHAPTER 16

Movement Analysis in Sporting Activities

Chapter Outline

- Throwing and striking
- Jumping
- Running
- Jogging
- Kabaddi
- Gymnastics
- Kicking
- Push ups
- Pull ups
- Swimming
- Cycling
- Biomechanics in dance

THROWING AND STRIKING

Anyone can throw a ball over-hand, but not everyone can do it well….

Phases

- Wind up
- Cocking
- Acceleration
- Deceleration
- Follow-through

Sequential Movements of the Body Segments

The movement that involves a sequential action body segments in a chain, leading to a high-velocity motion of external objects. It results in production of a summated velocity at the end of the chain of segment used.

Examples:

- A pitcher throwing a baseball
- A young adult spiking a volleyball
- Hitting a cricket ball in a batter way
- An elderly drives a golf ball
- A tennis player serves a tennis

Modification

- **Objectives:**
  - Skill
  - Speed
  - Accuracy
  - Distance
- **Components:**
  - Numbers of body segment used
  - Range of motion (ROM) used
  - Lever length used

Classification

Depending upon the nature of force application

- **Momentary contact:** The force imparted to an object through temporally contact with that object by a moving part of the body segment or by implementing held or attached on the body segment.

  The object may be either stationary or moving.

  Examples:
  - *On moving object:* Baseball striking, soccer heading or kicking, volleyball set, or tennis driving
  - *On stationary object:* Golf

- **Projection:** The force imparted to an object through the end of a chain of body segments in order to develop kinetic energy, followed by a high-velocity motion of that object.

  The object may be held in one hand or hands.

Examples:
- *For distance:* Shot put, javelin, or volleyball serving
- *For accuracy:* Baseball pitching or dart throw

• **Continuous application:** The force is imparted to an object with the force continuously applying to that object.

Examples:
- *Against large resistance:* Pushing a desk or lifting weight
- *Maintain a position while waiting for a release:* Archery

Biomechanics of Baseball Throwing

Patterns of Throwing (Figs. 16.1A to C)
- Overarm (overhead)
- Sidearm
- Underarm

Kinematics of Overarm Throwing
- **Windup (cocking) phase:**
  - Shoulder horizontal abduction and fully external rotation (closed-packed position)
  - Trunk left rotation
  - Prone to have shoulder impingement syndrome (**Fig. 16.2**)
- **Acceleration phase:** Shoulder internal rotation
- **Deceleration phase:** Checked by shoulder external rotators
- **Follow-through phase:** Trunk rotation

Kinematics of Sidearm Throwing
- **Preparation phase:**
  - Shoulder horizontal abduction only
  - Trunk right rotation
- **Acceleration phase:** Shoulder horizontal adduction
- **Deceleration phase:** Checked by deltoid posterior
- **Follow-through phase:** Opposite hip internal rotation

Kinematics of Underarm Throwing
- **Preparation phase:**
  - Shoulder extension
  - Elbow extension
- **Acceleration phase:** Shoulder flexion
- **Deceleration phase:** Checked by shoulder extensors
- **Follow-through phase:** Trunk rotation

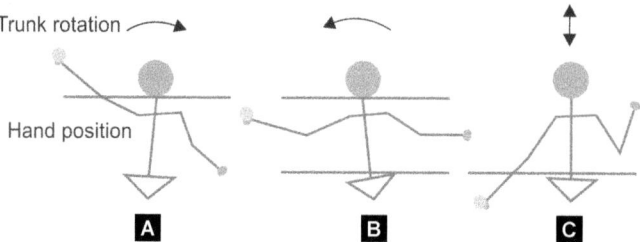

Figs. 16.1A to C: Patterns of throwing. (A) Overarm throwing; (B) Sidearm throwing; (C) Underarm throwing

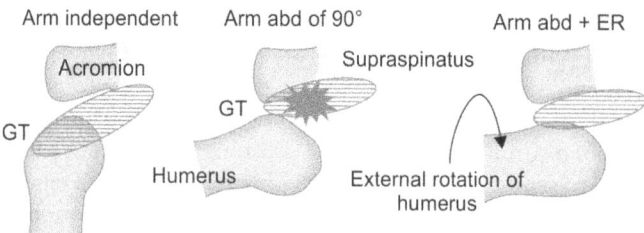

Fig. 16.2: Shoulder impingement syndrome

Mechanical Factors of Throwing

- Ballistic movement of one segment
- **Imparting force must overcome the inertial of an object:**
  - Mass of object
  - Internal resistance
  - Friction between object and supporting surface
  - Resistance to surrounding medium
- **Force needed dependent on:**
  - Speed of object
  - Distance of throwing
  - *Accuracy of target:* Related to direction of the object after its release
- **Direction of the object after release dependent on:**
  - *Direction of the object at the moment of release:* Path tangential to the arc of motion
  - Gravity
  - Air or water resistance
  - Spin of the object
- **Timing pattern of movement part:**
  - The slowest or the heaviest part must start to move first, and the quickest and the lightest one last.
  - To facilitate use of stretch reflex

Biomechanics of Striking

Forehand Drive in Tennis

- **Action:** The player takes the racket to hit the ball and send it into the opponent's court.
- **Type of movement:** Ballistic movement
- **Participating lever:** Racket, racket-side arm, and trunk
- **Location fulcrum:** The hip joint at nonracket side
- **Skill requirement:** High speed and moderate accuracy

Motion Description

- **Back swing phase:**
  - The player pivots his body to have the no racket side face forward.
  - The racket is taken back at the shoulder level.
  - The body weight is over the foot of the racket side.
  - The head of the racket is kept above the wrist.
- **Forward swing phase:**
  - The player lowers down his body by flexing the knee to have the racket below the intended contact point.
  - The trunk rotates forward to shift the weight to the foot of the nonracket side.
  - The racket is perpendicular to the ground at the moment of impact.
- **Follow-through phase:**
  - The body continues forward.
  - The racket arm swings across the body and up toward the chin.
  - The effect of body spinning
  - *Mechanical factors contributing the impact to the ball:* The greater impart force will impart more momentum to the ball, leading to speed up the ball on its return flight.
  - Increase the lever-arm length by using a long-arm racket, keeping the arm straight
  - *Firmness of grip depends on:*
    - Muscle strength of wrist and finger flexors
    - The angle of the racket faces at ball hitting because the angle of rebound is highly correlated to the angle of incidence.
    - Actually, the ball is not a rigid body so that the angle of rebound is slightly less than the angle of incidence.

Striking

Forehand Drive in Tennis

- **Action:** The player takes the racket to hit the ball and sends it into the opponent's court.
  - *Type of movement:* Ballistic movement
  - *Participating lever:* Racket, racket-side arm, and trunk
  - *Location fulcrum:* The hip joint at nonracket side
  - *Skill requirement:* High speed and moderate accuracy

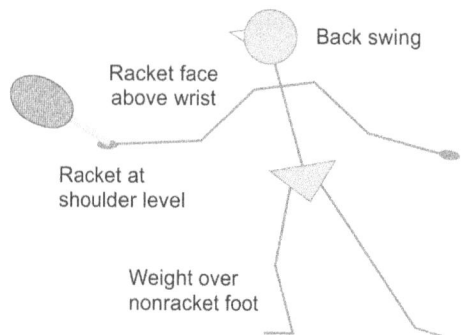

Fig. 16.3: Back swing phase

- **Motion description:**
  - *Back swing phase (Fig. 16.3)*
    - The player pivots his body to have the nonracket side face forward.
    - The racket is taken back at the shoulder level.
    - The body weight is over the foot of the racket side.
    - The head of the racket is kept above the wrist.
  - *Forward swing phase*
    - The player lowers down his body by flexing the knee to have the racket below the intended contact point.
    - The trunk rotates forward to shift the weight to the foot of the nonracket side.
    - The racket is perpendicular to the ground at the moment of impact.
  - *Follow-through phase*
    - The body continues forward.
    - The racket arm swings across the body and up toward the chin.
- The effect of body spinning
- **Mechanical factors contributing the impact to the ball:** The greater impart force will impart more momentum to the ball, leading to speed up the ball on its return flight.
  - Increase the lever-arm length by using a long-arm racket, keeping the arm straight
- **Firmness of grip depends on:**
  - Muscle strength of wrist and finger flexors
  - The angle of the racket faces at ball hitting because the angle of rebound is highly correlated to the angle of incidence.
    - Actually, the ball is not a rigid body so that the angle of rebound is slightly less than the angle of incidence.

JUMPING

It is the process of moving free from the ground, by muscular action of feet and legs. It is an act of raising one's center of gravity higher in the vertical plane solely with the use of one's own muscles. In vertical jumping, the maximum height is achieved by extending the proximal joint first and then the distal joints to a point of extension occur at the ankle joint. By the time the ankle joint is involved in the sequence, very high joint moments and extension velocities are required. Here the role of the two joint muscles becomes very important. The biarticular gastrocnemius muscle crosses both the knee and ankle joint. Its contribution to the jumping action is influenced by the knee joint. In the jumping action, the knee joint extends and optimizes the length of gastrocnemius. This keeps the contraction velocity of the gastro low even when the ankle is plantarflexed very quickly. With the velocity lowered, the gastrocnemius is able to produce more force in the jumping action **(Fig. 16.4)**.

Muscles involved: Fast twitch muscles
- **Overall:** Produce great amount of work in small amount of time
- Optimal balance between high velocity of contraction and force generated to maximize power
- Knees flex and muscles become increasingly stiff
  - Body halts the fast stretch of the muscle.
  - Great amount of force is produced in the muscle and a rise in elastic energy storage in the muscles.

BIOMECHANICS OF RUNNING

Running: Running is a locomotor activity which requires a greater amount of speed,

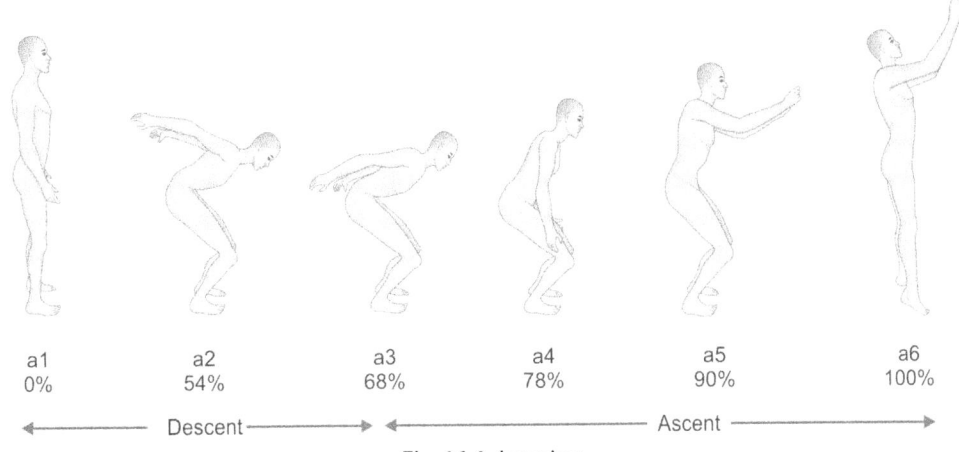

| a1 | a2 | a3 | a4 | a5 | a6 |
| 0% | 54% | 68% | 78% | 90% | 100% |

←——— Descent ———→ ←——————— Ascent ———————→

Fig. 16.4: Jumping

balance, and muscle strength to cover a distance in a shorter period of time compared to walking.

The major difference between walking and running is based on the contact of the foot on the ground. For walking, there will be periods of double support during the stance phase of the gait cycle (i.e., both feet will be simultaneously in contact with the ground). In case of running there will be double float at the beginning and the end of the swing phase of gait (i.e., neither foot will be touching the ground).

As the speed of running increases, the initial contact on the ground changes from being on the hindfoot to the forefoot which can further distinguish between running and sprinting.

- Running is performed over longer distances, for endurance, and with primarily aerobic metabolism. Example: Jogging, road racing, and marathons. Approximately 80% of distance runners are rearfoot strikers. The remaining is characterized as midfoot strikers. In case of distance running on the other hand, the body is moved at a more controlled rate in relation to the energy demand of the race.
- Sprinting activities are done over shorter distances and at faster speeds, with the goal of covering short distance in the shortest period of time possible without regard for maintaining aerobic metabolism. For sprinting the body and its segments are moved as rapidly as possible throughout the entire race.
- Elite sprinters (those who perform high intensity sprinting sessions) perform with a forefoot initial contact instead of hindfoot which may never contact the ground.

Gait Cycle (Figs. 16.5A to D)

A gait cycle begins when one foot comes in contact with the ground and ends when the same foot contacts the ground again.

The moment of time at which the foot comes in contact with the ground is referred to as initial contact (beginning of the stance phase). The stance ends when the same foot contacts the ground again. Toe off followed by the placement of the same foot again on the ground marks the beginning and end of the swing phase respectively.

In running, toe off occurs before 50% of the gait cycle is completed. There are no periods when both feet are in contact with the ground. Instead, both feet are airborne twice during the gait cycle, one at the beginning and one at the end of swing referred to as double float. The timing of toe off will be proportional to the speed. Whereas in walking, the stance phase will be longer than 50% of the gait cycle and there will be two

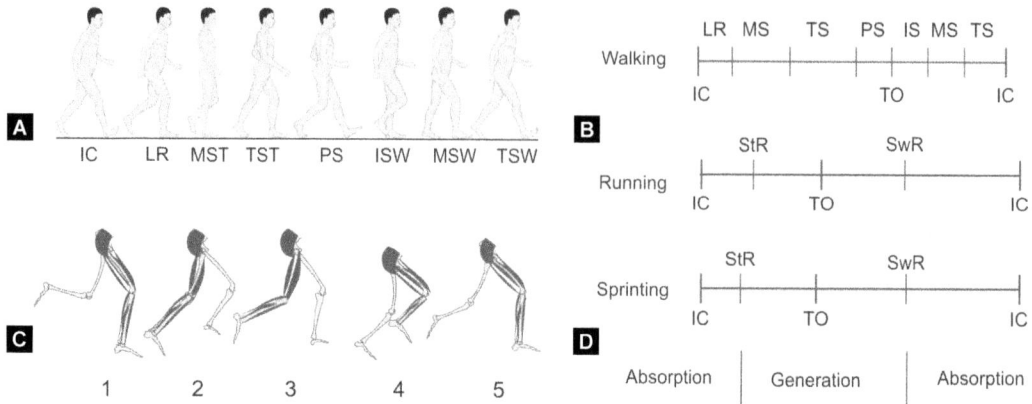

Figs. 16.5A to D: Gait cycle. (A) Walking figure; (B) Walking gait cycle: (IC, initial contact; LR, loading response; TO, toe off; MS, midstance; TS, terminal stance; PS, preswing; IS, initial swing; MS, midswing; TS, terminal swing). (C) Running figure: 1. Stance phase absorption. 2. Stance phase generation. 3. Swing phase generation. 4. Swing phase reversal. 5. Swing phase absorption. (D). Running gait cycle: for running and sprinting; IC, initial contact; TO, toe off; StR, stance phase reversal; SwR, swing phase reversal; absorption, from SwR through IC to StR; generation, from StR through TO to SwR

periods of double support when both feet are on the ground, one at the beginning and one at the end of stance phase. The alternate periods of acceleration and deceleration which occur during running, regardless of the speed are referred to as absorption and generation. During the period of absorption, the body's center of mass (COM) falls from its peak height during double float. This period is divided by initial contact (IC) into swing phase absorption and stance phase absorption. The velocity of the COM decelerates horizontally during this period. After stance phase reversal, the COM is propelled upward and forward during stance phase generation. Kinetic and potential energy increase. The limb is then propelled into swing phase after toe off (swing phase generation). The next period of absorption begins at swing phase reversal.

Kinematics

Kinematics is description of movement without considering the forces that cause the movement. Motion in all three planes will be considered.

- **Sagittal plane kinematics:** In sagittal plane motion, there will be a shift into flexion and the COM is lowered as the motion changes from walking to running to sprinting. Pelvic motion is minimized to conserve energy and maintain efficiency in running and sprinting. The position and acceleration of the runner's COM determine the direction and magnitude of the ground reaction force.

In running, during the absorption period of stance phase, the knee flexes to approximately 45° it reaches 10° of hyperextension after toe off. At the end of the swing phase, the hip extends to 50° in order to prepare for the next heel strike. About 40° of knee flexion will be there as the heel strikes, later flexes to 60° during loading response. This is followed by knee extension to an average of 25°–40° during the propulsion phase. During the initial part of the floating period of swing phase knee flexes to reach up to 125° during the mid-swing. Maximum knee flexion during swing is much less than the average of 90° in running. Initial contact during running occurs with heel. During the absorption phase of running, the ankle dorsiflexes for about 10° as body weight is transferred to the stance leg, later dorsiflexes to 25°.

- **Coronal plane:** The motion of knee and ankle is restricted by the coronal ligaments. Pelvis remains stationary as the limb is loaded. The hip adducts relative to the pelvis as a shock absorbing mechanism. Pelvis drops throughout the rest of the stance phase. During swing phase, the pelvis elevates in order to obtain foot clearance. The hip is adducted while the limb is loaded in stance phase and abducted during swing. A relatively minimal head and trunk motion allows the balance and equilibrium to be maintained.
- **Transverse plane kinematics:** The movement patterns in the transverse plane are more important in determining the energy efficiency. During running, maximum internal pelvic rotation occurs in mid-swing to lengthen the stride, later by the time of initial contact, the pelvis will be rotated exteriorly. This maximizes horizontal propulsion force and avoids the potential loss of speed. The pelvis also functions as a pivot between the counter-rotating shoulders and legs. For example, when the right leg is maximally forward in mid-swing, the left shoulder is rotated forward and the pelvis is neutral. The pronation of the foot occurs during the absorption phase while the limb is loaded and then the foot supinates during the generation phase which provides as a stable lever for push-off.

Kinetics

Kinetics explains about the forces that causes the movement which are basically by the muscles. The major tasks that the muscles performs are:
- Shock absorption and control of vertical collapse during any weight acceptance phase
- Balance and posture control of the upper part of the body
- Energy generation associated with forward and upward propulsion
- Control of direction changes of the COM of the body.

Muscles are most active in anticipation of and just after initial contact of the foot. Muscle contraction more important at the time of initial contact of the foot with the ground than it is for the preparation for or during the act of leaving the ground.
- **Sagittal plane kinetics:** During running, the ankle movement pattern is similar to walking. The forefoot is lowered to the ground under the control of eccentric contraction of the *anterior tibial muscles*. The anterior tibialis dorsiflexes the ankle to provide clearance in swing (concentric), to allow ground contact with the hindfoot initially, and to control the lowering of the forefoot to the ground during the first part of stance (eccentric). The onset of the ankle plantarflexion occurs at 5–10% of the running gait cycle. The period of power generation occurs soon after the period of absorption which provides energy for forward propulsion. The magnitude of the ankle power generation is proportional to the speed of the individual while running. The activity of *gastrocnemius* muscle starts just after loading at heel strike and also acts in the later swing phase.

The knee moment pattern is similar in running and sprinting. During the preparation for the initial contact, the *Hamstring* becomes dominant in the second half of swing producing a knee flexor moment. This controls rapid knee extension. Later after the initial contact, the *quadriceps* becomes dominant producing a knee extensor moment. As the magnitude of peak extensor moment is greater in running, there will be a greater degree of knee flexion as the limb is loaded. The *quadriceps* (eccentric contraction) and *rectus femoris* both fire from late swing to midstance to prepare the limb for ground contact and to absorb the shock of that impact during stance phase absorption. The *quadriceps* contracts concentrically during the second half of the stance phase where the power will be generated. The muscles absorb power to control the movement of the swinging leg. *Rectus femoris* contracts eccentrically to prevent the excessive knee flexion in the early swing. During the late swing phase, the *Hamstrings* contract eccentrically to control the momentum of the tibia and prevent knee hyperextension as the knee is rapidly extending.

For all the conditions of forward locomotion, the hip movement pattern is similar. The hip extensors *gluteus maximus* and *gluteus medius* just prior to and just after initial contact. Whereas the hip flexors mainly *iliopsoas* are dominant in the second half of stance through the first half of swing. Both the hip flexors and extensors are responsible for power generation. Peak hip flexion occurs in the second half of swing which follows the concentric contraction of the hip extensors in order to extend the hip for the preparation of initial contact. Later the hip flexors become dominant and decelerate the backward rotating thigh in preparation for swing. During this time, the psoas tendon is stretched. The energy absorbed in stretching the tendon is returned at toe off.

- **Coronal plane kinetics:** There is minimal motion in the coronal plane compared with sagittal plane therefore have less power generation and absorption. The *gluteus medius* along with *tensor fascia lata (TFL)* produces a continuous hip abductor moment during the stance phase. *TFL* is also active between early and mid-swing. During the absorption phase, hip adducts as the ground reaction force falls medial to the hip and the hip abductor moment is less than the external adduction moment due to gravitational and acceleration loads. The *gluteus medius* contracts eccentrically to control this motion. During the propulsion phase, the gluteus medius contracts concentrically abducting the hip and generating power. The adductor muscle, *adductor magnus* will be active from the late stance to early part of swing phase.

Potential and Kinetic Energy (Fig. 16.6)

The two are in phase in running. Running has varying energy needs in order to propel oneself from a low point during the middle portion of stance (stance phase reversal) to a peak during double float. In running, the effective interchange between the potential and kinetic energy is not possible as they are in phase. So, the efficiency is maintained in two ways:

1. The storage and later return of elastic potential energy by the stretch of elastic structures (especially tendons)
2. The transfer of energy from one body segment to another by two joint muscles such as the rectus femoris and the hamstrings.

The potential and kinetic energies are peak in mid-swing. While landing to the ground, as the COM falls toward the ground, potential energy is lost and as soon as the foot contacts the ground, kinetic energy is lost. Some of the lost potential and kinetic energy is converted into elastic potential energy and stored in the muscles, tendons, and ligaments. During the generation phase, the COM accelerates upward which increases both potential and kinetic energy. The active contraction of the muscles supplies energy for this movement and the elastic potential energy

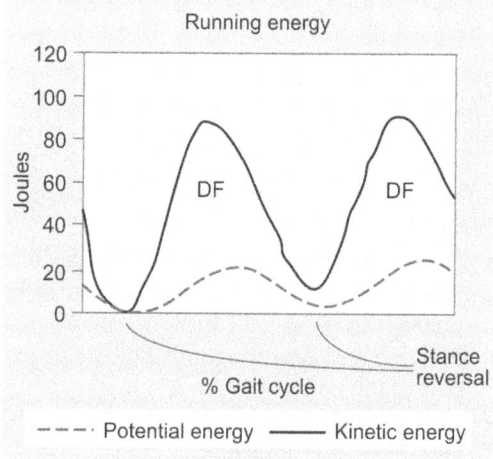

Fig. 16.6: The relationship between potential and kinetic energy in running

stored in the ligaments and the tendons are released.

JOGGING

Definition

Jogging is running at slow pace, it is a form of aerobic exercise. It can be preferably, be a warm up and cool down before a run.

Classification of long-distance runners (Brody, 1980):
- **Jogger:** Run 3–20 miles per week at a rate of 9–12 minutes per mile
- **Sports runner:** Run 20–40 miles per week and participate in "fun runs" or races of 3–6 miles
- **Long-distance runner:** Run 40–70 miles a week at a pace of 7–8 minutes per mile and may compete in 10,000 m races or marathons
- **Elite marathoner:** Run 70–200 miles a week with a pace of 5–7 minutes per mile

Characteristics of Jogging

- Stance phase decreases to 31%
- Should prevent repetitive impact stresses
- Heel strike or midfoot strike
- Medial and lateral flares
- Better material for heel pad

KABADDI

Kabaddi is a traditional contact sport played between two teams of seven players, with an objective is for the player on offence (raider) in the defender's court and tag out the defenders without being tackled out and return home court with a span of 30 seconds. And also the role of the defenders is to tackle the raider returning to his court. Every touch point for the raiding team and tackle point for the defending team will revive a player to the team. It is an indoor as well as outdoor game that demands tremendous physical stamina, agility, individual proficiency, neuromuscular coordination, lung capacity, quick reflexes, intelligence, and presence of mind on the part of both raiders and defenders.

Court Dimensions (Fig. 16.7)

The seven players of each team will occupy opposite halves of a court of total dimension of 13 m and 10 m. Each side of the court has 2 lobby where a raider or defender can enter after contact between the raider and defender. The raider has to touch the baulk line (touch line) to consider as a legal raid. The Bonus line (second line) is active for the raider to score a point when there are six or more defender in the defending court. End line (last line) is the boundary, if touched considered as out before any contact between the defenders and raider.

Kabaddi being contact sport, its powerful nature is prone to injuries. Sports injuries becoming more prevalent in the field around the world. Stress injuries account for maximum injuries which an athlete encounters. Improper techniques, mishap, or overload are some of the factors responsible for the injuries. In kabaddi, raiders sustain sudden turning and twisting movements put them at high risk of injuries at the knee joint. To prevent from tackling, the raiders performs quick reflexive

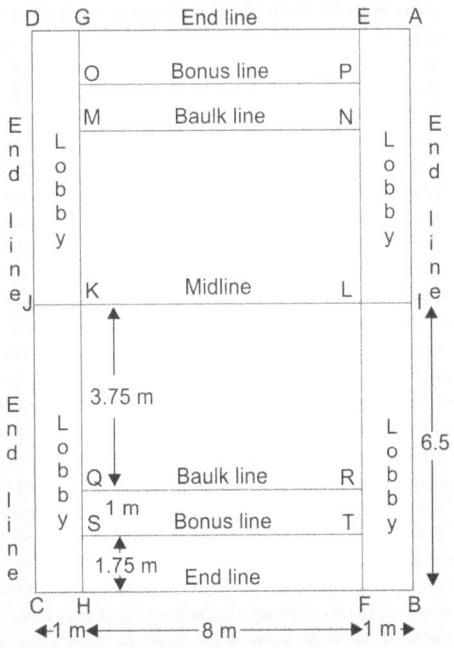

Fig. 16.7: Court dimensions

actions such as starting, stopping, bending, twisting, and changing direction exert extreme force on the knee resulting in knee injuries. From the literature, it is found that anterior cruciate ligament (ACL) and calf strains are common in knee joint. Contusions, blunt trauma, shoulder injuries, and head collisions are found to be more during the highly intensive phase of the game. An effort made by the defender to tackle the raider, they try to immobilize one or both the lower limbs. The defenders usually performs thigh hold, ankle hold, and front block, and rarely double thigh hold or double ankle hold. The raider tries to free the tackle by rolling or jumping over the defender.

Common technique to score a point by the raider:
- **Running hand touch:** The athlete sprint in the court and stretches his both hands and legs to maximum to the defender and score a point.
- **Toe touch:** The athlete will be in full squat position on one knee and other leg in complete extended at hip, knee and ankle joint and hands touching the ground to propelling himself and free from getting tackled.
- **Kick:** The athlete uses his one of the leg to kick front during sprinting or planned back kick.
- **Scorpion kick:** The athlete will maintain the balance of the body in one leg and two hands and sweeps his other leg like a scorpion tail with an attempt to score a point.

Common technique to score a point by the defender:
- **Thigh hold:** The athlete uses the technique of holding the thigh of the raider with 2 hands clasped each other.
- **Ankle hold:** The athlete grabs the ankle of the raider and tackles for the point.
- **Front block:** The defender stops the movement of the raider in the defender's court by blocking the waist of the raider by the help of shoulder and clasping the hands behind the waist.
- **Dash:** The defender pushes the raider out of the court before touching the entry line (midline).

Biomechanics acts as tool to understand the human movements that helps to enhance the player's performance and thus reduces the risk of sports injuries. It provides conceptual and mathematical tool that kinesiology professional improve movements and reduce the risk of injuries. Sports biomechanics is a diverse interdisciplinary field that deals with the physical anthropology, orthopedics, bioengineering, and human performance. The role of the sports biomechanics is to understand the mechanical cause effect relationship of the athlete's motions in the space.

Knee injuries can be prevented by changing body's position with a combination of features such as balance, coordination, speed, reflexes, and strength. It is also very advantageous to adapt certain exercise programs that integrate exercises to stabilize knee joints. Thigh and calf muscles are large muscles that are under maximum stress during sprinting during the game of kabaddi. Adapting exercise program that reinforces these muscles will deliver superior control and diminish the frequency of knee injury.

Strategies to reduce the risk of injuries:
- Warm up prior to matches and training is thought to reduce muscle stretch injuries because the muscle is more extensible when the tissue temperature has been increased by one or two degrees.
- Range-of-motion exercises can help to maintain normal joint function by increasing and preserving joint mobility and flexibility.
- Maintaining good muscle strength and flexibility may help prevent muscle strains.
- Tight muscles are associated with strains. Stretching is therefore practiced to maintain muscle length and prevent injury.
- Diet can have an effect on muscle injuries. If a player's diet is high in carbohydrate in the 48 hours before a match there will be an adequate supply of the energy that is necessary for muscle contractions.

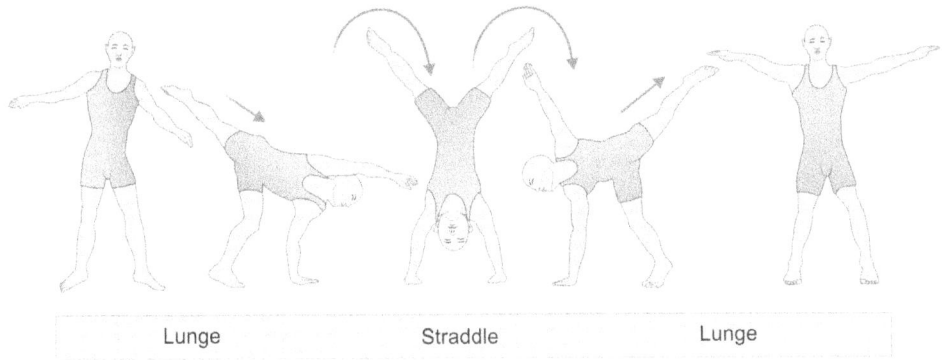

Fig. 16.8: Gymnastics poses

- Recovery after training sessions and matches can be enhanced by performing a cool down and stretching exercises.

BIOMECHANICAL ANALYSIS OF GYMNASTICS (FIG. 16.8)

Gymnastics is a sport that involves the performance of exercises requiring balance, strength, flexibility, agility, endurance, and control.

Gymnastics is derived from Greek word "gym nazo" that means to "train naked," "train in gymnastic exercise."

It is a combination of exercises that includes flexibility as the key along with balance, strength, agility, endurance, and coordination. The movement involved utilizes arms, legs, shoulders, back, chest, and abdominal muscles.

This is performed on event floors using many props such as vault, ball, hoop, ribbon, rings, beams, uneven bars, parallel, and horizontal bar, etc.

Phases:
- Preparation
- Action
- Recovery

Equipment Considerations

Women's gymnastics composed of four events:
1. Floor exercise
2. Balance beam
3. Uneven parallel bars
4. Vault/equestrian vaulting

Male gymnastics compete on:
1. Rings
2. Floor exercise
3. Parallel bars
4. Pommel horse
5. Horizontal bar

Vault

- Both men and women participate in vaulting and floor exercises but they perform it differently.
- The key differences in vaulting are the height and position of the horse.
- Men place the horse at a height of 5.5 feet.
- Women place the horse at a height of 4.5 feet
- For men, the horse is placed in the line of direction of the run, hence the name long-horse vaulting **(Fig. 16.9)**.
- In women, horse is placed perpendicular to the run, hence the name side-horse vaulting **(Fig. 16.10)**.

Technique

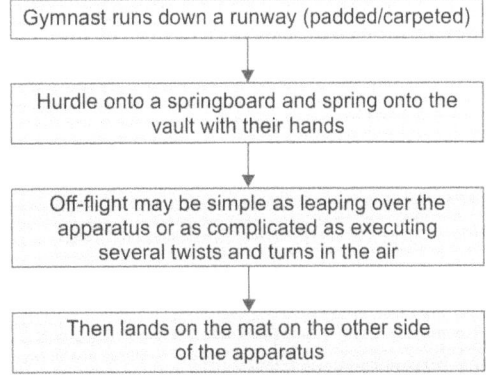

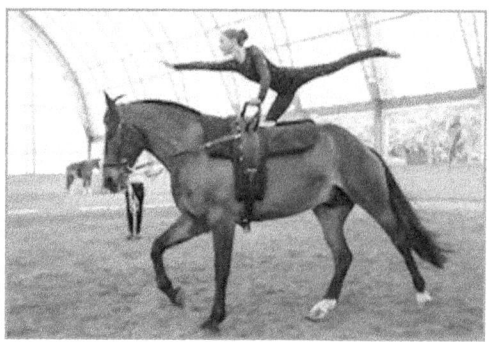

Fig. 16.9: Long-horse vaulting

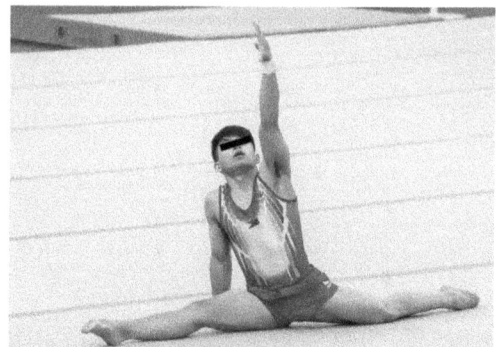

Fig. 16.11: Floor exercises

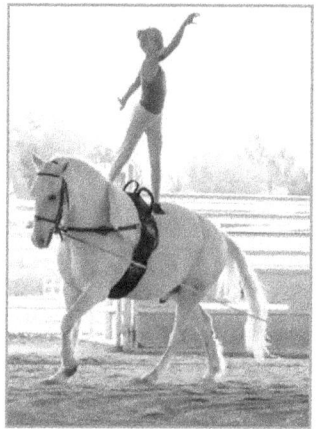

Fig. 16.10: Side-horse vaulting

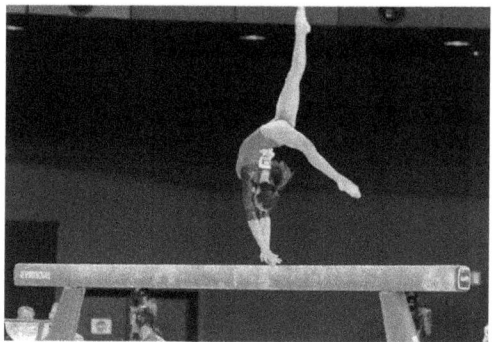

Fig. 16.12: Balance beam

Floor Exercises (Fig. 16.11)

Same floor dimensions are used for males and females. However, the time of the event differs for males and females. Men compete for 50–70 seconds and women compete for 70–90 seconds.

Women's routines are performed with music. Floor exercises are performed either with metal springs under plywood or a material called Ethafoam, which provides softer surface for landing. It reduces the number of injuries.

Balance Beam (Fig. 16.12)

Balance beam is a 16.5 feet long, slightly less than 4 inches wide and 4 feet off the floor.

It is made from hardwood with a thin rubber coating for shock absorption. The gymnast must perform both dance and tumbling skills on the beam.

Uneven Parallel Bars (Fig. 16.13)

- Uneven parallel bars, compensated for the lesser upper extremity strength in females, incorporating swinging into the routine.
- The two rails are adjustable. Lower rail is approximately 4.5–5 feet from the floor and upper rail is 7–7.5 feet from the floor. Rails are made of fiber glass to avoid splitting and cracking.
- They are 7 feet, 9 inch long and provide for some spring.
- Routine consists of a series of grasp and release moves as well as large swings.

Parallel Bars (Fig. 16.14)

It consists of two parallel foot long rails, 5 feet, 9 inches off the floor.

Event requires great upper extremity strength because upper extremity functions mainly as a closed kinetic chain throughout a series of swinging and support moves.

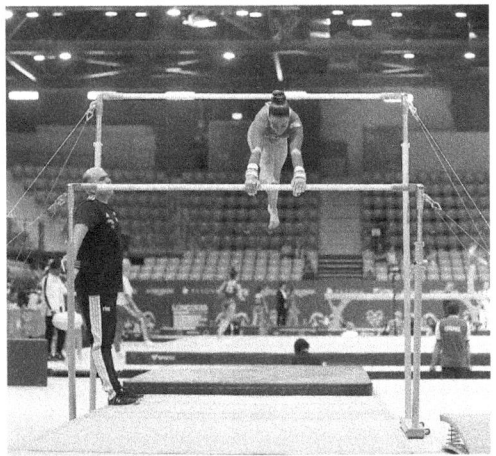

Fig. 16.13: Uneven parallel bars

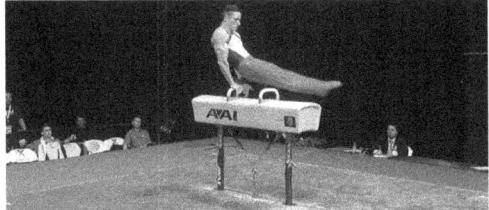

Fig. 16.15: Pommel horse

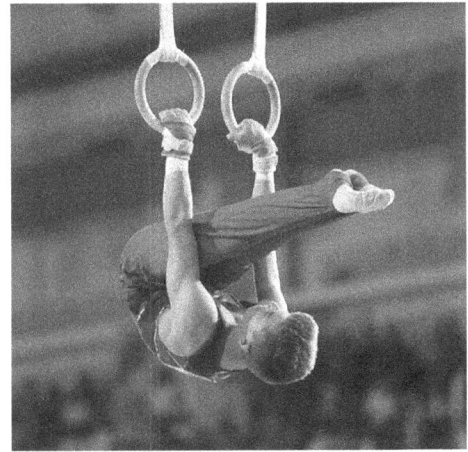

Fig. 16.16: Still rings

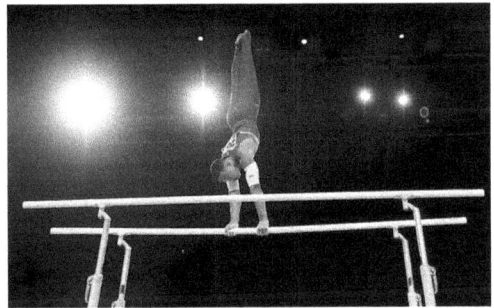

Fig. 16.14: Parallel bars

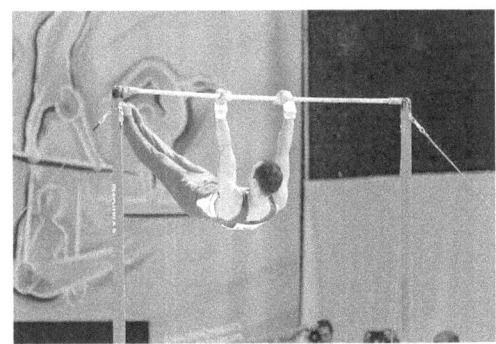

Fig. 16.17: Horizontal bars

Pommel Horse (Fig. 16.15)

Pommel horse stands approximately 3 feet, 8 inches from the floor. The pommel adds 5 inches to the height. The gymnast must maintain himself on the horse while performing both support and swinging moves. Along with physical strength, the athlete should have good body control in order to maintain oneself on the pommels saddle.

Still Rings (Fig. 16.16) and Horizontal Bars (Fig. 16.17)

Still rings and horizontal bar require the gymnast to begin a routine from a hanging position. Still rings are 8.5 feet from the floor.

Horizontal Bars

Made of tempered steel and is 8.5 feet from the floor. Mainly concerned with grasping, releasing, and regrasping the bar making the event one of timing and strength. It must control 5–7 times body weight while swinging.

Injuries most common in lower extremity with sprains being the most common type (acute) and chronic injury is patellofemoral pain syndrome. Lower extremity injuries are more common in women and upper extremity injuries are more common in men. Greater number of injuries are during floor exercises (45%) and balance beam (12%).

Upper extremity injuries are:
- **Hand injuries:**
  - Skin tears
  - Dorsal wrist pain
  - Distal radius stress fracture
  - Scaphoid fracture
  - Ulnar impaction syndrome
- **Shoulder injuries:**
  - Supraspinatus strain
  - Impingement syndrome
  - Shoulder instability
  - Subluxation and dislocations
  - Bicipital tendinitis
- **Elbow injuries:**
  - Fractures
  - Dislocations
  - Triceps tendinitis
  - Medial and lateral epicondylitis
  - Osteochondritis dissecans
- **Knee injuries:**
  - Chondromalacia patella
  - Patellar dislocations/subluxations
  - Meniscus tear
  - ACL injuries
  - Patellofemoral pain
  - Jumpers knee/patellar tendinitis
  - Osgood-Schlatter disease
- **Low back injuries:**
  - Scheuermann disease
  - Herniated nucleus pulposus
  - Spondylolysis
  - Spondylolisthesis
- **Ankle injuries:**
  - Ankle sprains
  - Anterior ankle impingement syndrome
  - Achilles tendinitis
  - Plantar fasciitis

KICKING

It involves acceleration from proximal to distal. Two techniques:
1. Straight on technique
2. Soccer style technique

Stages of Kicking Motion (Fig. 16.18)

- **Approach:** It involves 45° angle of approach and produces maximum peak ball velocity.
- **Swing limb loading:**
  - Lower leg is cocked back to prepare for upcoming downward swing.

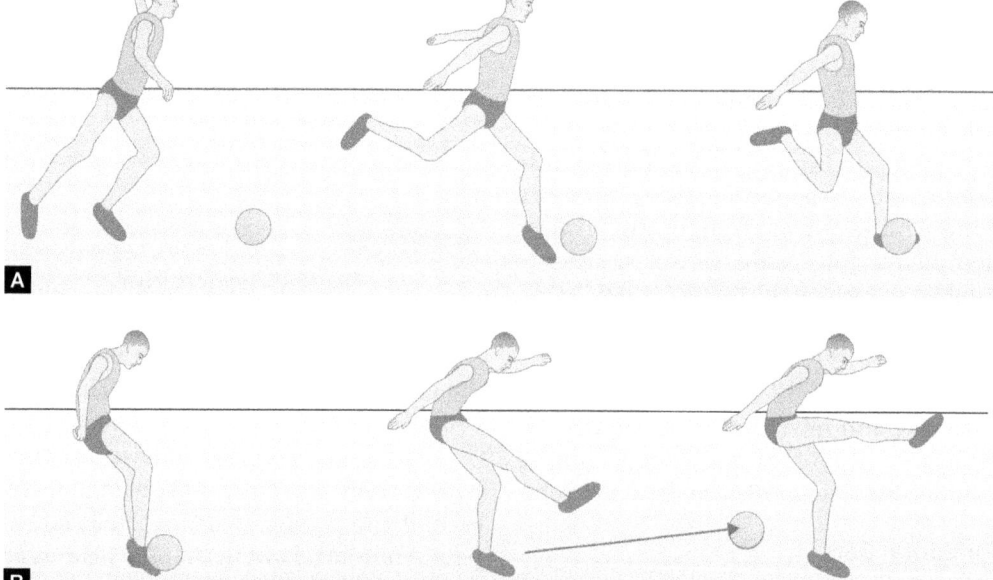

Figs. 16.18A and B: Stages of kicking a ball

- Knee extensor muscles are key as the knee flexes and stores elastic energy.
- **Plant:**
  - Force and orientation of plant foot are crucial.
  - Plant should be about a foot's length away from the ball and directionally facing the target.
  - Incorrect placement of the plant foot will drastically affect both distance and direction of kick.
- **Hip flexion and knee extension:**
  - From its loaded position, the thigh quickly swings forward as the lower leg drives downward toward the ball.
  - Knee extensors help propel leg forward, releasing built up elastic energy.
- **Contact:**
  - Knee is extended, ankle is plantar flexed.
  - Hamstrings act in eccentric contraction to slow down the lower leg.
  - Kinetic energy is transferred from moving leg to stationary football.
- **Follow through:**
  - Longer time of contact improves transfer of momentum, increases ball speed
  - Proper follow through should improve both distance and accuracy, as well as help to prevent injury.
  - Skipping through the kick provides power and helps the kicker stayed aligned with the target.

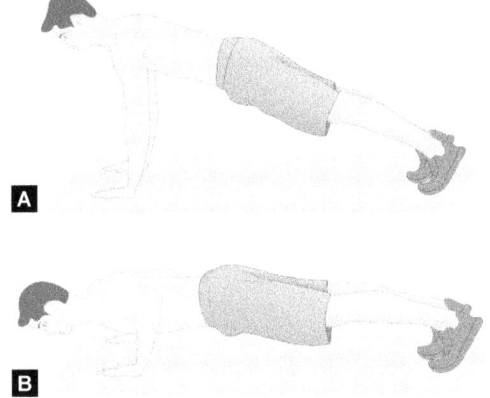

Figs. 16.19A and B: (A) Push up phase; (B) Push ups in down phase

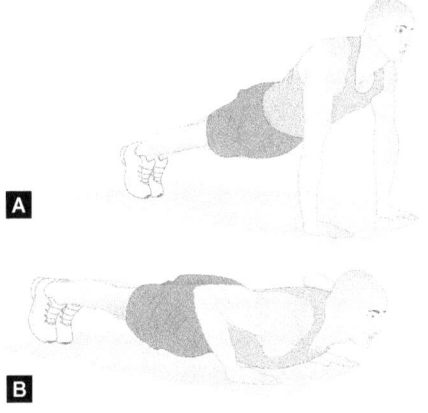

Figs. 16.20A and B: (A) Push ups in up phase; (B) Push down phase

PUSH UPS

It is a callisthenic activity which includes lowering and rising of body simultaneously from prone on hand plank position.

The whole body muscles are exercised and majorly it involves pectoral muscles, triceps, deltoid, serrates anterior, and coracobrachialis. There are two phases:
1. Down phase **(Figs. 16.19A and B)**
2. Up phase **(Figs. 16.20A and B)**

PULL UPS

A pull up is an upper body strength exercise where the body is suspended by hands grasping a horizontal bar.

Phases:
- Raising the body **(Fig. 16.21)**
- Lowering the body **(Fig. 16.22)**

Position:
- **Arms:** Pronated
- **Head:** Held high
- **Scapula:** Drawn downward
- **Trunk and leg**—straight
- **Heels:** Together
- **Ankle:** Plantar flexed

Muscle work and uses:
- Flexors of fingers—to grasp the bar
- Wrist musculature—reduce joint strain, acts as synergists for flexors of fingers
- Elbow flexors—reduce joint strain
- Shoulder adductors—lift the body on arm

- Plantar flexors—points the toes toward floor

SWIMMING

It is a form of exercise that includes trained physical movements, through the water in terms of stroke, start, and turn. It relies on proposition through water using both upper and lower limbs. Approximately, 90% of the force is generated by upper limb **(Fig. 16.23)**.

Stroke length, frequency, velocity, and sprinting speed define the efficiency of a swimmer.

Swimming Strokes
- Front crawl
- The backstroke
- Breast stroke
- Butterfly

Four Phases
1. **The reach:** The arm reaches forward to entry of water.
2. **The catch:** The elbow flexes to 100°, shoulder extends, horizontally abducts, and medially rotates.
3. **Pull:**
   - Varies slightly with each stroke
   - Swimmer pushes water the propulsion phase.
4. **Recovery:**
   - Out of the water phase
   - Arm returns to start the pull again.

CYCLING

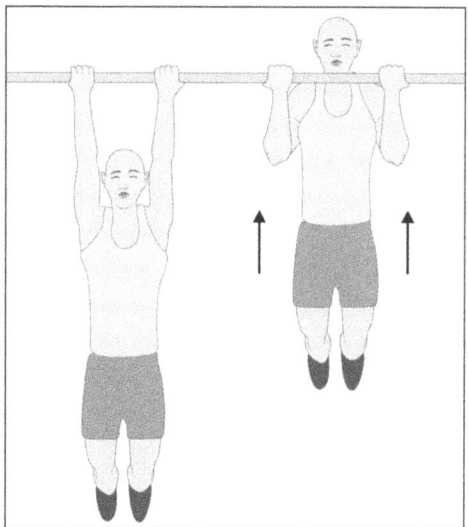

Fig. 16.21: Raising the body

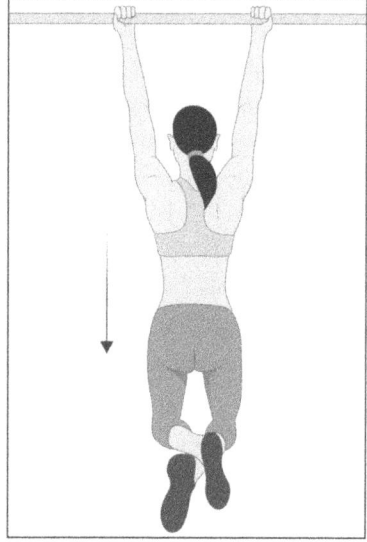

Fig. 16.22: Lowering the body

- Depressors, retractors, and lateral rotator of scapula—to stabilize the scapula and brace the upper back
- Prevertebral and postvertebral neck muscles—work reciprocally to keep the head and neck in position
- Flexor of lumbar spine and hip extensors—correct the tendency to arch back
- Adductors of hip—keep the legs together
- Knee extensors—maintain full flexion

Cycling is an exercise performed on either a static or movable machine, which consists of two wheels, connected to a plank, via rubber device and pedals for forward propulsion. It is a combination of extreme postural inertia of the upper and lower body together with excessive repetitive load on lower limb **(Fig. 16.24)**.

There are three points of contact:
1. Pelvis → saddle
2. Hand → handlebars
3. Foot → pedal

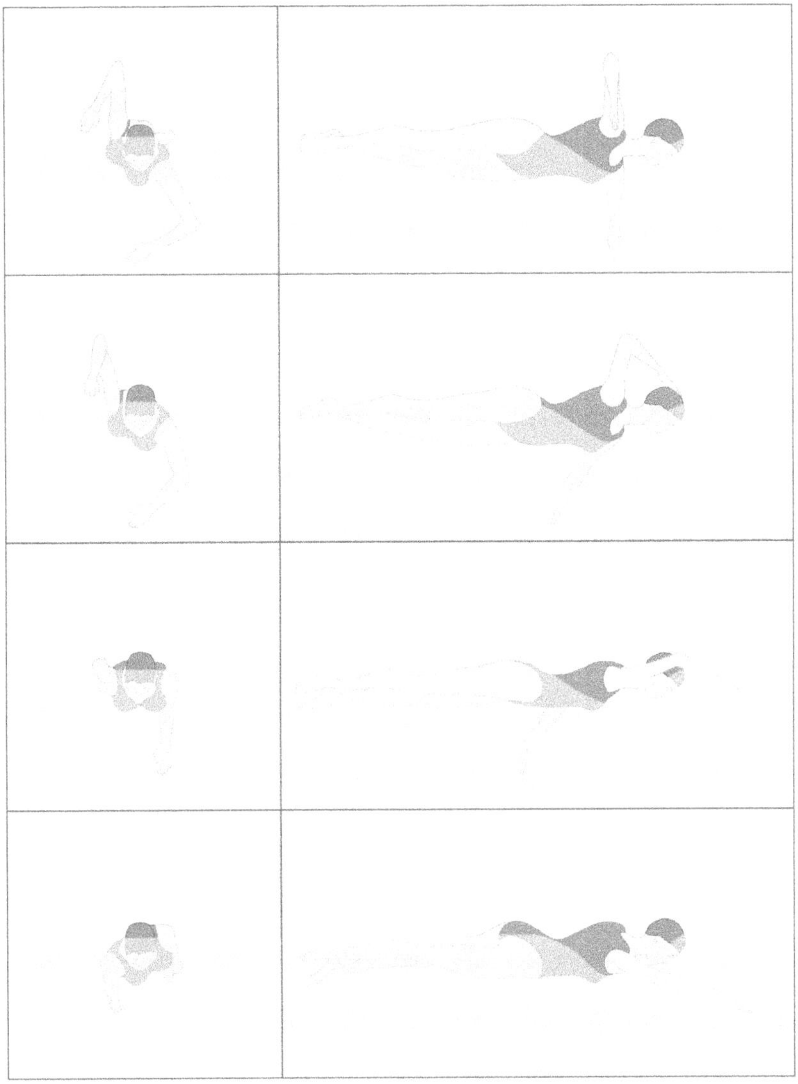

Fig. 16.23: Swimming

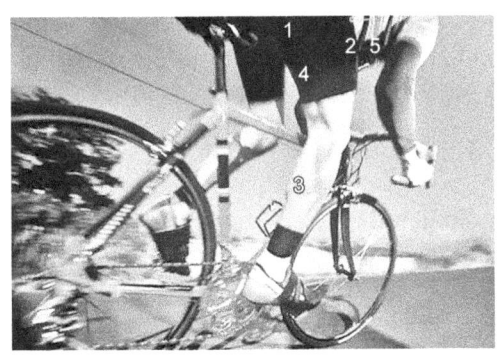

Fig. 16.24: Cycling

Two Phases (Fig. 16.25)

1. **Power phase**
   - It is the downward stroke on pedal.
   - Moves the pedal from 12'o clock position to the 6'o clock position.
   - These two positions are referred as 0–180°, respectively.
   - It has two segments: 0–90° and 90–180°
   - *Position:*
     - Initial: Hip and knee flexion, ankle in neutral

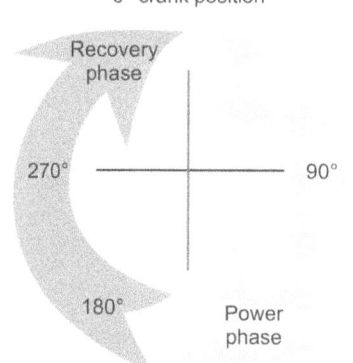

Fig. 16.25: Phases of cycling

- Middle: Hip extension
- End: Hip extension and knee flexion

2. **Recovery phase**
   - Upward stroke on the pedal
   - Moves the pedal on crank from 180° perpendicular to the start of rotation at 0°
   - It is divided into two segments: 180–270° and 270–360°
   - At the initial segment of recovery, the muscles are relaxed while the later the muscle activity increases, where in quadriceps and tibialis anterior muscles play an active role.

Position on the Bike

- **Seat height:** Improper seat height can alter the length tension relationship between muscles resulting in excessive stress on joints.
- **Cleat position:** Cleat should allow the base of the 1st metatarsal to sit over the pedal axis to facilitate maximum leverage through the foot. The main aim of the cleat is to align the hip, knee, and ankle. Pedal and cleat systems work together. Seats should be horizontal.
- **Reach:** Reach depends on flexibility of the rider, experience, comfort, desired bike handling, and desired aerodynamics.

Peddling Techniques

- Pedal stroke should be smooth and continuous.
- The rider has to avoid upstrokes as it leads to injuries.
- Cleats assist in stopping the foot from slipping during fast peddling, through proprioception.

WICKET KEEPING

It is a part of cricket game. In this the player on the fielding side is standing behind the stumps. He works in the game to take a catch, run out a batsman, and to stump the batsman out.

Position: When the ball is bowled the wicket-keeper crouches himself in full squatting position while partly in standing position when the ball is received.

Phases: There are three phases (**Fig. 16.26**):
1. Wicket
2. Keeping
3. Crouch

BIOMECHANICS IN DANCE

Dance is a conscious effort to create visual designs in space by continuously moving the body through a series of poses and pattern training. Dancing is one of the most physically strenuous activities on the musculoskeletal system. Dancers are a unique blend of artist and athlete particularly susceptible to musculoskeletal injuries and pain.

The lower back seems to be the most frequently injured anatomical site, which together with pelvis, legs, knees, and feet account for more than 90% of injuries. Overwork, unsuitable floors, difficult choreography, inadequate flexibility, and aspects related to muscle imbalances and body composition are thought to contribute to such injuries.

Different Styles of Dance

- Ballet
- Indian Classical (Bharatanatyam, Kuchipudi, Kathak, Kathakali, Odissi, Manipuri)
- Hip Hop
- Shuffle
- Latin/ballroom
- Contemporary

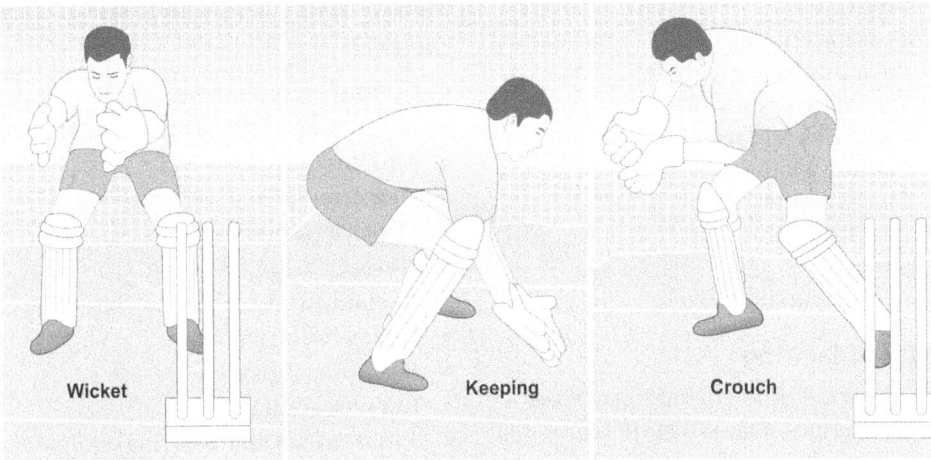

Fig. 16.26: Three phases of wicket keeping

Each of these dance forms has their own styles and techniques.

Biomechanics of Dance

Biomechanics of dance is defined as the science examining internal and external forces acting on a dancer, points out mechanical and physiological effects produced by these. Biomechanics may enhance dancer's ability to detect the root cause of faults during particular movement, avoid movements that may potentially cause injury, and secure the best possible use of their natural abilities.

Dance training is characterized by a systematic progression of repeated motions. Biomechanics observes forces acting on the body, which contributes to an understanding of the technical demands and artistry of dance.

Most dance movements can be categorized as one or two body parts moving in relation to, and supported by, the rest of the body. The movement of one segment has an effect on rest of the body as well as the movement as a whole.

Looking at the interaction between the gesture leg and pelvis, it is found that skilled dancers had greater range of motion in the pelvis accompanying the range of motion for the gesturing leg. In other words, after the leg has reached a certain height the pelvis must move to accommodate further range of motion. Movements to the front and side past 90° of flexion involve the pelvis in the three-dimensional movement. To the back, anterior tilting of the pelvis is seen after 15° of hip hyperextension. This research clarifies the role of pelvis in movements at the hip joint that requires large range of motion. To move the leg fully the pelvis must follow the leg, even though the illusion advocated is to keep the pelvis immobile.

The role of pelvis in facilitating gesture leg motion, and the related "cost" of the muscles involved. The skilled dancers are working more efficiently in their standing leg to support the pelvis and gesture leg, whereas the less-skilled dancers are mostly using the muscles in the gesturing leg. When working on movements where one leg is moving fully, a strategy to focus on the standing leg will help balance the necessary movement in the pelvis and spine.

The strategies that dancers use for balance and counterbalance are based on neuronal and reflex adjustments that develop with dance training. It is found that dancers use (subconscious) motor program to maintain the vertical orientation of the head when the leg is moving.

Factors those are responsible for dance injuries:
- **Extrinsic risk factors**
  - Technique demands
  - Dance styles

- Exposure
- Training errors
- Environmental conditions
- Shoes and costumes
- **Intrinsic risk factors**
  - Age and gender
  - Previous injury
  - Joint laxity
  - Strength
  - Aerobic conditioning

Benefits of Dancing

- Improved condition of heart and lungs
- Increased muscular strength, endurance, and motor fitness
- Increased aerobic fitness
- Improved muscle tone and strength
- Weight management
- Stronger bones and reduced risk of osteoporosis
- Better coordination, agility, and flexibility
- Improved balance and spatial awareness
- Increased physical confidence
- Improved mental functioning
- Improved general and psychological wellbeing
- Greater self-confidence and esteem
- Better social skills

Preventing Musculoskeletal Injury for Dancers

- Controlling over training or burnouts
- Monitoring physical fitness and flexibility
- Muscle strength
- Dance on sprung floors
- Dance in warmer studios
- Warm up before dancing
- Remain aware of dancers' limitations
- Rest between workouts
- Rest when injured
- Get proper nutrition
- Avoid strain when carrying equipment

CONCLUSION

By applying principles from mechanics, engineering and electronics, biomechanics is able to provide data on the forces that act upon the body and the effects they produce. In dance, biomechanical methodologies are used to improve aspects of dance technique which, in turn, may help dancers to prevent disabling injuries, to assess fitness levels and control over training (or burnout) and to plan effective scheduling of practice and exercise sessions.

CHAPTER 17

Goniometry

Chapter Outline

- Definition
- Principles
- Types of goniometry
- Indications
- Contraindications
- Precautions
- Measurement procedure
- Measurement
- Recording of the measurement

DEFINITION

The instrument which is used for measuring range of motion (ROM) of a joint is called goniometer.

The term goniometer is derived from Greek word "gonio" means angle and "metron" means measurement. Therefore, goniometer refers to the measurement of angles created at the joints by the bones of the human body.

- **ROM:** This is the amount of motion that is available at a joint.
- **Active ROM (AROM):** This is the ROM the joint can move by the person voluntarily.
- **Passive ROM (PROM):** This is the ROM attained by a joint when the movement done by the therapist.

PRINCIPLES OF GONIOMETRY

- Explanation and instruction
- Patient position
- Therapist position
- Therapist hand placement
- Trick movements
- Stabilization

Explanation and Instructions

Briefly explain about the effects, uses, and measurement procedure of joint ROM.

Before measuring the ROM, the therapist must demonstrate the movement to be performed and proper instructions have to be given before starting the measurement procedure.

Patient Position

The patient positioned in a comfortable and well supported with the joint to be assessed in the anatomical position, i.e., to allow only the desired movement of the joint by stabilizing the proximal segment of the joint.

Therapist Position

The therapist must stand near the patient facing the joint which has to be measured; the therapist can stand in stride/walk stance position based on the joint measuring.

Therapist Hand Placement

With one hand, the therapist must stabilize the proximal segment of the joint by holding the stable arm of goniometer and another hand is used to perform the movement of the distal segment of the measuring joint by holding the movable arm of the goniometer.

Trick Movements

While measuring the joint ROM, the therapist must make sure the patient is not going for any trick/substitute movements, thus giving the appearance of having greater ROM than the actual ROM of the joint.

To eliminate/prevent the trick movements, the therapist must give proper instruction to the patient regarding the actual movement to be performed and the about the trick movement done in that particular joint, comfortable and relaxed positioning of the patient, adequate stabilization of the proximal segment of the joint, and the therapist must know and recognize all the trick movements the patients could use.

Stabilization

Stabilize the proximal segment of the joint for accurate joint ROM measurement. Stabilization can be done by patients own body weight, comfortable position of the patient, and by external forces.

Measurement

The method used for measuring the joint ROM is called as "Neutral zero method." All the joints range of motions are measured form their zero positions.

Positioning the patient in a relaxed manner and the joint measuring should be free from any obstructions like pillows, couch, tight clothings, etc.
- **Goniometer placement:** The ideal placement of the goniometer is lateral to the joint, but it can also be placed on the top of the joint with a light contact between the joint and the skin.
- **Axis:** The axis of the goniometer is placed on the axis of the movement of the joint. A specific bony prominence or anatomical landmark can be used to represent the axis of the joint.
- **Stable arm:** Usually the stable arm of the goniometer is placed parallel to the longitudinal axis of the proximal segment of the joint.
- **Movable arm:** Usually the movable arm of the goniometer is parallel and longitudinal to the axis of the moving distal segment of the joint.

Recording of the Measurement

Numerical charts can be used to record ROM. The ROM is recorded by writing the no. of degrees the joint has moved away from the zero-degree point.

TYPES

- Universal
- Gravity dependent/fluid goniometer
- Pendular goniometer
- Electro goniometer

Universal Goniometer (Fig. 17.1)

It is the most used variety of goniometer. It is designed by Moore. Universal goniometer has body, stationary arm, and movable arm.

Body

Body of the goniometer resembles full or half protractor. Half circle protractor consists of 0–180°/180–0°; full circle protractor body consists of 0–360°/360–0° of reading.

In the middle of the body, axis/fulcrum screw is present, which connects the movable and stable arm.

The axis of goniometer placed over the axis of the joint, which must be measured.

Stable Arm

This is the extension from the body of goniometer. The stable arm does not have any motion. This will be aligned with a proximal segment of the measuring joint.

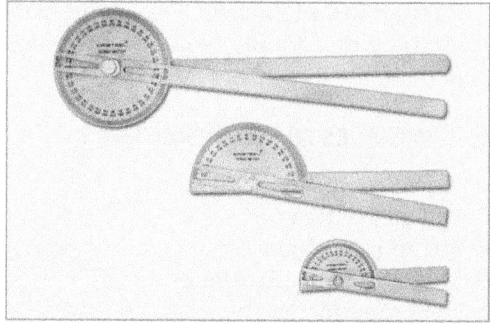

Fig. 17.1: Types of universal goniometer

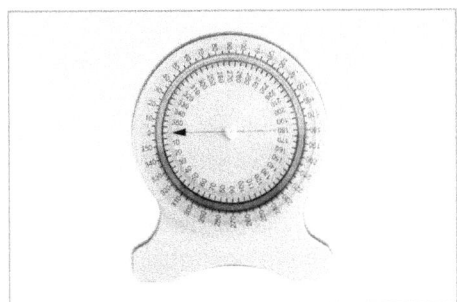

Fig. 17.2: Inclinometer

Movable Arm

This is the additional attachment with the body of the goniometer in the axis.

The movable arm is aligned with the distal segment of the measuring joint.

Gravity Dependent/Fluid Goniometer (Fig. 17.2)

It was designed by "Sckenkas" in 1956; it is having a gravity affecting pointer and the fluid-filled chamber with air bubble. It is mostly used for measuring the pelvic inclination/tilt/drop. It is also called as pelvic inclinometer.

Pendular Goniometer (Fig. 17.3)

It is designed by "Fox and Van Breemen" in 1934. It consists of 360° protector with a weighted pointer.

Electro Goniometer

It is designed by "Karporich" in 1959. It consists of two arms; one is attached to the proximal segment and the other is attached to the distal segment of the measuring joint.

The potentiometer is connected with these 2 arms, changing in the joint position, shows the angulation in the potentiometer.

Factors Affecting Joint ROM

- **Soft tissue tightness:** When soft tissues like muscles and ligaments become taut they restrict the range of motion. The soft tissue tightness might be due to prolonged immobilization of the joint, injury around the joint, joint diseases like osteoarthritis, rheumatoid arthritis, tuberculosis arthritis, etc.
- **Adhesion formation:** Adhesion formation of the joint reduces ROM of the joint due to lack of mobility that leads to reduction of flexibility, nourishment, and blood circulation around the joint. Prolonged immobilization of the joint causes increasing in the collagen fibers and reduction in elastic property of the fibers of the connective tissues and the soft tissues of the joint.
- **Muscle bulk:** Increase in muscle bulk may cause the reduction of the active or

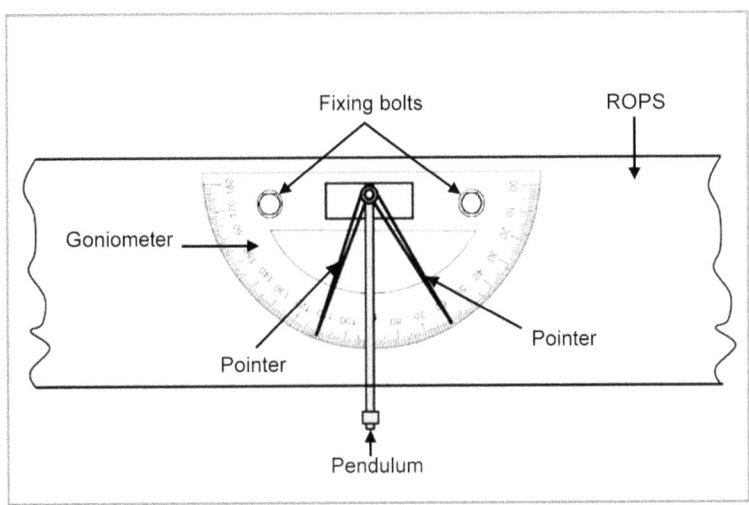

Fig. 17.3: Pendular goniometer

passive ROM of the joint, e.g., for a normal individual, the elbow flexion ROM is 125–135°, but it is very much less body builder due to their huge biceps bulk.
- **Sex:** The ROM will vary with the sex. Generally female will have more flexibility than the males.
- **Age:** The ROM of the joint will be more in infants and childhood due to nonfusion of the bones. Day-by-day ROM reduces with ages difference while reaching the adulthood; ROM reduces while comparing with childhood and late childhood. The ROM again increases in age due to hypotonicity of muscles and reduction of the muscle bulk.
- **Nervous system:** Sometimes ROM may vary with the pathological changes, i.e., diseases process in the nervous system. The spasticity of the muscle, which is the result of the motion neuron session, will be reducing the ROM and the joint is said to be hypomobile.

The lower motor neuron which causes the flaccidity results in hypermobile joints. If the musculoskeletal disorders rise due to lesions of any part of nervous system like cerebellum, basal ganglion, cerebral cortex, thalamus, internal capsule, midbrain, and pons result in the decreasing or increasing ROM.

Indications

- Stiffness of soft tissues and joints
- Pain
- Muscular weakness
- Postoperative fracture conditions
- Neurological conditions

Contraindications

Active or passive ROM must not be measured if any contraindications are present.
- The region of dislocation or unhealed fractures
- Immediately following surgical procedures to general tendons, ligaments, muscles, joint capsule, and skin
- The presence of myositis ossificans (formation of bone in the muscle)

Precautions

- Presence of infections or inflammatory changes in and around the joint.
- In patients on medications for muscle relaxants, as the patient may not be able to respond appropriately and movement may be performed vigorously.
- In the region of osteoporosis PROM must be performed with extreme care.
- While measuring a hypermobile or subluxed joint
- In painful conditions of the joints, the assessment should be taken with care.
- Patients with hemophilia
- Presence of deep vein thrombosis (DVT) or hematoma
- Suspected case of ankylosis/spondylosis
- Immediately after injury

Measurement Procedure

- Patient clothes should be loose where the joint measurement is taken.
- Position the patient in relaxed manner and joint to be measured should be free from any obstructions such as pillows, couch, etc.
- Measuring joint must be in 0° position.
- Total procedure is explained to the patient.
- The therapist must stand near the patient and facing the joint which must be measured.
- The axis/fulcrum of the goniometer is placed over the joint axis to be measured.
- Stable arm is fixed to the proximal segment of the measuring joint.
- Movable arm is fixed to the distal segment of the measuring joint.
- The therapist must move the distal segment of the joint along with the movable arm of the goniometer to measure the joint range of motion.
- The type of goniometer must be selected based on the measuring joint, if the measuring joints are big, bigger goniometer, i.e., bigger length movable and stable arm are used, and for smaller joints in vice versa.
- Complete ROM of the joint must be permitted.

MEASURING OF ROM IN UPPER EXTREMITY

Shoulder Flexion (Fig. 17.4)
- **Position of patient:** The patient is in supine lying or in sitting position, arm at the side and palm facing medially.
- **Axis:** The axis is placed approximately 2.5 cm inferior to the lateral aspect of the acromion process.
- **Stable arm:** Parallel to the lateral midline of the trunk.
- **Movable arm:** Parallel to the longitudinal axis of the humerus pointing toward the lateral epicondyle of the humerus.
- **End position:** The humerus is moved in an anterior direction to the limit of motion.
- **Trick movement:** When sitting, trunk extension and shoulder abduction
- **Normal ROM:** 0–180°

Shoulder Extension (Fig. 17.5)
- **Position of patient:** The patient is in siting or in prone position. The arm is at the side, with the palm facing medially.
- **Axis:** The axis is placed approximately 2.5 cm inferior to the lateral aspect of the acromion process.
- **Stable arm:** Parallel to the lateral midline of the trunk.
- **Movable arm:** Parallel to the longitudinal axis of the humerus pointing toward the lateral epicondyle of the humerus.
- **End position:** The humerus moves posteriorly to the limit of emotion 60°.

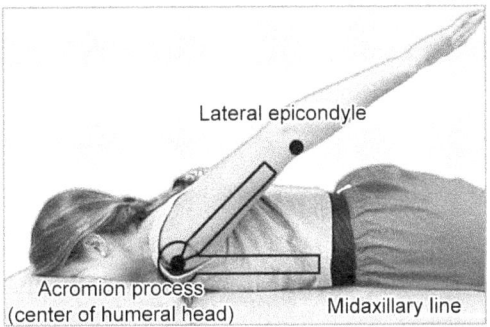

Fig. 17.5: Shoulder extension

- **Trick movement:** Scapular elevation and shoulder abduction. The patient may flex the trunk while sitting.
- **Normal ROM:** 0–60°

Shoulder Abduction (Fig. 17.6)
- **Position of patient:** The patient is supine or sitting. The arm is at the side in adduction and external rotation.
- **Axis:** The axis is placed at the midpoint of the anterior/posterior aspect of the glenohumeral joint, approximately 1.3 cm inferior and lateral to the coracoid process.
- **Stable arm:** Parallel to the clavicle
- **Movable arm:** Parallel to the longitudinal axis of the humerus
- **End position:** Humerus moves lateral to the limit of 180°
- **Trick movement:** Contralateral trunk flexion, scapular elevation, and shoulder flexion
- **Normal ROM:** 0–180°

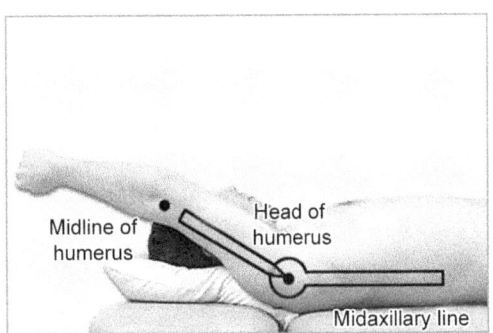

Fig. 17.4: Shoulder flexion

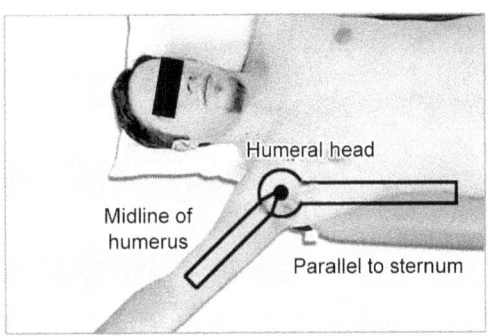

Fig. 17.6: Shoulder abduction

Shoulder Adduction

- **Position of patient:** The patient is in sitting position; the shoulder is on 90° abduction. The therapist supports the arm in abduction.
- **Axis:** The axis is placed on the top of the acromion process.
- **Stable arm:** Perpendicular to the trunk
- **Movable arm:** Parallel to the longitudinal axis of the humerus.
- **End position:** The humerus moves anteriorly across the chest to the limit of motion in horizontal adduction 125°.
- **Trick movement:** Contralateral trunk rotation
- **Normal ROM:** 0–125°

Shoulder Medial/Lateral Rotation (Figs. 17.7A and B)

- **Position of patient:** The patient is in supine lying with the shoulder at 90° of abduction and elbow at 90° of flexion. Forearm is in mid prone position.
- **Axis:** The axis is placed on the olecranon process.
- **Stable arm:** Perpendicular to the floor.
- **Movable arm:** Parallel to the longitudinal axis of the ulna, pointing toward the ulnar styloid process.
- **End position:** The palm of the hand is moved toward the ceiling to limit of internal rotation.
- **Trick movement (medial rotation):** Elbow extension, scapular elevation and abduction.
- **Trick movement (lateral rotation):** Elbow extension, scapular depression and adduction.
- **Normal ROM:** Medial rotation—0–90°/lateral rotation—0–90°

Elbow Flexion/Extension (Figs. 17.8A and B)

- **Position of patient:** The patient is in supine or sitting, the arm is in anatomical position with the elbow in extension.

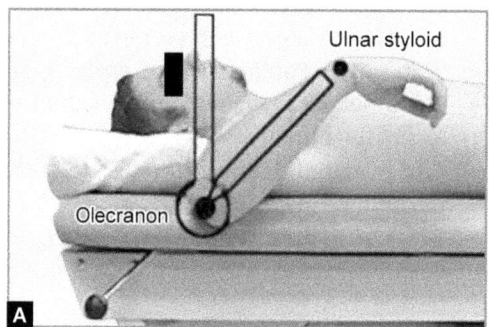 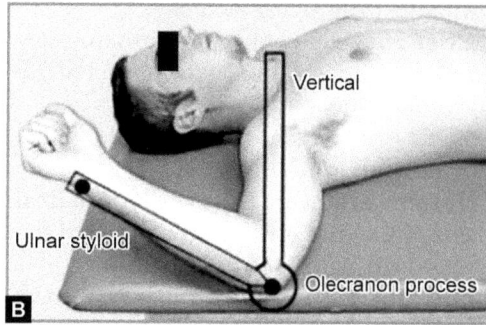

Figs. 17.7A and B: (A) Shoulder medial rotation; (B) Shoulder lateral rotation

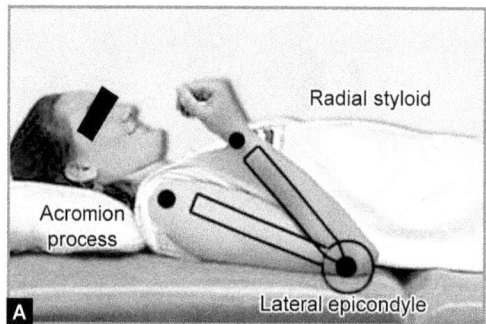 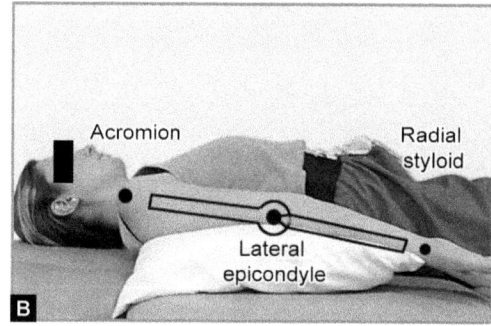

Figs. 17.8A and B: (A) Elbow flexion; (B) Elbow extension

- **Axis:** The axis is placed over the lateral epicondyle of the humerus.
- **Stable arm:** Parallel to the longitudinal axis of the humerus, pointing toward the tip of the acromion process.
- **Movable arm:** Parallel to the longitudinal axis of the radius pointing toward the styloid process.
- **End position (flexion):** From the start position of the elbow extension, the forearm is moved in an anterior direction so that the hand approximates the shoulder to the limit of elbow flexion.
- **End position (hyperextension):** The forearm is moved in a posterior direction beyond 0° of extension. Hyperextension of 10–15° is common in females because of the smaller olecranon process.
- **Normal ROM:** Flexion—0–125°/Extension—0°

Radioulnar Joint Supination/Pronation (Figs. 17.9A and B)

- **Position of patient:** The patient is sitting, the shoulder is adducted, and elbow is flexed to 90° with the forearm in mid position. A pencil is held in the tightly closed fist with the pencil protruding from the radial aspect of the hand.
- **Axis:** The axis is placed over the head of the 3rd metacarpal.
- **Stable arm:** Perpendicular to the floor
- **Movable arm:** Parallel to the pencil
- **End position (supination):** The forearm is rotated externally from mid position so that the palm faces toward the ceiling.
- **End position (pronation):** The forearm is rotated internally so that the palm faces downward toward the floor.
- **Trick movement (supination):** Wrist extension or radial deviation, adduction, and external rotation of shoulder, ipsilateral trunk flexion.
- **Trick movement (pronation):** Wrist flexion and ulnar deviation, addiction and internal rotation of shoulder, contralateral trunk flexion.
- **Normal ROM:** Supination—0–90°/pronation—0–90°

Wrist Flexion/Extension (Figs. 17.10A and B)

- **Position of patient:** The patient position is sitting, the forearm is resting on stable in pronation, and the wrist is in neutral position. The hand is over the end of the table.
- **Axis:** The axis is placed at the level of the ulnar styloid process.
- **Stable arm:** Parallel to the longitudinal axis of the ulna

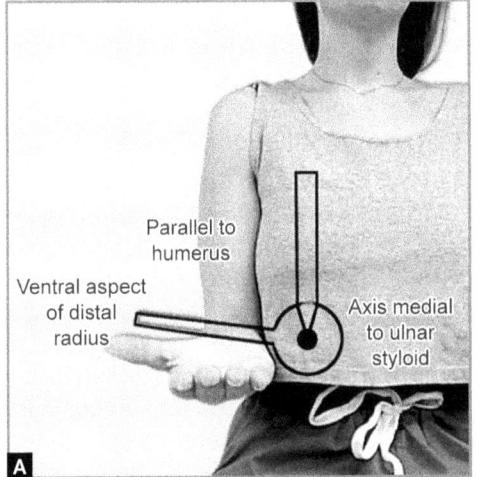 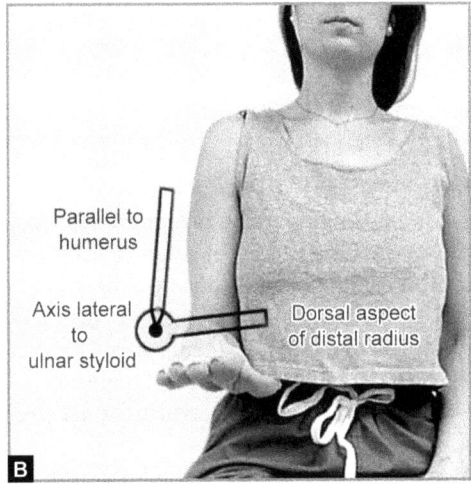

Figs. 17.9A and B: (A) Forearm supination; (B) Forearm pronation

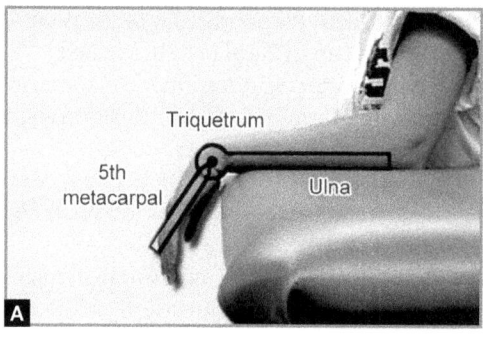
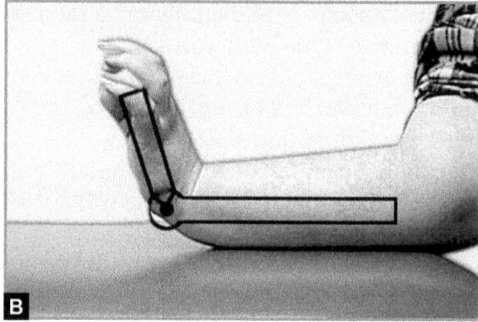

Figs. 17.10A and B: (A) Wrist flexion; (B) Wrist extension

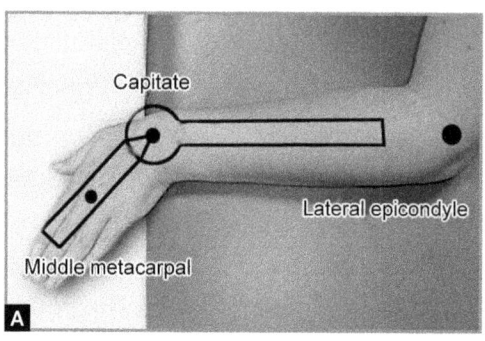
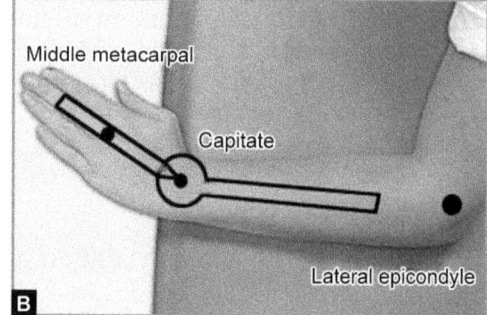

Figs. 17.11A and B: (A) Wrist ulnar deviation; (B) Wrist radial deviation

- **Movable arm:** Parallel to the longitudinal axis of the 5th metacarpal
- **End position (flexion):** The wrist is moved in avower direction.
- **End position (extension):** The wrist is moved in a dorsal direction.
- **Trick movement:** Wrist deviations
- **Normal ROM:** Flexion—0–80°/Extension—0–70°

Wrist Ulnar/Radial Deviation (Figs. 17.11A and B)

- **Position of patient:** The patient is in sitting position, the forearm is pronated, and the plane surface of the hand is resting on a table. Wrist is in neutral position and fingers are relaxed.
- **Axis:** The axis is placed on the dorsal aspect of the wrist joint over the capitate bone.
- **Stable arm:** Along the midline of the forearm
- **Movable arm:** Parallel to the longitudinal axis of the shaft of the 3rd metacarpal

- **End position:** During ulnar deviation, wrist is adducted to the ulnar side to the limit of motion 30°.
- **End position:** During radial deviation, wrist is abducted to the radial side to the limit of motion 20°.
- **Trick movement:** Wrist flexion and extension
- **Normal ROM:** Ulnar deviation—0–30°/Radial deviation—0–20°.

Metacarpophalangeal Flexion

- **Patient position:** The patient is in sitting with elbow flexed and forearm supported on the table, the wrist is slightly extended and the MCP joint of the finger being measured is at 0° of extension.
- **Axis:** The axis is placed over the dorsal aspect of the MCP being measured.
- **Stable arm:** Parallel to the longitudinal axis of the shaft of the metacarpal.
- **Movable arm:** Parallel to the longitudinal axis of the proximal phalanx.

- **End position:** All fingers are moved toward the palm to the limit of motion 90°. The range may increase from index finger to fifth finger. The proximal IP joint is allowed to flex and distal IP joints remain in extension.
- **Normal range:** 0–90°

Metacarpophalangeal Extension

- **Patient position:** The patient is in sitting with elbow flexed and forearm supported on the table, the wrist is slightly extended and the MCP joint of the finger being measured is at 0° of extension.
- **Axis:** The axis is placed over the volar surface of the MCP joint being measured.
- **Stable arm:** Parallel to the longitudinal axis of the shaft of metacarpal.
- **Movable arm:** Parallel to the longitudinal axis of the proximal phalanx.
- **End position:** The fingers are moved in dorsal direction to the limit of motion 40°. The IP joints are allowed to flex.
- **Normal range:** 0–40°

Metacarpophalangeal Abduction and Adduction

- **Patient position:** Patient is sitting with elbow flexed at 90°; forearm is pronated and resting on the table, wrist in neutral position, and fingers in anatomical position.
- **Axis:** The axis is placed over the dorsal surface of the MCP joint being measured.
- **Stable arm:** Parallel to the longitudinal axis of the shaft of metacarpal.
- **Movable arm:** Parallel to the longitudinal axis of the proximal phalanx.
- **End position:** The finger is moved away from the midline of the hand to the limit of motion in abduction. The finger is moved toward the midline of the hand to limit of motion in adduction.
- **Normal range:** Abduction—0–20°/ adduction—0–15°

Interphalangeal Flexion and Extension

- **Patient position:** Patient is sitting with forearm supported on the table in mid pronation, the wrist and fingers are in anatomical position.
- **Axis:** The axis is placed over the dorsal surface of the proximal or distal IP joint being measured.
- **Stable arm:** During proximal interphalangeal (PIP) measurement, parallel to the longitudinal axis of the proximal phalanx.
- During distal interphalangeal (DIP) measurement, parallel to the longitudinal axis of the middle phalanx.
- **Movable arm:** In PIP, parallel to the longitudinal axis of the middle phalanx.
- In DIP, parallel to the longitudinal axis of the distal phalanx.
- **End position:** The PIP and DIP joints are flexed to the limit of motion 100°, 90°, respectively.
- **Normal range:** Flexion—0–100°/Extension—0°

Thumb CMC Flexion and Extension

- **Patient position:** Patient is sitting, forearm is supported with elbow in flexion, forearm in mid-prone position, wrist slightly in ulnar deviation, fingers are in anatomical position, and the thumb is in contact with metacarpal and the proximal phalanx of the index finger.
- **Axis:** The axis is placed over the CMC joint.
- **Stable arm:** Parallel to the longitudinal axis of the thumb.
- **Movable arm:** Parallel to the longitudinal axis of the thumb metacarpal bone.
- **End position:** During flexion, the thumb is placed across the palm to the limit of motion 20°.
- During extension, the thumb is extended away from the palm to the limit of motion 15°.
- **Normal range:** Flexion—0–20°/Extension—0–15°

Thumb CMC Abduction and Adduction

- **Patient position:** Patient is sitting, forearm is supported with elbow in flexion, forearm in mid-prone position, wrist slightly in ulnar deviation, fingers are in anatomical

position, and the thumb is in contact with metacarpal and the proximal phalanx of the index finger.
- **Axis:** The axis is placed at the function of the base of the 1st and 2nd metacarpals.
- **Stable arm:** Parallel to the longitudinal axis of the 2nd metacarpal.
- **Movable arm:** Parallel to the longitudinal axis of the 1st metacarpal.
- **End position:** Thumb is abducted to the limit of 60°.
- **Normal range:** Abduction 0–60°

MEASURING OF ROM IN LOWER EXTREMITY

Hip Flexion (Fig. 17.12)
- **Position of patient:** The patient is in supine position, the hip and knee on the test side are in the neutral position and the other hip and knee may be flexed or extended.
- **Axis:** The axis is placed over the greater trochanter of the femur.
- **Stable arm:** Parallel to the midaxillary line of the trunk.
- **Movable arm:** Parallel to the longitudinal axis of the femur pointing toward the lateral epicondyle of the femur.
- **End position:** The hip is flexed to the limit of motion 125°, while flexing the knee the patient is instructed to keep the pelvis on the surface of the plinth.
- **Trick movement:** Flexion of the lumbar spine.
- **Normal ROM:** 0–125°

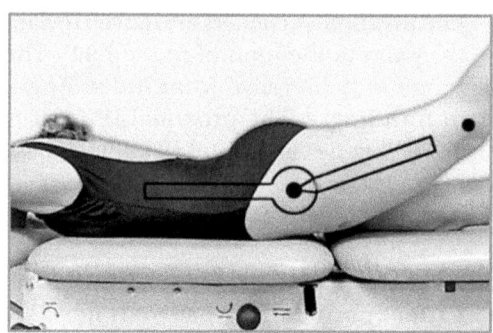

Fig. 17.13: Hip extension

Hip Extension (Fig. 17.13)
- **Position of patient:** The patient is in prone position; the hips and knees are in neutral position. The feet are over the end of the plinth.
- **Axis:** The axis is placed over the greater trochanter of the femur.
- **Stable arm:** Parallel to the midaxillary line of the trunk.
- **Movable arm:** Parallel to the longitudinal axis of the femur pointing toward the lateral epicondyle of the femur.
- **End position:** The hip is extended to the limit of motion 30°. The patient is instructed to keep the knee extended and the pelvis on the surface of the plinth.
- **Trick movement:** Extension of the lumbar spine
- **Normal ROM:** 0–30°

Hip Abduction (Fig. 17.14)
- **Position of patient:** The patient is supine with the lower extremities in neutral position.

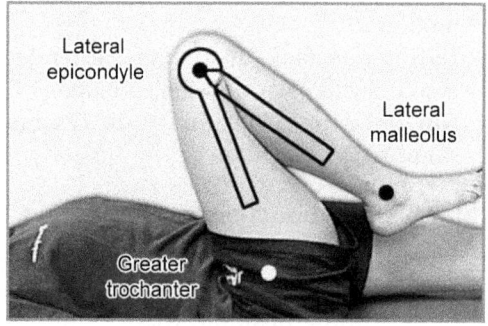

Fig. 17.12: Hip fllexion

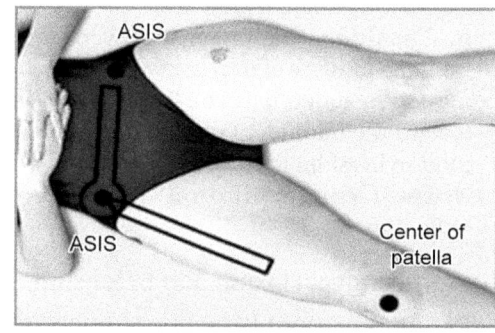

Fig. 17.14: Hip abduction

Chapter 17 | Goniometry

- **Axis:** The axis is placed over the anterior superior iliac spine (ASIS) on the side of hip being measured.
- **Stable arm:** Along a line between the 2 anterior superior iliac spines.
- **Movable arm:** Parallel to the longitudinal axis of the femur
- **End position:** Hip is abducted to the limit of motion 45°.
- **Trick movement:** External rotation of the hip.
- **Normal ROM:** 0–50°

Hip Adduction (Fig. 17.15)
- **Position of patient:** The patient is supine with the lower extremities in neutral position.
- **Axis:** The axis is placed over the anterior superior iliac spine (ASIS) on the side of hip being measured.
- **Stable arm:** Along a line between the 2 anterior superior iliac spines.
- **Movable arm:** Parallel to the longitudinal axis of the femur.
- **End position:** The hip is adducted to the limit of motion 30°.
- **Trick movement:** Hip internal rotation
- **Normal ROM:** 0–30°

Hip Medial/Lateral Rotation (Figs. 17.16A and B)
- **Position of patient:** The patient position is sitting. The hip being measured is in 90° of flexion and neutral rotation with the knee flexed to 90°. The contralateral foot

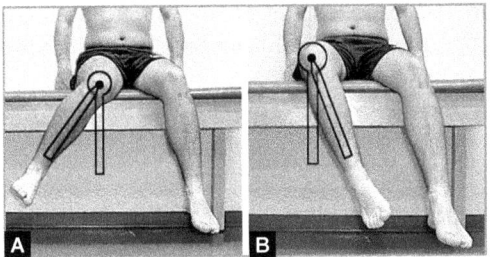

Figs. 17.16A and B: (A) Hip medial rotation; (B) Hip lateral rotation

is abducted, and the foot is placed on the stool.
- The alternative patient position is prone lying with knee flexed to 90°.
- **Axis:** The axis is placed over the midpoint of the patella.
- **Stable arm:** Perpendicular to the floor
- **Movable arm:** Parallel to the anterior midline of tibia
- **End position:** The hip is internal rotated to the limit of 45° so that leg and foot move in a lateral direction.
- During external rotation, the hip is externally rotated to the limit of motion 45° so that the leg and foot move in medial direction.
- **Normal ROM:** Medial rotation—0–50°/ Lateral rotation—0–45°

Knee Flexion (Fig. 17.17)
- **Position of patient:** Patient is supine, the hip is anatomical position, and the knee is in 0° of extension.
- **Axis:** The axis is over the lateral epicondyle of the femur.

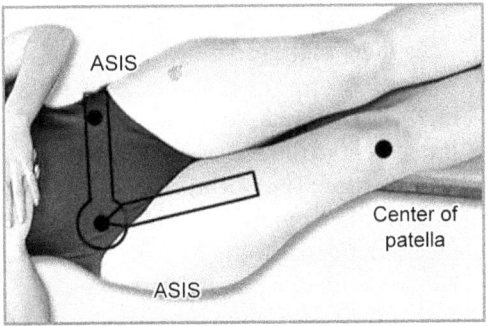

Fig. 17.15: Hip adduction

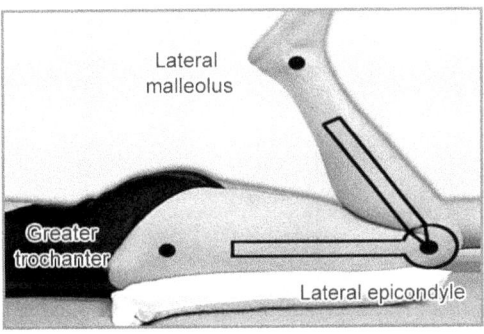

Figs. 17.17: Knee flexion

- **Stable arm:** Parallel to the longitudinal axis of the femur pointing toward the greater trochanter.
- **Movable arm:** Parallel to the longitudinal axis of the fibula pointing toward the lateral malleolus.
- **End position:** From the start position of knee extension the hip and knee are flexed, the heel is moved toward the buttocks to the limit of knee flexion 135°.
- **Normal ROM:** 0–135°

Knee Extension

The femur is stabilized, and the lower leg is moved in an anterior direction beyond 0° of extension. Hyperextension from 0–10° may be present.

Ankle Dorsiflexion/Plantar Flexion (Figs. 17.18 and 17.19)

- **Position of patient:** The patient is in sitting or in supine lying, in sitting knee is flexed to 90°. In supine, the knee is flexed to approximately 20–30° with a towel roll placed under the knee joint. The foot is in neutral position.
- **Axis:** The axis is placed approximately 1.5 cm inferior to the lateral malleolus.
- **Stable arm:** Parallel to the longitudinal axis of the fibula.
- **Movable arm:** Parallel to the longitudinal axis of the 5th metatarsal.
- **End position:** During dorsiflexion, the ankle is flexed with the dorsal aspect of the foot approximately the anterior aspect of the lower leg.
- During plantar flexion, the ankle is extended to the limit of motion 50°.
- **Trick movement:** Inversion and eversion of the foot.
- **Normal ROM:** Dorsiflexion—0–20°/Plantar flexion—0–50°

Foot Inversion and Eversion (Figs. 17.20A and B)

- **Patient position:** Patient is supine lying with a towel roll placed under the knee to maintain slight knee flexion. The ankle is in neutral position. A piece of paper is placed under the foot; a flat surface object (pad, book, cardboard, etc.) is placed against the full sole of the foot with line drawn parallel on the flat surface.
- **Axis:** The goniometer is placed on the line graphics to obtain measure the movement of the arch.
- **Stable arm:** The goniometer is placed on the line graphics to obtain measure the movement of the arch.
- **Movable arm:** The goniometer is placed on the line graphics to obtain measure the movement of the arch.
- **End position:** The foot is placed in inversion to the limit of motion; the book is placed in positioned against the full sole of the foot with a line drawn parallel to the book.
- **Normal range:** Inversion—0–20°/Eversion—0–20°

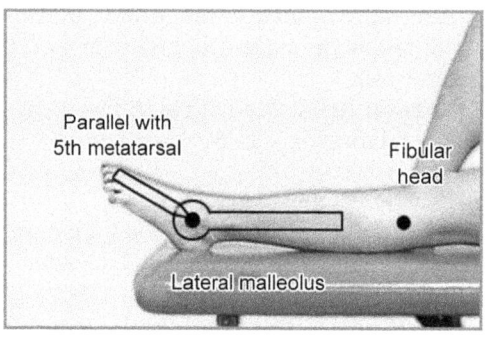

Fig. 17.18: Ankle plantar flexion

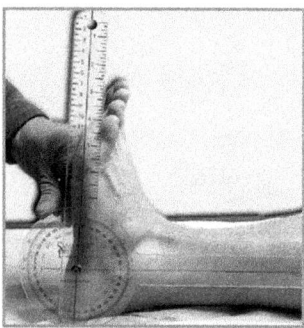

Fig. 17.19: Ankle dorsiflexion

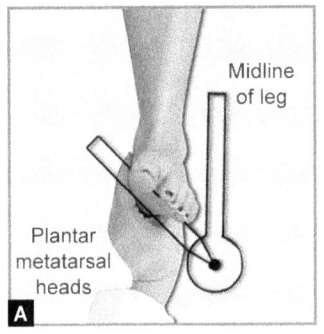
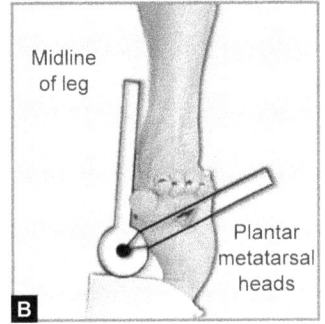

Figs. 17.20A and B: (A) Foot inversion; (B) Foot eversion

Metatarsophalangeal Flexion

- **Patient position:** Patient is supine with knees slightly flexed or in sitting position. The ankle and toes are in neutral position.
- **Axis:** The axis is placed over the dorsal of the MTP joint. Or alternatively the axis can also be placed over the lateral aspect of the great and 5th toe.
- **Stable arm:** Parallel to the longitudinal axis of the metatarsal of the toe being measured.
- **Movable arm:** Parallel to the longitudinal axis of the proximal phalanx of the toe being measured.
- **End position:** The MTP joint is flexed to the limit of motion 45° for the great toe 40° for the lateral 4 toes.
- **Normal range:** 0–45°

Metatarsophalangeal Extension

- **Patient position:** Patient is supine with knees slightly flexed or in sitting position. The ankle and toes are in neutral position.
- **Axis:** The axis is placed over the medial or plantar aspect of the foot.
- **Stable arm:** Parallel to the longitudinal axis of the metatarsal of the toe being measured.
- **Movable arm:** Parallel to the longitudinal axis of the proximal phalanx of the toe being measured.
- **End position:** The MTP joint of the toe being measured is extended to the limit of motion 0° for the great toe and 40° for the lateral 4 toes.
- **Normal range:** 0–40°

Joint	Movement	Patient position	Axis	Stable arm	Movable arm	Normal range
Shoulder	Flexion	Supine	Acromion process	Parallel to midaxillary line	Lateral midline of humerus, along lateral epicondyle	0–180°
	Extension	Prone	Acromion process	Parallel to midaxillary line	Lateral midline of humerus, along lateral epicondyle	0–60°
	Abduction	Supine	Anterior to acromion process	Parallel to midline of sternum	Parallel to midline of humerus anteriorly, along medial epicondyle	0–180°
	Adduction	Supine	Anterior to acromion process	Parallel to midline of sternum	Parallel to midline of humerus anteriorly, along medial epicondyle	0–30°

Contd...

Contd...

Joint	Movement	Patient position	Axis	Stable arm	Movable arm	Normal range
	Medial/internal rotation	Supine with shoulder abducted and elbow flexed to 90°	Olecranon process of ulna	Perpendicular to floor	Along shaft of ulna, along styloid process of ulna	0–90°
	Lateral/external rotation	Supine with shoulder abducted and elbow flexed to 90°	Olecranon process of ulna	Perpendicular to floor	Along shaft of ulna, along styloid process of ulna	0–90°
Elbow	Flexion	Supine	Lateral humeral epicondyle	Parallel to lateral midline of humerus	Along lateral midline of forearm, in line with radial styloid process	0–125°
	Extension	Supine	Lateral humeral epicondyle	Parallel to lateral midline of Humerus	Along lateral midline of forearm, in line with radial styloid process	125–0°
Forearm	Supination	Sitting with forearm supported	Medial to ulnar styloid process	Parallel to anterior midline of humerus	Across ventral aspect of wrist, proximal to ulnar and radial styloid process	80–90°
	Pronation	Sitting with forearm supported	Lateral to ulnar styloid process	Parallel to anterior midline of humerus	Across dorsal aspect of wrist, proximal to ulnar and radial styloid process	80–90°
Wrist	Flexion	Sitting with forearm supported	Distal to ulnar styloid process	Parallel and over lateral midline of ulna	Lateral midline of 5th MC	80–90°
	Extension	Sitting with forearm supported	Distal to ulnar styloid process	Parallel and over lateral midline of ulna	Lateral midline of 5th MC	60–70°
	Ulnar deviation	Sitting with forearm supported	Dorsal to wrist, over capitate	Dorsal aspect of forearm, along lateral epicondyle of humerus	Midline of dorsal surface of 3rd MC	0–35°
	Radial deviation	Sitting with forearm supported	Dorsal to wrist, over capitate	Dorsal aspect of forearm, along lateral epicondyle of humerus	Midline of dorsal surface of 3rd MC	0–20°

Contd...

Contd...

Joint	Movement	Patient position	Axis	Stable arm	Movable arm	Normal range
Hip	Flexion	Supine	Lateral aspect of hip, over greater trochanter	Parallel to lateral midline of pelvis	Along lateral midline of femur, along lateral femoral epicondyle	0–125°
	Extension	Prone	Lateral aspect of hip, over greater trochanter	Parallel to lateral midline of pelvis	Along lateral midline of femur, along lateral femoral epicondyle	0–30°
	Abduction	Supine	ASIS	Horizontal line connecting both ASIS	Anterior midline of femur, along midline of patella	0–50°
	Adduction	Supine	ASIS	Horizontal line connecting both ASIS	Anterior midline of femur, along midline of patella	0–30°
	Medial/internal rotation	High sitting	Anteriorly over patella	Parallel to floor	Anterior tibial surface	0–50°
	Lateral/external rotation	High sitting	Anteriorly over patella	Parallel to floor	Anterior tibial surface	0–45°
Knee	Flexion	Supine/prone	Lateral femoral epicondyle	Parallel to lateral midline of femur	Lateral to midline of fibula	0–130°
	Extension	Prone	Lateral femoral epicondyle	Parallel to lateral midline of femur	Lateral to midline of fibula	130–0°
Ankle	Plantar flexion	High sitting	Inferior to lateral malleolus	Lateral to midline of fibula	Parallel to 5th MT	0–50°
	Dorsiflexion	High sitting	Inferior to lateral malleolus	Lateral to midline of fibula	Parallel to 5th MT	0–20°
Subtalar joint	Inversion	High sitting	Midway between two malleoli, anteriorly	Anterior midline of tibia	Anterior midline of 2nd MT	0–20°
	Eversion	High sitting	Midway between two malleoli, anteriorly	Anterior midline of tibia	Anterior midline of 2nd MT	0–20°

(MC: metacarpal; MT: metatarsal)

CHAPTER 18

Walking Aids

Chapter Outline
- Introduction
- Indications
- Classification of walking aids

INTRODUCTION

It is an assistive device which helps during walking. The person may use walking aids either to compensate the inability to walk properly or enhance the walking pattern.

INDICATIONS

- Problem of balance
- Weakness
- Muscle fatigue
- Pain
- Joint instability
- Excessive skeletal loading

CLASSIFICATION OF WALKING AIDS

It is divided into three types:
1. Crutches
2. Walker
3. Cane

The biomechanical functions of walking aids are to eliminate weight bearing either fully or partially on the lower extremity.

Crutches

It is used to improve the balance or to relieve weight from lower extremity. They are usually use bilaterally. There are three types:
1. Axillary crutches
2. Elbow crutches
3. Gutter crutches

Axillary Crutches

It consists of either light weight wooden or aluminum pipe or iron pipe. There are two vertical uprights connected by single vertical upright with axillary pad and rubber tip at the distal end. It is available in different sizes. Axillary pad is placed two inches below the axilla (or two finger clinically). The single vertical upright allows the lengthening of the crutch. Biomechanically, rubber tip prevents frictions and avoids slippage. Hand grip is positioned such a manner, elbow should be placed 15° to 20° when weight is not taken, when weight is taken elbow is extended.

Prolonged compression of axilla by axillary pad can lead to neuropraxia of radial nerve or brachial plexus injury

Measurement procedure:
- **Supine lying position**
  - *With shoes off:* Measurement is taken from base of axilla to tip of lower margin of medial malleolus
  - *With shoes on:* From two inches from base of axilla to 20 cm lateral to the heel of shoes
- **Standing position**
  - Two inches from base of axilla to two inches lateral and six inches anterior to the little toe
  - *One more method:* Total weight of the person minus 16 inches.

Measurement of hand grip: Two inches from base of axilla to ulnar styloid process with elbow flexed (15° to 20°)

Uses:
- Increases base of support
- Increase lateral stability
- Allows upper extremity to transfer the weight to the ground.

Forearm/Elbow Crutches

It consists of a forearm band or cuff, handgrip and vertical upright with rubber tip. Length is adjusted by means of press button or screw button. This type of crutch is advised for the patient who has good arm muscles, weight transmission is same as axillary crutches.

Positioning: Placed upper one-third of forearm approximately 1-1.5 inch below elbow joint axis.

Advantages:
- It can early be adjusted by press button mechanism.
- It allows good functional activities during stair climbing.

Disadvantages:
- It provides less lateral stability.
- Cannot use for a patient having less arm power.

Measurement procedure
- It is taken with patient in supine lying with shoes on.
- Taken from ulnar styloid process to 20 cm lateral to the heel of the shoe.

Gutter Crutches

It consists of a forearm support with adjustable handgrip.

The height can be adjusted by means of press button mechanism. It is specially advised for rheumatoid arthritis patients who cannot take the weight through the wrist and hand due to pain or deformity.

Measurement procedure:
- If the patient is able to stand, taken from elbow to floor.
- In supine lying position, taken from the elbow joint to 20 cm lateral to the heel of the shoe.

Gait Patterns for Use of Crutches

Gait patterns are selected on the basis of patient's balance, coordination, muscle function, and weight bearing status. Some important points should be taught to the patients before crutch walking.

Precrutch Training
- The body weight must be borne on the hand, not on the axillary pads. If it is borne on axillary crutch, it may damage nerves and vascular structures in the axilla.
- The lower end of the axillary crutch should be at least four inches lateral and four inches anterior too little toe (optimal position).
- Axillary pads should be close to the chest wall, as a result increases lateral stability.
- The patient should be taught holding head and tail positions.

Crutch Muscles
- **In upper extremity:**
  - *At shoulder:* Extensor and adductors should be assessed and strong enough
  - *At hand:* Finger flexors should be assessed.
- **In lower extremity:**
  - *In nonweight bearing:* Hip joint-hip extensors and abductors (gluteus maximus, medius, minimus)
  - *At knee joint:* Knee extensors (quadriceps)
  - *At ankle joint:* Ankle plantar flexors (gastro-soleus).
- **Gait patterns:**
  - Three point/nonweight bearing
  - Partial weight bearing
  - Four point gait patterns
  - Two point gait patterns

Three Point Gait Patterns

In this gait patterns, three points are in contact with the ground. It is required when nonweight bearing status is required in the one lower extremity. Weight is borne on axillary crutches not on the affected body.

Sequences

Three point gait pattern

1. **Starting position:** In **Figure 18.1**, the left lower extremity is nonweight bearing (affected). The position should always be triangular base.
2. Weight is shifted to the unaffected lower extremity and the crutches are advanced
3. Weight is shifted through the upper extremities on to the crutches and unaffected limit advances to the level of crutches
4. Cycle is repeated.

Progression of Three Point Gait Pattern

- **Three point swing to:** In which unaffected limb advances to the level of crutches
- **Three point swing through:** In which unaffected limb advanced beyond the level.

Partial weight bearing gait pattern: This is the modification of three point gait pattern. In this gait pattern, weight is borne on both the crutches and some amount on the affected limb.

Sequences:
- In **Figure 18.2,** left lower extremity is partially weight bearing
- Weight is shifted on to the unaffected limb. Both the crutches and affected limb moves forward simultaneously.
- Weight is shifted into the crutches and partially to the affected extremity and unaffected limb advances
- Cycle is repeated.

Four point gait pattern (Fig. 18.3): In this, always three points are in contact to the ground. This is not stable type of gait pattern. It is always due to poor balance, muscle weakness, and incoordination. Weight is borne both the crutches and both the limbs.

Sequences
- **Starting position:** Weight is borne on both the crutches and both the limbs.
- Right crutch is advanced.
- The left limb is advanced.
- The left crutch is advanced.
- The right extremity is advanced.
- Cycle is repeated.

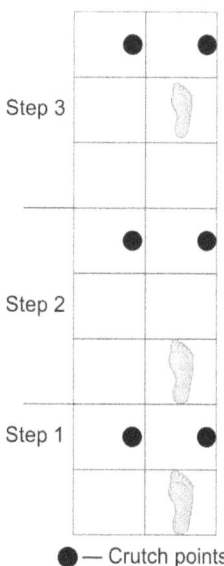

Fig. 18.1: Three point gait pattern

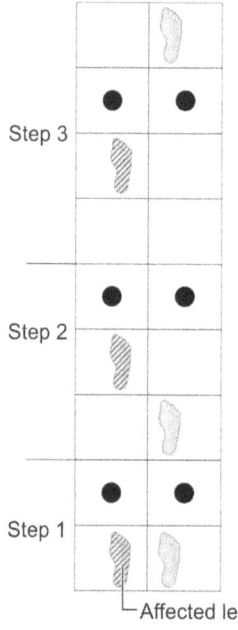

Fig. 18.2: Partial weight bearing gait pattern

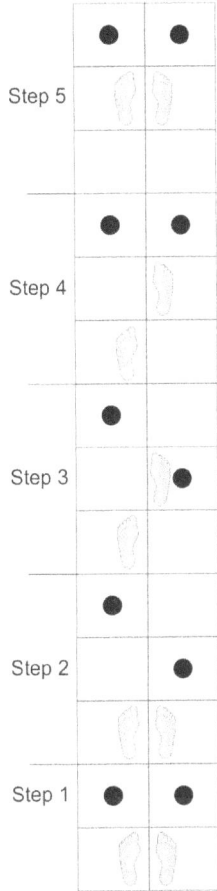

Fig. 18.3: Four point gait pattern

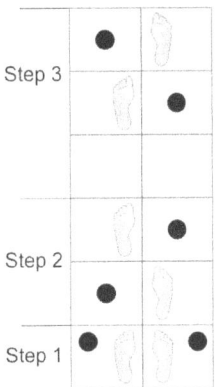

Fig. 18.4: Two point gait pattern

Two point gait pattern (Fig. 18.4)
In this, two points are in contact to the ground. This is less stable than four points gait pattern. It is similar to normal walking because opposite extremity and upper extremity move together.

Sequences
- **Starting position:** Weight is borne on both the extremities and both the crutches.
- The left crutch and right leg is moved together.
- The right crutch and left leg moved together.
- Cycle repeated.

Apart from these gait patterns, two more gait patterns are less commonly used are:
1. Swing to gait pattern
2. Swing through gait pattern

These types are especially advised in spinal cord injury patients, such as paraplegia.

Swing to Gait Patterns
Sequences
- Starting position
- Both the crutches are advanced.
- Both lower extremities are advanced up to the level of crutches.
- Cycle is repeated.

Swing Through Gait Patterns
Sequences
- Staring positions
- Both the crutches are advanced.
- Both the lower extremities are advanced beyond the level of crutches.
- Cycle is repeated.

CANES

Cane is made up of either wood, aluminum or stainless steel with half circle handle. Length is adjusted by press button mechanism. At the distal end, there is a rubber fitter that increases friction.

Functions of Cane
- It increases base of support.
- It improves the balance.
- It provides lateral stability.

Cane is always advised to hold opposite to the affected side or side of pain. Biomechanically, when cane is held opposite to the base of support it increases the distance from the affected side joint to the distal end of cane and reduces joint reaction force (compressive force) produced by abductor muscles.

If same cane is held on the same side of the deformity only reduces 50% or half of the joint reaction force produced by high abductor muscles.

Types of Cane

- **Unipod:** It has one point of contact to the ground.
- **Bipod:** It has two points of contact to the ground.
- **Tripod:** It has three points of contact to the ground.
- **Tetrapod:** It has four points of contact to the ground.

Functions of cane/advantages/uses
- Light weight
- It is easily adjusted.
- It is advised where space is limited or in narrow spaces in case of stair climbing.

Measurement procedure: Measurement is taken when patient is in standing position. Measurement is taken from ulnar styloid process to 15 cm (six inches)

Lateral to the heel of patient with slight elbow flexion.

Biomechanical importance of elbow flexion
- It allows shortening and lengthening of arm driving different phases of gait cycle.
- It provides shock absorbed mechanism due to sudden pressing down on cane.

Clinically it is checked, superior end of cane should coincide with greater trochanter.

Precane training (Fig. 18.5)
- It is advised to hold the cane opposite to the affected side.
- It should remain close to the body.
- If it is placed too far laterally or anteriorly, it may cause anterior trunk bending or lateral trunk bending.

WALKER

Walker is made up of either aluminum or iron with vinyl hand grips. Height can be adjusted

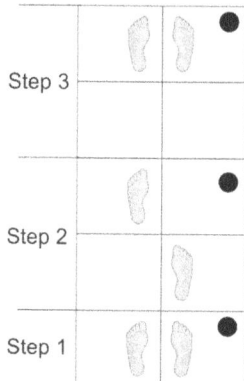

Fig. 18.5: Cane gait pattern

by coarse mechanism. At the distal end, there is rubber fitter as that provides friction. Out of three assistive devices, walker provides the greatest stability.

Types of Walker

Walkers are modified from standard walker (nonholding walker).
- **Folding walker:** Especially advised for them who usually travel frequently.
- **Reciprocal walker:** It is designed in such a manner that half of the walker moves in the unilateral progression. It is advised for the patient who is unable to lift the walker.
- **Rollator:** It is advised for CP (cerebral palsy) or ataxia patient.

Functions of Walker

- Increases base of support
- Improves anterior and lateral stability
- Allows upper extremity to transfer body weight to the floor

Prewalker Training

- Patient is advised to stand at center of base of support of walker. Walker is picked up and moved forward about an arm length and placed down all four legs at a time.
- Patient should be taught to hold head off and maintain good posture.
- Patient should not stand close to the stand bar. As a result overall base of support decreases, the patient may fall backward.

Gait Patterns
- Three points/nonweight bearing gait pattern
- Partial weight bearing gait pattern
- Four points gait pattern
- Two points gait pattern

Full Weight Bearing Gait Pattern
- **Starting position:** Patient is allowed to stand at center of base of support of walker.
- Walker is moved forward about an arm length.
- One of the extremities moved forward, the other extremity is moved forward beyond the first extremity.
- Cycle is repeated.

Partial Weight Bearing Gait Pattern
- **Starting position:** Patient is allowed to stand at the center of base of support of walker.
- Walker is moved about an arm length.
- Affected leg is moved forward.
- Body weight is transferred partially to the affected side and partially to the walker through upper extremity.
- Unaffected leg is advanced beyond the affected leg.
- Cycle is repeated.

Nonweight Bearing Gait Pattern
- **Starting position:** Patient is allowed to stand at the center of base of support of the walker with one leg.
- Walker is moved about an arm length.
- Body weight is transferred to the walker through upper extremities.
- The unaffected leg is advanced forward.
- Cycle is repeated.

Measurement Procedure
Same as cane measurement. Clinically checked, superior border of walker should coincide with greater trochanter.

CHAPTER 19

Orthotics and Prosthetics

> **Chapter Outline**
> - General classification
> - Common internal fixators
> - Biomechanical principle of orthosis
> - Spinal orthosis
> - Upper extremity orthosis
> - Lower extremity orthosis

INTRODUCTION

Bioengineering: It is a branch of engineering field that deals with the study of prosthesis and orthotics.
- **Prosthesis:**
  - It is the study of prosthesis.
  - It is a mechanical device that replaces or substitutes the anatomical lost part of the body, It is always advised in amputation cases, e.g., above knee (AK), below knee (BK), above elbow (AE), and below elbow (BE).
- **Orthotics:** The study of orthosis is called as orthotics.
- **Orthosis:** It is a mechanical device that is fitted to any part of body in order to maintain maximum anatomical and functional position, e.g., cervical collar.

GENERAL CLASSIFICATION

- External orthosis
- Internal orthosis, e.g., dental clips, internal fixators.

External Orthosis
- Lower limb orthosis
- Upper limb orthosis
- Spinal orthosis

Lower Limb Orthosis
- Foot orthosis
- Ankle foot orthosis (AFO)
- Knee ankle foot orthosis (KAFO)
- Knee orthosis (only knee joint)
- Hip knee ankle foot orthosis (HKAFO)
- Hip orthosis (only hip joint)

Upper Limb Orthosis
- Hand orthosis
- Wrist hand orthosis (wrist drop)
- Elbow orthosis (tennis elbow, cubitus varus, and valgus)
- Shoulder orthosis

Spinal Orthosis
- Lumbar sacral orthosis
- Thoracolumbar sacral orthosis
- Cervicothoracolumbar sacral orthosis
- Sacral orthosis

Advantages
- It helps in locomotion/walking.
- It supports the weaker part of body.
- Prevents and corrects the deformity

Disadvantages
- Discomfort to the patient
- Difficult to operate
- Cost is very high.
- Causes muscle wasting to some extent.

Indication
- To relieve pain

- To relieve axial load
- To align the abnormal part, e.g., limbs
- To correct/to protect the deformity

Contraindication

- When the limbs are paralyzed.
- Severe mentally retarted person.
- Noncooperative patient.

COMMON INTERNAL FIXATORS

- **Austin–Moore prosthesis:** For fracture of neck of femur
- **Baksi's prosthesis:** For elbow replacement
- **Buttress plate:** For condylar fractures of tibia
- **Charnley prosthesis:** For total hip replacement
- **Condylar blade plate:** For condylar fracture of femur
- **Dynamic compression plate**
- **Ender's nail:** For intertrochanteric fracture
- **Grosse–Kempf (GK) nail:** For tibial or femoral shaft fracture
- **Harrington rod:** For fixation of the spine
- **Hartshill rectangle:** For fixation of the spine
- **Insall Burstein prosthesis:** For total knee replacement
- **Interlocking nail:** For femoral or tibial shaft fractures
- **Kirschner wire:** For fixation of small bones
- **Kuntscher nail/Intramedullary nail:** For fracture shaft femur
- **Luque rod:** For fixation of the spine
- **Moore's pin:** For fracture of the neck of femur
- **Neer's prosthesis:** For shoulder replacement
- **Rush nail:** For diaphyseal fractures of long bone
- **Smith Peterson (SP) nail:** For fracture of neck of femur
- **Smith Peterson nail with McLaughlin's plate:** For intertrochanteric fracture
- **Seidel nail:** For fracture of the shaft of humerus
- **Souter's prosthesis:** For elbow replacement
- **Steffee plate:** For fixation of the spine.
- **Steinmann pin:** For skeletal traction
- **Swanson prosthesis:** Replacement of joints of fingers
- **Talwalkar nail:** For fracture of radius and ulna
- **Thompson prosthesis:** Fracture of neck of femur

BIOMECHANICAL PRINCIPLE OF ORTHOSIS

Three Points Pressure/Force Principle

Two forces should be acting on the concave side of curve and 3rd force/counter force should be acted on convex side of curve. As a curve is straightened.

- **Supportive:** To support a weakened body and prevent unwanted motion of body, e.g., cervical collar, femoral, tibial brace, taylor brace.
- **Corrective:** Used to correct the deformity e.g., genu valgum/varum brace, Milwaukee brace.
- **Protective:** Protect the deformed joint and align the part in normal anatomical position, e.g., foot drop splint, cockup splint, lumbo-sacral corset, medial arch support (pes planus).
- **Functional:** It is used to prevent the deformity and replaces the lost function of joint. It is dynamic in nature, e.g., dynamic cock-up splint.

SPINAL ORTHOSIS

Cervical Orthosis

Cervical orthoses are those that apply over cervical spine restrict the movement, such as flexion, extension, lateral flexion, and rotation. These are available in any surgical or medical store. Custom-made is made according to patients size and requirement.

Cervical collar: Type—soft and hard
- **Soft collar:** The materials used in this collar are polyethylene sponge and stockinette.
- **Hard cervical collar:** The materials used in this collar are polyethylene.
- The thickness varies 1–3 mm and selected on the patients age.

- The advantages of hard collar are the length and height can be easily adjusted.

Functions:
- It restricts some amount of flexion and extension and lesser amount of lateral flexion and rotation.
- As the sensory feedback, it reminds the patient to restrict the head and neck motion.
- It retains the body heat and helps in healing of soft tissue injury and reduces muscle spasm.

Indication:
- Cervical spondylosis
- Cervical disc diseases
- Wry neck or torticollis (paralysis of sternocleidomastoid)
- Early rheumatoid changes

Philadelphia collar

It has got two parts, anterior and posterior part connected laterally by means of Velcro. It is prepared from either polyethylene or ethaflex.

Functions:
- It restricts greater amount of flexion, extension, lateral flexion, and rotation than cervical collar.
- It provides more stability.

Location:
- Anterosuperiorly extend up to chin.
- Posterosuperiorly extend up to the occipital protuberance
- Inferiorly (anterior and posterior) extend up to the mid thorax.

Indication:
- When fracture at cervical spine.
- Severe neck pain

SOMI Brace: (Sterno-occipital mandibular immobilizer)

It controls flexion, extension, and rotation.
- **Design:** It consists of sternal plate mandibular support, occipital support, one anterior upright, and two posterior upright on which occipital support is attached to over shoulder bands with straps anterior upright is to connect between mandibular support and sternalplate.

- **Function:** It controls the maximum amount of flexion, extension at cervical spine.
- **Indication:** Multiple and severe fracture of cervical spine, TB of cervical spine.

Flexible Spinal Orthosis

Sacroiliac Corset

This is prepared from foam or elastic materials which are adjusted circumferentially by means of Velcro.

Location:
- Anterior superior at the level of iliac crest.
- Anterior inferior half inch above the symphysis pubis.
- Posterior superior at the level of iliac crest
- Posterior inferior extends up to the gluteal fold.

Indication: Post-traumatic stabilization of sacroiliac joint or pubic symphysis.

Abdominal Corset

It is prepared from elastic materials and available in different sizes. It is applied over abdomen and provides compression to abdominal muscle.

Indications:
- Postoperative surgical condition
- Postdelivery
- Pseudotummy reduction

Lumbosacral Corset (LS Corset): This is a flexible spinal orthosis which is prepared from cloth as well as elastic materials adjusted circumferentially by means of Velcro and placed over lower part of trunk and hip.

Location:
- **Anterior-superior:** 1/2 inch below the xiphoid process.
- **Anterior-inferior:** 1/2 inch to 1 inch above symphysis pubis
- **Posterior-superior:** 1 inch below inferior angle of scapula.
- **Posterior-inferior** extends up to the gluteal fold.

Functions:
- Anterior and lateral part of corset increase intra-abdominal pressure so it reduces weight on vertebra and intervertebral disc.

- Depending up on the placement number and rigidity of vertical upright.
- It is based on three points force system (or three points pressure system restrict the spinal motion).
- In all cases, corset acts as a remainder to restrict spinal motion.

Indication:
- Low back pain
- Intervertebral disc prolapse (IVDP)
- Lumbosacral strain
- Osteoporotic pain at lumbar spine

Thoracolumbosacral corset: This is prepared from cloth and elastic material adjusted circumferentially by means of Velcro. It extends upper part of trunk.

Location:
- Anterior-superior and anterior inferior same as LS corset.
- Posterior-superior extends up to the spine of scapula.
- Posterior-inferior same as LS Corset.

Function: It stabilizes the trunk. The rest of the function are same as LS corset.

Indication:
- Osteoporosis pain at thoracic spine
- Intervertebral disc prolapse (IVDP) at thoracic spine
- Mild pain at thoracic spine

UPPER EXTREMITY ORTHOSIS (SPLINT)

They are classified according to the regionwise, such as hand, wrist, hand, and shoulder orthosis. Orthosis applied to hand is called splint.

Splint may be:
- Static
- Dynamic

Static Splint

Static splint does not allow any movement at joint and maintain body in a stable position.

Dynamic Splints

Dynamic splints are those that allow movement at joint. It is also called final splint.

At the hand level commonly used short opponent and long opponent splint.
- **Short opponent splint (SOS):** It consists of palmar, dorsal bar, radial extensor, wrist band, and wrist bar.
  - *Indication:* When finger is paralyzed or involved.
- **Long opponent splint (LOS):** Where a forearm bar and hand are connected to the SOS then it is converted into Los.
  - *Indication:* To maintain a stable wrist position with paralysis or weakness of finger.
- **Cock-up splint:** Types: (1) Static; (2) Dynamic
  - *Static cock up splint:* It is made up of either aluminum or thermoplastic material. It maintains the wrist 30° of extension. It does not allow movement at wrist joint.
  - *Dynamic cock up splint:*
    - It consists of forearm hand with strap, wrist band with strap, and rigger attachment leather loops.
    - It maintains the wrist in extension.
    - It allows the movement at MCP, PIP, and DIP joint.
  - *Indication:* Wrist drop or radial nerve injury.
- **Knuckle bender:**
  Indication:
  - Allow hand deformity
  - It consists of dorsal pad, palmar pad, and finger pad which are connected by wire.
  - **Force system:** Anteriorly directed force by finger and dorsal pad posteriorly directed force from palmar pad.
- **Elbow turn buckle splint:**
  Indication: Soft tissue contracture of elbow.

LOWER EXTREMITY ORTHOSIS

Ankle Foot Orthosis

Indications: AFO is commonly used in order to prevent or correct deformities of ankle and foot. It is also indicated if a subject suffers from muscle weakness at the ankle and subtalar joint. In addition, AFO helps in distributing the weight bearing forces equally.

Parts of AFO

- Proximal calf band with leather straps
- Media and lateral bands articulates with medial and lateral ankle joints that help in controlling plantar and dorsiflexion.
- Stirrups anchor the uprights to the shoe.

Prescription

- AFO prescription is based on the power of muscles controlling the ankle.
- Free ankle is given for normal ankle power.
- Limited ankle joint is prescribed when the ankle is totally flail.
- 90° foot drop stop is prescribed when there is foot drop.
- Reverse 90° ankle joint is prescribed to prevent calcaneus deformity.
- Fixed ankle joint protects the foot from weight bearing.

Indications

- **Subject suffering from foot drop:**
  - The main aim is to prevent contractures of Achilles tendon.
  - A plastic posterior leaf spring AFO is attached to assist in dorsiflexion. The spring prevents the foot from dragging during swing and prevents slight plantarflexion during early stance. This allows the subject to achieve a foot flat position without doing knee flexion.
  - In addition, the Achilles tendon gains tension thus counteracts any tendency to form contractures.
- **Paralysis of plantar flexors:**
  - AFO with limited motion ankle joints and rigid rocker sole shoe enables the wearer to pivot over the rocker. Thus reducing the gait deviations
  - Prescription of a metal and leather AFO with an anterior stop that is set in slight plantar flexion or reverse 90° foot drop stop
- **Subject with ankle and foot paralysis:**
  - The main aim is to provide stability and reduce gait deviations during stance and swing phases.
  - Polypropylene solid ankle AFO is worn with a resilient heel.
  - Hinged AFO can be prescribed which enables the therapist to alter the range of ankle excursion.
  - Limited ankle joint can be prescribed that permits ankle movement about a small range usually 10–15° of dorsiflexion and plantar flexion.
  - Third option is prescription of metal and leather AFO with adjustable ankle joints for plantarflexion and dorsiflexion and corrective straps for valgus and varus deformities. Thus mediolateral stability is achieved.
- **Spastic foot:** A plastic solid AFO is prescribed to prevent plantarflexion, thus stopping toe drag during swing phase. It also stabilizes the foot during early stance.
- **Limited weight bearing (e.g., fracture calcaneus):**
  - AFO with weight bearing brim at the patellar tendon and fixed ankle joints are prescribed.
  - Heel of foot does not come in contact with the inner sole.

Knee Ankle Foot Orthosis

- It stabilizes the knee, ankle, and foot.
- It is same as the metal AFO. The only difference is that there are uprights extended to the knee joint and lower thigh band.
- The KAFO has calipers at the knee joint that enable the subject to sit down. In weight bearing position example standing the joint is locked for stability.

The three types of knee joints:
1. **Straight knee joint:** Provides rotation about single joint axis. It permits knee flexion and prevents hyperextension. It can be used along with drop lock to give further stability. It is cheap and easy to repair.

2. **Polycentric knee joint:** Uses double axis system to produce flexion/extension movements of femur and tibia at knee joint.
3. **Posterior offset knee joint:** Commonly prescribed for subject with weak knee extensor strength and good hip extensor strength.

The commonly used locks are:
- Drop lock—the drop lock drops over the knee joint when the knee is fully extended.
- Spring loaded lock—it provides automatic locking.
- Cam lock with spring loaded cam—it provides good stability. It provides simultaneous locking and unlocking thus providing maximum rigidity.
- Dial lock—can be adjusted 6° for control of knee flexion.
- Plunger type lock—indicated in persons having hand weakness.

Indications
- **Muscle weakness:** It is indicated in subjects who suffer from spinal cord damage, lower motor neuron disease, such as poliomyelitis or injury to a nerve. Mostly indicated in subjects who have muscle weakness in knee and hip muscles
- **Upper motor neuron lesion:** There is locomotor impairment. Extension synergy is present that is used by the hemiplegic to achieve stance stability. The orthotic device incorporates the knee joint which limits hyperextension.
- **Loss of structural integrity:** Loss of structural integrity could be due to injuries to the ligaments of the knee and joint diseases, such as inflammatory (septic arthritis) or degenerative (osteoarthritis).

Hip-Knee-Ankle-Foot Orthosis

- The hip-knee-ankle-foot orthosis is composed of a pelvic band that is mainly used to control hip joint rotational movement. The pelvic band is padded rigid steel band that covers the hips posteriorly and laterally. It fits between the iliac crest and greater trochanter. It has a front closer with Velcro or buckle strap fastener. It is connected to the KAFO by lateral uprights. It has permits uniaxial hip joint movements which allows only hip flexion and extension.
- It is also used as an ischial weight relieving caliper in which patient bears weight on the ischial seat and the weight is transmitted from ischial seat through metal uprights and shoe sole to the ground. It improves patients balance and provides a better forward leg swing in subjects with weak hip musculature.
- Disadvantage of HKAFO is difficulty in donning and doffing, decreased step length and increased lumbar spine movements to compensate for limited hip motion.

Components
The components are same as KAFO except it has an drop lock at the hip joint and a pelvic band which surrounds the iliac crest and greater trochanter.

Uses
- Commonly prescribed when the muscles around the hip is weak and poor stability is seen.
- It has hip rotation control straps that reduces gait deviations particularly toeing. It controls amount of hip internal and external movements.

CHAPTER 20

Ergonomics

Chapter Outline

- Ergonomics of desk job
- Ergonomic chair
- Ergonomics of sitting
- Ergonomics of driving
- Ergonomics of standing job
- Ergonomics of lying down

INTRODUCTION

Ergonomics is derived from the Greek words "Ergon" meaning work and "Nomoi" meaning natural laws which together means science of work.

Ergonomics is mainly concerned with the interactions of human body with the surrounding elements of the professional setup design in order to optimize human well-being and overall system performance.

It helps to:
- Enhance comfort
- Increase productivity
- Improve job satisfaction and morale
- Reduce musculoskeletal discomfort, work injuries/illnesses

Ergonomic hazards, such as faulty workstation layout, incorrect work methods and postures, improper lifting, and overuse of poorly designed tools along with job design problems that include aspects of repetitive workflow, excessive speed demands, poor postures, force requirements, and the lack of work or rest cycles will decrease the outcome of the profession along with serious health issues.

ERGONOMICS OF DESK JOB

Sitting jobs which are usually in front of the computers provide harmful effects on the body. Arrangements should be made in order to decrease the discomfort to the back, shoulders, and arms by avoiding awkward postures and positions.

Good work practices include:
- Avoiding mechanical stresses to the arms (for example, avoid resting hands or forearms on the sharp table edge).
- Taking rest between tasks that require hand grasping or pinch gripping (such as grasping large files, or stapling).
- Rest and stretch after repetitively performing the same motion or motion pattern, such as every few seconds for more than two hours continuously or four hours daily.
- Avoid working in a position that requires maintaining an unsupported fixed or awkward posture for more than one hour continuously, or four hours daily. These postures include raised elbows and arms, bent wrists, or hands.
- Avoid using vibrating or impact tools or equipment for more than one hour continuously or two hours daily.
- Avoid using forceful hand exertions for more than two hours daily.
- Unassisted frequent or heavy lifting should be avoided also. A person may be able to lift heavy loads, but the potential for back injury increases with each lift.

PREVENTION

Prevention is the key to reducing and eliminating the risk of a person developing a repetitive injury. Prevention includes the use of good body mechanics, good ergonomic design (engineering controls), and the use of administrative controls. Early intervention makes a difference for employees who complain of pain, numbness, tingling, or tenderness in the fingers, hands, or arms or pain in the back, shoulders, or legs from lifting or other body motions.

- Workplace must be evaluated to identify ergonomic risk factors and potential sources of accidents. Avoid awkward motions and postures.
- Encourage employee awareness and provide education.
- Use ergonomically appropriate work habits and require the same of employees.
- Take frequent breaks, stretch, and move around to keep muscles flexible. Workplace exercises relieve physical discomfort.
- Use ergonomically designed hand tools and furniture. The preferred furniture provides flexibility for adjustments and allows for preferred individual posture. Furniture and the workplace should be adjusted to the user.
- Perform five minutes of alternative work activity, or resting for every 30 minutes of continuous, high intensity, and repetitive work. For example, after two hours of continuous keyboarding, devote 15 minutes to nonrepetitive motion activities, such as returning phone calls or filing.
- Avoid the constant repetition of any one particular task.
- Evaluate and intervene when the employee complains of repetitive motion injury symptoms or when the employee complains of back pain. Prompt corrective action is required to allow for the body to recover from overexertion.

Work Surfaces (Fig. 20.1)

- Adjust the work surface (table) so that the keyboard is at the correct height to maintain

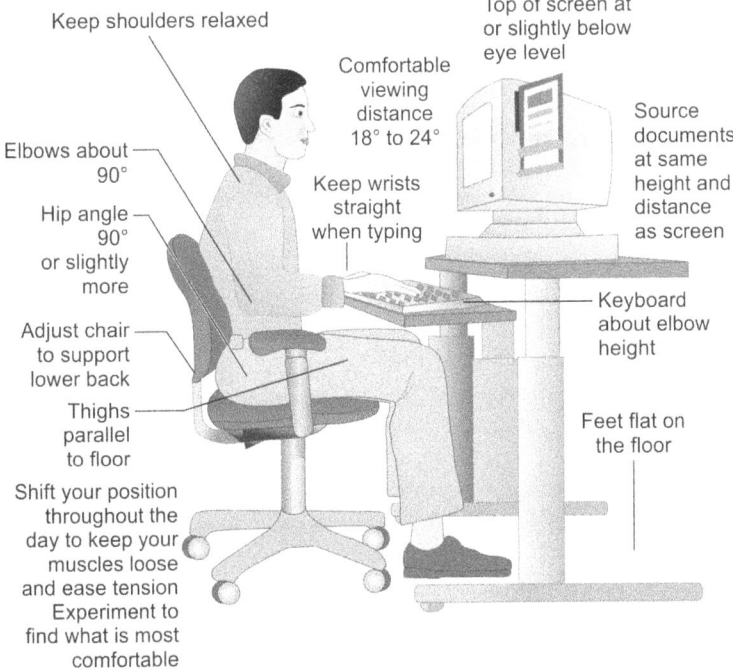

Fig. 20.1: Preferred posture at a computer workstation

the best posture as the elbows at keyboard height with the forearms parallel to the floor.

- A split-level design table that has an adjustable top height can be used in which the lower level for the keyboard and mouse or trackball, and the upper level for the video display terminal or video display terminal (VDT) which is usually used for computer display or monitor. The height of each level must be adjusted separately.
- Use a table large enough to hold the keyboard, monitor, wrist rest, mouse or trackball, and a document holder or all necessary documents.
- Adequate clearance must be kept under the table for leg length, knee height, and thighs.

Chairs

- Use a chair that is stable, mobile, and allows for operator movement.
- Substantial lower back support must be provided by the chair. The back support should be easy to adjust backward, forward, up, and down. A properly adjusted chair is important to help reduce or prevent discomfort on the back and should support the inward curve of the back.
- Use a chair that has an adjustable seat height. Raise or lower the chair to a comfortable height such that the thighs are parallel to the floor and the knees are at a 90° angle. Rest the feet flat on the floor or use a footrest.
- Use the armrests if they allow maintaining elbows at a 90° angle. If the armrests obstruct sitting posture, then adjust the armrests, use a chair that allows an erect posture, or use a chair without armrests.

Guidelines for using the correct work surfaces and chair height according to persons height is shown in **Table 20.1**.

▌ERGONOMIC CHAIR (FIG. 20.2)

Sitting can lead to a hard effect on the back as it transfers the full weight of the upper body onto the buttocks and thighs. Sitting for long periods

◢ **Table 20.1:** Guidelines for work surfaces and chair heights.

Person's height	Standing surface (inch)	Seated (inch)
5.2"	37.1	22.3
5.3"	38.2	22.4
5.4"	38.8	23.0
5.5"	39.6	23.8
5.6"	40.1	24.4
5.7"	40.7	25.3
5.8"	41.9	26.4
5.9"	42.5	27.0
5.10"	43.3	27.6
5.11"	43.5	27.8
6.0"	44.2	28.3
6.1"	45.4	29.5

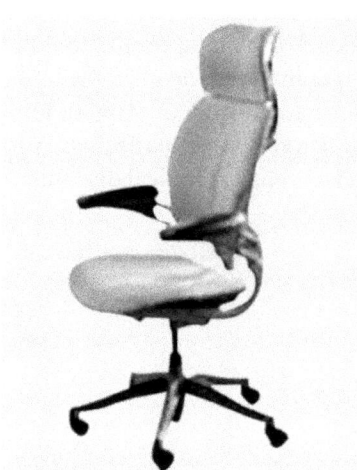

Fig. 20.2: The back office chair

of time can also cause increased pressure on the intervertebral discs—the springy, shock-absorbing parts of the spine. Improper sitting posture can cause physical discomfort and also contributes to serious health problems, including:

- Back pain
- Neck pain
- Eye strain
- Abdominal pain
- Leg pain
- Repetitive movement disorders

Ergonomic chairs are used at a computer workstation or in front of a machine on the factory floor. It can help to reduce fatigue and discomfort, increase blood flow, reduce the risk of injury, and increase productivity.

In order to increase the comfort and reduce the risk of injury, the ergonomic chairs with the following settings can be used:

- **Casters:** Use a chair with casters (a pivoting roller or wheel attached to the bottom of the chair) and a 5-point base to make movement easier and minimize tipping. Rubber locking casters are useful on stools to prevent tipping.
- **Seat pan:** The seat pan is the part of the chair that supports the majority of the weight. Its cushion is made from dense, small-cell foam padding, or spring coils. The seat pan should be at least one inch wider than your hips and thighs on either side. The front part of the seat should slope down slightly and allow a fist size gap between the back of your knees and the front edge of the seat pan to reduce pressure on the back of your thighs. Tilt adjustments allow for a forward working posture or a reclined posture and a sliding mechanism in the chair allows small and tall users to adjust the distance of the seat pan from the backrest.
- **Backrest:** Backrest gives adequate lumbar support. Inadequate lumbar support places excess pressure on the spine leading to back pain. The backrest should either be small enough to fit into the small of the back, clearing the pelvis and back of the rib cage, or curved to provide adequate support. Many chairs come with a built-in lumbar adjustment, which can be adjusted by turning a knob on the side of the chair. This is the best if more than one person will be using the chair.
- **Armrests:** The armrest should be made of a soft material and should be at least 2" wide to provide adequate surface area for comfortable positioning of the arms on the chairs.
- **Seat height:** In most of the chairs seat, height adjustments help the feet to rest properly on the floor while the upper body is properly aligned with the tools, such as a computer, display monitor, or keyboard. Pneumatic adjustments allow you to adjust the seat height while sitting on the chair. The mechanism to adjust the seat height must be easy to reach.
- **Chair recline or tilt adjustability:** The chair reclines or tilt adjustment changes the angle of the entire seat relative to the floor.
- **Foot rest:** Foot rest chooses a free-standing floor-mounted support that allows to rest your feet in front in a comfortable position.

PRECAUTIONS WHILE SITTING

To minimize discomfort and injury while sitting the following precautions are taken:
- Not sitting on one position for prolonged periods of time.
- Alternate between sitting and standing.
- Make sure your feet are flat on the floor.
- Sit upright with your back and shoulders against the backrest.
- Keep the arms properly on the arm rests. Elbows and lower arms should rest lightly to avoid circulatory problems or nerve pressure.
- Make sure your shoulders are relaxed and slightly dropped while keyboarding.

Monitors

- Position the monitor directly in front and in line with the keyboard.
- Position the monitor at a comfortable viewing distance (18-24 inch from the eyes), viewing height at the top of the display screen at or slightly below eye level, and viewing angle 10-15° below the horizontal line of sight.
- Use a monitor that tilts and rotates and has adjustable contrast and brightness. Adjust the contrast to a high level and the brightness to a low level to minimize or prevent eyestrain.

Keyboards

- Position the keyboard directly in front of your torso approximately at the elbow height.
- The keyboard angles must be kept in a comfortable position which keep the wrists straight and in line with the forearm.
- When using a mouse, trackball, or special keypads, place the wrist in a neutral position. Rest the arm and hand close to the body and at the natural elevation.
- A mousepad rest or wrist pad is provided with cushion in order to keep the wrist in the comfortable position.

Exercises

- Look away from the work to a distant point at least every hour in order to relax the eyes.
- Stretch the neck, shoulders, back, legs, arms, and fingers at least twice a day. Stand up and walk around often to increase blood flow circulation. Warm up exercises are recommended in the morning, prior to commencing work, and after lunch, to recondition for data entry work.

ERGONOMICS OF SITTING

- Sit up with your back straight and your shoulders back. Your buttocks should touch the back of your chair.
- All three normal back curves should be present while sitting. A small, rolled-up towel or a lumbar roll can be used to help you maintain the normal curves in your back.
- Here's how to find a good sitting position when you are not using a back support or lumbar roll:
  - Sit at the end of your chair and slouch completely
  - Draw yourself up and accentuate the curve of your back as far as possible.
  - Hold for a few seconds
  - Release the position slightly (about 10°). This is a good sitting posture.
- Distribute your body weight evenly on both hips.
- Bend your knees at a right angle. Do not sit with your knees crossed. Keep your knees even with or slightly higher than your hips.
- Keep your feet flat on the floor.
- Try to avoid sitting in the same position for more than 30 minutes.
- At the office, practice good ergonomic principles by adjusting your chair height and work station so you can sit up close to your work and tilt it up at you. Rest your elbows and arms on your chair or desk, keeping your shoulders relaxed.
- When sitting in a chair that rolls and pivots, do not twist at the waist while sitting. Instead, turn your whole body.
- When standing up from the sitting position, move to the front of the seat of your chair. Stand up by straightening your legs. Avoid bending forward at your waist. Immediately stretch your back by doing 10 standing backbends.

ERGONOMICS OF DRIVING

Normal sitting is different from that of sitting in a driving seat while driving. While a vehicle is in motion the body is subjected to different forces—to accelerations and decelerations, to lateral swaying from side to side, and to whole-body up and down vibrations. During driving, the feet are actively being used, the right foot on the accelerator pedal, the left on the brake, and in a stick-shift also on the clutch. When the feet are active they cannot be used to support and stabilize the lower body as normally happens when they are placed on the floor during normal sitting in a chair.

An ideal car seat design should have:

- Adjustable seat back incline (100° from horizontal is optimal)
- Changeable seat bottom depth (from seat back to front edge)
- Adjustable seat height
- Adjustable seat bottom incline
- Seat bottom cushion with firm (dense) foam
- Adjustable lumbar support (horizontally and vertically adjustable)

- Depth pulsating lumbar support, to reduce static load
- Adjustable bilateral arm rests
- Adjustable head restraint with lordosis pad
- Seat shock absorbers to dampen frequencies between 1 and 20 Hz.
- Linear front-back seat travel to allow differently sized drivers to reach the pedals.
- Seat back damped to reduce rebounding of the torso in rear-end impacts.

ERGONOMICS OF STANDING JOB

Standing jobs are mostly done by security guards, machine operators, policemen, teachers, and sales people. Standing for a longer period can lead to particular health issues, such as varicose veins, swelling of the legs, muscular fatigue, decreased venous return which can eventually lead to dizziness or fainting, low back pain, and stiffness of the neck and shoulders.

Ergonomic changes to reduce the physical discomfort can be:

- Changing the working positions frequently within short duration gaps.
- Take suitable rest periods in-between, such as sitting for a few minutes and returning back to standing.
- In case of standing in front of a work table, the height of the work table must be appropriate to the person according to his/her body dimensions and elbow heights.
- A footrest can be used in order to shift the body weight to each of the legs.
- Few stretching of the body, upper extremities, and lower extremities must be done remove the strain on the muscles.
- Trunk turning and bending can also release the strain on the back.

ERGONOMICS OF LYING DOWN/SLEEPING

The ideal position differs from person to person. No matter what position you lie in, the pillow should be under your head, but not your shoulders, and should be a thickness that allows your head to be in a normal position.

- Try to sleep in a position which helps you maintain the curve in your back (such as on your back with a pillow under your knees or a lumbar roll under your lower back; or on your side with your knees slightly bent). Do not sleep on your side with your knees drawn up to your chest. You may want to avoid sleeping on your stomach, especially on a saggy mattress, since this can cause back strain and can be uncomfortable for your neck.
- Select a firm mattress and box spring set that does not sag. If necessary, place a board under your mattress. You can also place the mattress on the floor temporarily if necessary. If you have always slept on a soft surface, it may be more painful to change to a hard surface. Try to do what is the most comfortable for you.
- Try using a back support (lumbar support) at night to make you more comfortable. A rolled sheet or towel tied around your waist may be helpful.
- When standing up from the lying position, turn on your side, draw up both knees, and swing your legs on the side of the bed. Sit up by pushing yourself up with your hands. Avoid bending forward at your waist.

CHAPTER 21

Starting and Derived Positions for Exercise

Chapter Outline
- Standing
- Kneeling
- Sitting
- Lying
- Hanging

INTRODUCTION

- The posture from which movements are initiated is known as starting positions.
- They may be either active or passive in character.
- Equilibrium and stability are maintained in these positions by a balance of forces acting upon the body and when the force of muscular contraction is used for this purpose the contraction is isometric.

Fundamental positions: There are five basic or fundamental starting positions and all others are derived from them.
1. Standing
2. Kneeling
3. Sitting
4. Lying
5. Hanging

STANDING (FIG. 21.1)

This is the most difficult of the fundamental position to maintain, as the whole body must be balanced and stability in correct alignment on a small base by the coordination work of many muscle groups.

Description: The position may be descried as follows:

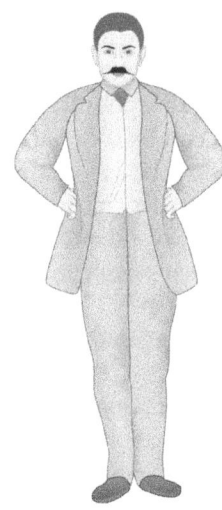

Fig. 21.1: Erect standing

- The heels are together and on the same line, the toes slightly apart.
- The hips are extended and slightly laterally rotated.
- The knees are together and straight.
- The pelvis is balanced on the femoral heads.
- The spine is stretched to its maximum length.
- The vertex is thrust upward, the ears are level, and eyes look straightforward.
- The shoulders are down and back.
- The arms hang loosely to the sides, palms facing inward toward the body.

Muscle Work

The muscle work required to maintain the position varies with the circumstances.

The muscle groups involved are:
- The intrinsic muscles of the feet working to stabilize the feet and to prevent curling of the toes so that the flexors of the IP joints can press the balls of the toes to the ground.
- The plantar flexors of the ankle, working to balance the lower leg of the foot.
- The dorsiflexors of the ankle, working to counterbalance the action of the plantar flexors and to support the medial longitudinal arch of the foot.
- The extensors of the hip, working to maintain hip extension and to balance pelvis on the femoral heads. Slight action of the lateral rotators of the hip is associated with a bracing of the legs and of the arches of the foot.
- The extensors of the spine, working to keep the trunk upright.
- The flexors of the lumbar spine working to prevent over action of the extensors of this region.
- The prevertebral neck muscles, working to control excessive extension of the neck and to straighten the cervical spine.
- The flexors and extensors of the atlanto-occipital joint, working reciprocal to balance the head. The elevators of the mandible close the mouth.
- The retractors of the scapula, working to draw the scapula backward so that the glenoid cavity faces more or less laterally.

Effects and Uses
- This position is suitable as starting position.
- Muscle work is minimum when perfect balance is achieved.
- In erect position, the thorax is free and the abdominal viscera are well supported.
- Feeling of joy and efficiency.

Positions Derived from Standing
By alteration of the arms:
- **Wing standing (Fig. 21.2):**
  - The hands are rest on the iliac crest, the fingers are extended and adducted, being anterior and the thumb is posterior. The wrist is extended, forearm pronated, elbow flexed, shoulder abducted, and the elbow point straight sideways.
  - *Muscle work:* The adductors of the shoulder and extensors of the elbow work to press the hands to the trunk.
- **Low wing standing:** This is similar to the wing standing but the fingers are placed across the front of the hip joint.
- **Bend standing (Fig. 21.3):**
  - The shoulders are laterally rotated and adducted strongly, elbows are flexed, forearm is supinated with wrist, and

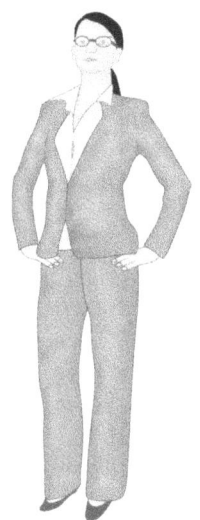

Fig. 21.2: Wing standing

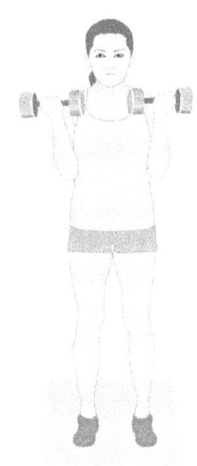

Fig. 21.3: Bend standing

finger flexed to rest above the lateral border of the acromion process.
  - *Muscle work:* The lateral rotators and adductors of the shoulder work strongly.
  - The retractors and depressors of the scapula work strongly as fixators.
  - The flexors of the elbow and the supinators of the forearm work to maintain the position of the forearm. The flexors of the wrist and fingers may work slightly.
- **Reach standing:**
  - The shoulders are flexed and the elbows are extended so that the arms are held parallel, shoulder width apart and at right angles to the body.
  - *Muscle work:* The shoulder flexors maintain the position against the gravity.
  - The transverse muscle of the back controls the forward movement of the scapula around the chest wall which is associated with shoulder flexion.
  - The extensors of the elbow, radial flexors of the wrist, and extensors of the fingers work slightly to keep the arms straight.
- **Yard standing (Fig. 21.4):**
  - The arms are straight and elevated sideways to a horizontal position.
  - *Muscle work:* The abductors and lateral rotators of the shoulder and the rotators of the scapula to stabilize the arms.

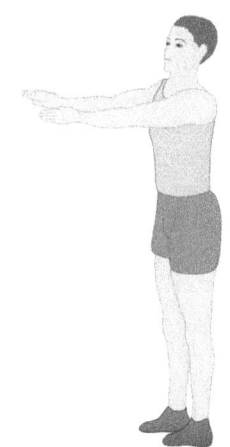

Fig. 21.5: Stretch standing

  - The extensors of the elbows, wrist, and fingers work to hold the limbs in straight line.
- **Stretch standing (Fig. 21.5):**
  - The arms are fully elevated so that they are in line with the body, parallel to each other, and palm facing each other.
  - *Muscle work:* The abductors and lateral rotators of the shoulder work strongly.
  - The lateral rotators of the scapulae to hold the arms in position.
  - The wrist and fingers are kept in alignment by interplay between the muscles working over the wrist and by the extensors of the fingers.

By alteration of the legs:
- **Close standing:**
  - The legs are rotated inward at the hip, so that the medial border of the feet is adjacent.
  - *Muscle work:* Medial rotators of the hip and lower limb muscles work strongly.
- **Toe standing (Fig. 21.6):**
  - The heels are pressed together and raised from the floor.
  - *Muscle work:* Plantar flexors and lower limb muscles work strongly.
- **Stride standing (Fig. 21.7):**
  - Legs are abducted, so that the heels are forward, two feet lengths apart, feet remain as in the fundamental position and weight is distributed equally.

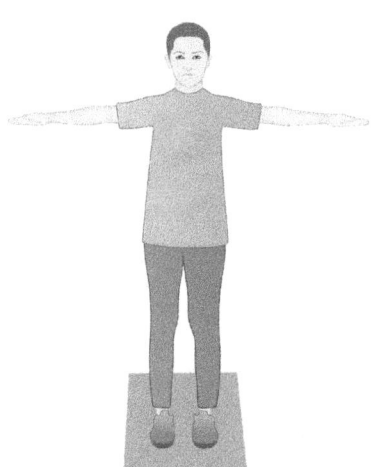

Fig. 21.4: Yard standing

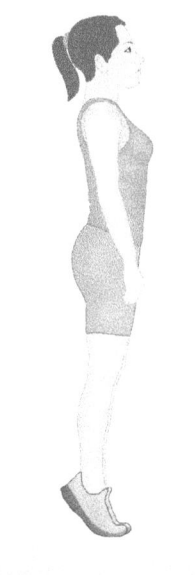

Fig. 21.6: Toe standing

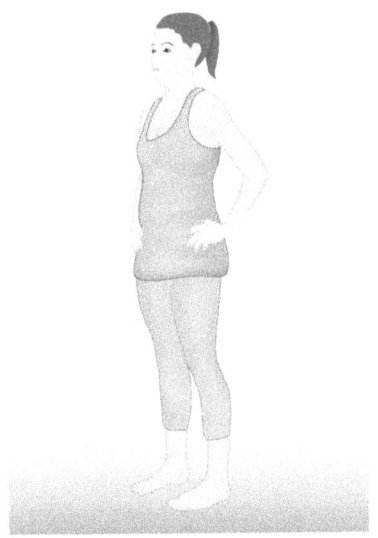

Fig. 21.7: Stride standing

- *Muscle work:* Adductors of the hip work to prevent from leg sliding on the floor.
- **Walk standing (Fig. 21.8):**
  - One leg is placed directly forward, so that the heels are two feet lengths apart and on the same line.
  - *Muscle work:* Extensors of the hip and knee.

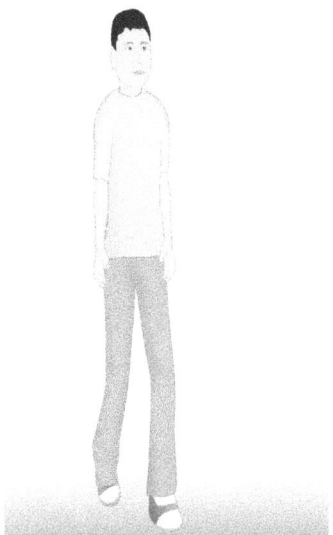

Fig. 21.8: Walk standing

- **Half standing (Figs. 21.9 and 21.10):**
  - The whole weight of the body is supported on one leg, the other leg may be free or supported in a variety of position.
  - *Muscle work:* Abductors of the hip of standing leg work to maintain the center of gravity over the base by slight lateral tilting of the pelvis.
  - The lumbar side flexors of the opposite side work to bring the trunk into alignment.
  - All the muscles of supporting leg work more strongly than on standing to sup-

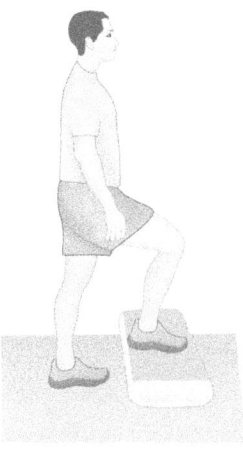

Fig. 21.9: Half standing

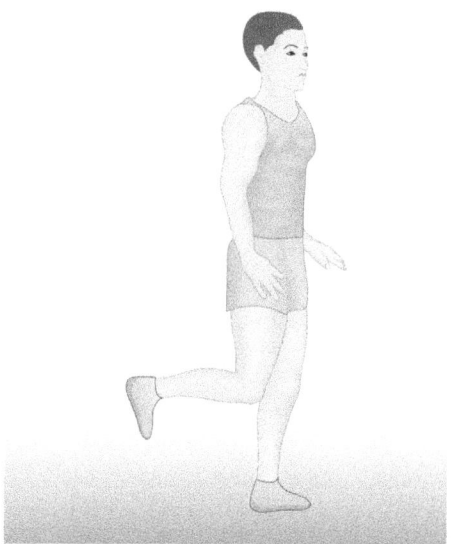

Fig. 21.10: Single leg standing

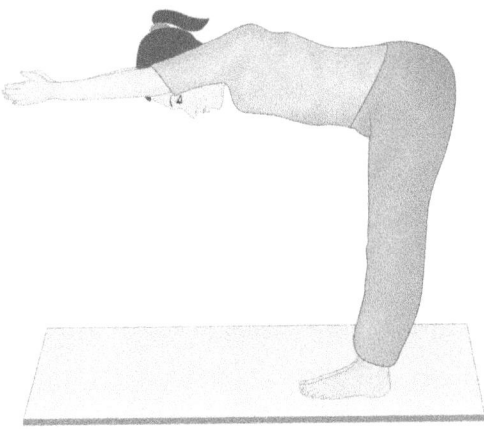

Fig. 21.12: Stoop standing

port the additional weight and preserve balance.
- **Step standing:** Leg on the stool with hip and knee bent, foot supported forward, and outward standing knee is extended.

By alteration of the trunk:
- **Lax stoop standing (Fig. 21.11):**
  - *Knee bent standing:* Hips are flexed when knees are allowed to bent in the position, tension on hamstrings, and lumbar muscles is reduced giving a feeling of relaxation right through the body.

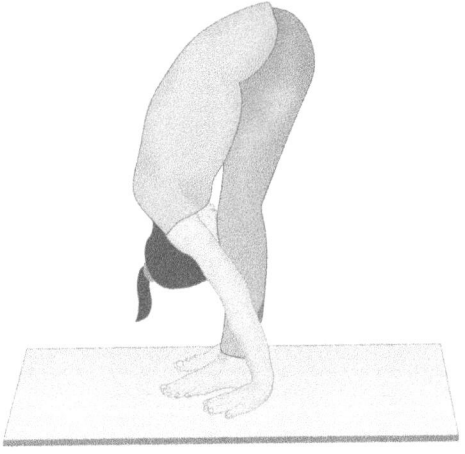

Fig. 21.11: Lax stoop standing

- *Muscle work:* Dorsiflexors of ankle stabilize the position of joint, while intrinsic foot muscle grips the floor.
- **Stoop standing (Fig. 21.12):**
  - The hip joints are flexed while the trunk, head, and arms remain in alignment and are inclined forward.
  - *Muscle work:* Dorsiflexors stabilize the position of the joint while the intrinsic foot muscles grip the floor. The extensors of knees may work to counteract the tension of hamstrings.
  - The longitudinal and transverse back muscles and the extensors of shoulders and elbows maintain the position against the pull of gravity. The posterior neck muscles controlled by prevertebral muscles support the head.

By alteration of the legs and trunk:
- **Fallout standing (Fig. 21.13):**
  - One leg is placed directly forward to a distance of three feet length and this knee is bent, the back leg remains straight and the body is inclined forward in line with it.
  - *Muscle work:* The extensors and foot muscles of forward leg, extensors of back leg, and dorsiflexors of this footwork to keep the heel on ground. Balance is maintained by action of trunk rotators and lumbar muscles on the side.
- **Lunges (Fig. 21.14):** These positions are similar with regard to the placing of legs,

Chapter 21 | Starting and Derived Positions for Exercise

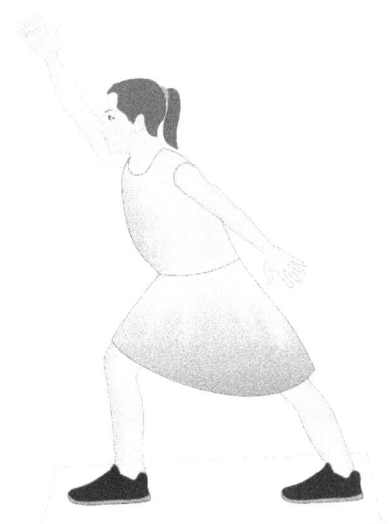

Fig. 21.13: Fallout standing

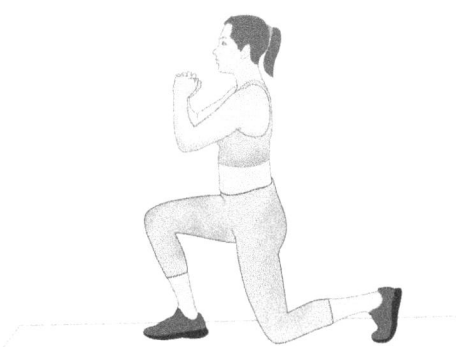

Fig. 21.14: Lunges

but the body always remains in a vertical position.

KNEELING

The body is supported on the knees which may be together or slightly apart.

The lower legs rest on the floor with the feet plantar flexed and rest of the body is held in standing position.

Muscle work:
- The lower leg is released; the body must be stabilized on knees.
- There is interplay between the flexors and extensors of knee to balance the femur vertically on knees.
- The extensor of hip and flexors of lumbar spine work more strongly to maintain correct angle of pelvic tilt.

Effects and Uses

It is used as a starting position for backward movements and for preparation of starting position during which feet are pressed to floor by extensors of knees and dorsiflexors, so that the lower legs act as brackets.

Derived Positions of Kneeling

- **Half kneeling (Fig. 21.15):**
  - One knee supports most of the body weight and other leg is bent to a right angle at the hip, knee, and ankle so that the foot is supported on the ground on forward direction.
  - *Muscle work:* Abductors of hip joint of supporting leg and the lumbar side flexors of opposite side. Extensors of hip and knee of forward leg.
- **Knee sitting (Fig. 21.16):** The knees and hips are flexed so that the patient sits on his knees.
- **Prone kneeling (Fig. 21.17):**
  - The trunk is horizontal, supported on shoulder by the arms and at the pelvis by the thighs, which must be held vertical.
  - *Muscle work:* Muscles round the shoulders and hip joints. Flexors of lumbar spine, extensors of head and neck.

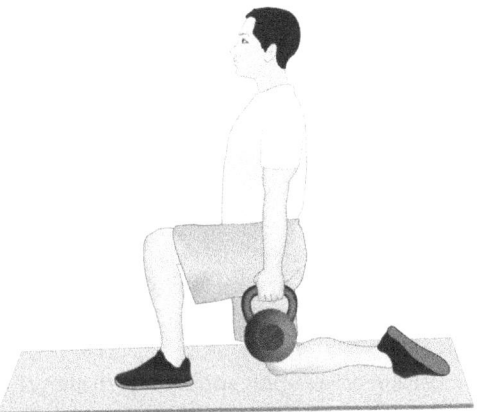

Fig. 21.15: Half kneeling

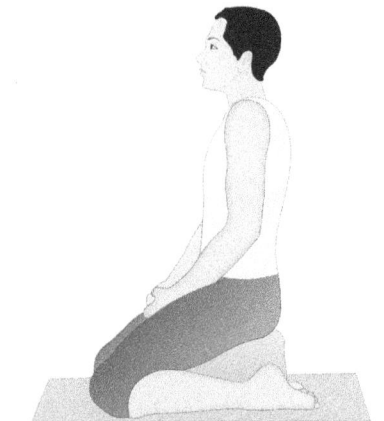

Fig. 21.16: Knee sitting

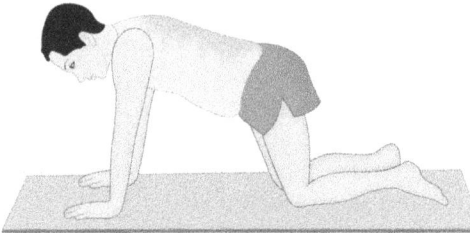

Fig. 21.17: Prone kneeling

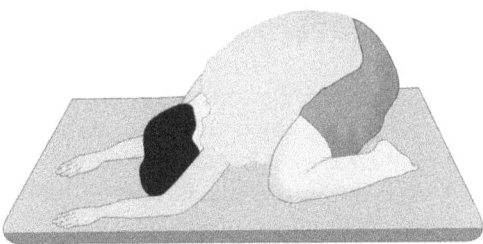

Fig. 21.18: Inclined prone kneeling

Muscle work:
- There need not be muscle work to hold the position of the legs.
- The flexors of hip work to maintain at the right angles at these joints.

Effects and Uses
- Comfortable, natural, and very stable position.
- Lateral and rotatory mobility of pelvis is eliminated by weight of body and position of legs and can be localized to spine.
- Many nonweight bearing exercises are advised for knees and feet.

Derived Positions of Sitting
General (position of legs):
- **Stride sitting (Fig. 21.19):** Similar to fundamental position, legs are abducted, so that the feet are up to two feet length apart.
- **Ride sitting (Fig. 21.20):** The person sits astride suitable apparatus, such as gymnastic form, which may be gripped between knees by adductors muscles of the hip.
- **Crook sitting (Fig. 21.21):** When siting on the floor, the knees are bent so that the feet are together and flat on the floor. The knees may be together or part.

- **Inclined prone kneeling (Fig. 21.18):** The body is inclined forward and downward by abduction of shoulder and bending of elbows.

SITTING

The position is taken on a chair or stool, the height and width of which allow the thighs to be fully supported and allows the knees and hips to flex to right angles.

The knees are apart sufficiently to allow the femur to be parallel and the feet rest on floor with heels vertically below knees.

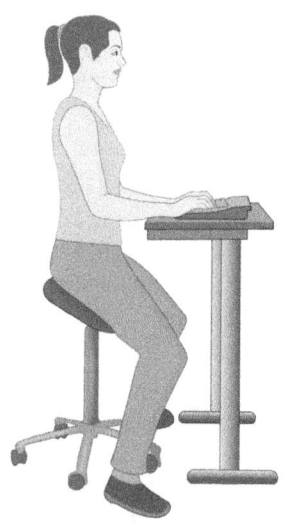

Fig. 21.19: Stride sitting

Chapter 21 | Starting and Derived Positions for Exercise

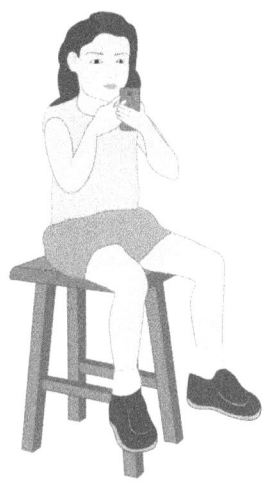

Fig. 21.20: Ride sitting

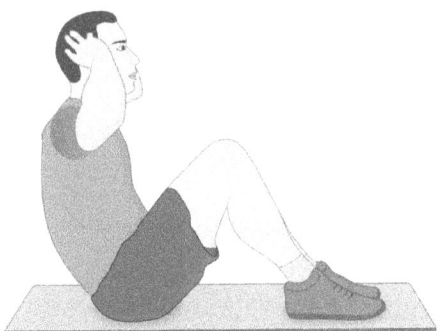

Fig. 21.21: Crook sitting

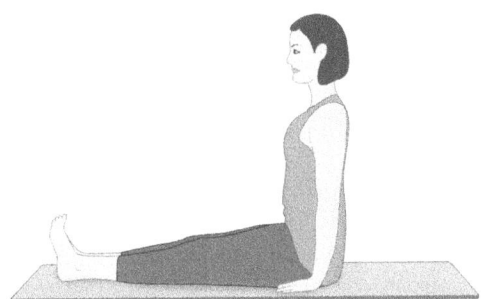

Fig. 21.22: Long sitting

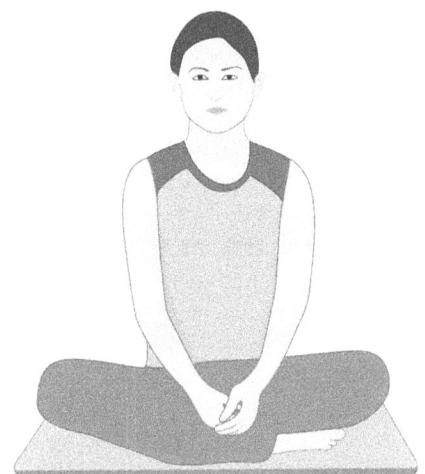

Fig. 21.23: Cross sitting

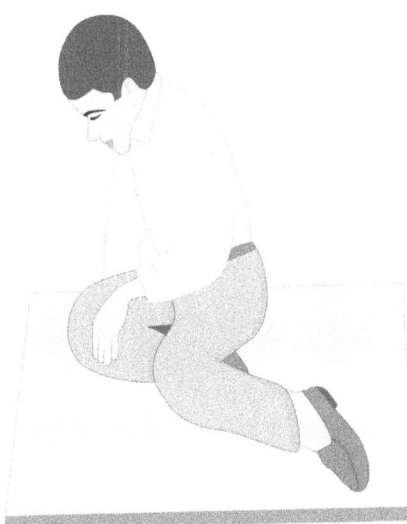

Fig. 21.24: Side sitting

- **Long sitting (Fig. 21.22):**
  - This is similar to previous position, but the knees are extended so that the whole leg is supported.
  - *Muscle work:* Extensors of knee work to counteract the increased tension of hamstring muscles.

- **Cross sitting (Fig. 21.23):** Similar to crook sitting but ankles are crossed and hips strong abducted and laterally rotated, so that the lateral aspect of knee is pressed to the floor.

- **Side sitting (Fig. 21.24):**
  - For left side sitting, the left leg remains as in cross sitting and this hip supports main weight of trunk, while the right leg is abducted and medially rotated, so that lower leg is bent and to the side.

- *Muscle work:* Pelvis is tilted laterally to left and lumbar side flexors on right side work to keep trunk upright.
- **High sitting:** Fundamental sitting position is taken on high table, but the feet remain unsupported.
- **Position of trunk:**
  - *Stoop sitting* (**Fig. 21.25**)*:* This is similar to, but easier and more stable than stoop standing position and is therefore very useful for arm and upper back exercises when hallowing of lumbar region is to be avoided.
  - *Muscle work:* The arms may be folded and supported on a plinth or table (arm lean sitting) allowing back muscles relax.
- **Fallout sitting (Fig. 21.26):** This position is same as fallout standing except that the hip and thigh of forward leg are supported across a stool, balance is therefore easier and the patient is able to concentrate on movements which may be added.

LYING

This is the easiest of fundamental positions as the body can be completely supported in supine position and is as stable as is possible.

Muscle work:
- Head rotators of both sides work reciprocally to stabilize the position of the head.
- Extensors of hips and flexors of lumbar spine work to combat the tendency to hallow the back.
- The medial rotators of hips work to keep the legs in the neutral position. So that the knees and inner borders of the feet are held together.

Effects and Uses

Treatment of spinal deformities.

Positions Derived from Lying

- **Crook lying (Fig. 21.27):**
  - From lying, the hips and knees are bent so that the feet rest on the floor or plinth provided the feet are fixed by friction.
  - *Muscle work:* Little muscle work is required apart from that of the adductors and medial rotators of hips to prevent the knees from falling apart.
- **Crook lying with pelvis lifted:** From the previous position, the pelvis is elevated so that the trunk rests on the shoulders and is brought into line with the thighs.
  A firm pillow may be used to support the buttocks or the extensors of hips may work to hold the position.
- **Half lying:** The trunk is supported in oblique position by inclination of long

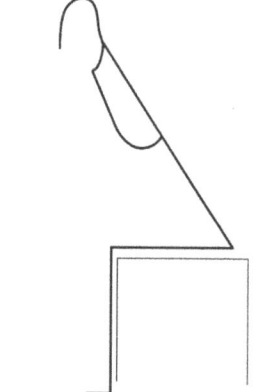

Fig. 21.25: Stoop sitting

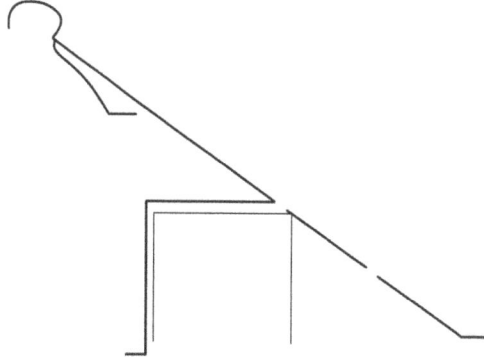

Fig. 21.26: Fallout sitting

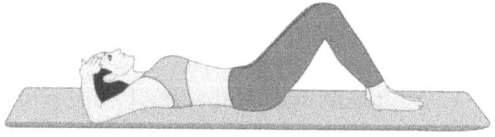

Fig. 21.27: Crook lying

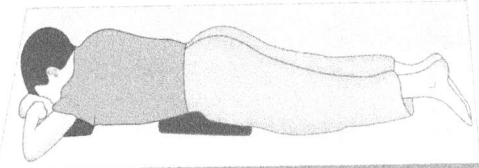

Fig. 21.28: Prone lying

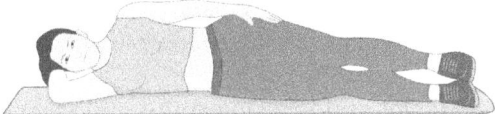

Fig. 21.29: Side lying

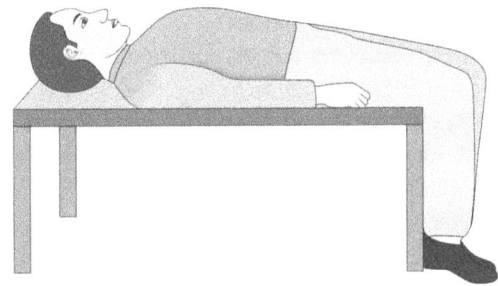

Fig. 21.30: Sit lying

end of plinth or by arrangement of pillows, while the legs are supported horizontally.

It is important to see that the trunk is in alignment to avoid slumping and so impeding respiration.

- **Crook half lying:** Knees may be bent to increase relaxation of abdominal wall or lower leg may hang over the end of the plinth with the feet resting on the floor.
- **Prone lying (Fig. 21.28):** Lying face downward, the body is fully supported anteriorly on the plinth or floor.
  The position may be active or relaxed.
  - *Muscle work:* Pre-post vertebral neck muscles maintain position of head.
  - Retractors and depressors of scapulae work to brace the upper back.
  - Lateral rotators of hip keep the heels together.
- **Leg prone lying:**
  - This is taken on a high plinth, the leg being supported from the anterior superior spines to the feet and stabilized by a strap.
  - The body is held in line with the legs and is unsupported the over the end of the plinth.
  - A stool is in position under trunk to afford support by arms in resting position.
  - *Muscle work:* Prevertebral and post neck muscles, the extensors of hips and longitudinal and transverse back muscles work strongly to maintain the position of trunk against gravity.
  - Extensors of shoulders and elbows hold the arms to the sides.
  - Flexors of the lumbar spine control the lumbar region which tends to become hallowed.
- **Side lying (Fig. 21.29):**
  - Patient rolls on to the side from lying or prone lying using the under arm to support the head. It is an unsteady position sometimes for strong trunk side bending exercises.
  - *Muscle work:* Alternatively, the shoulder may be stabilized by support from the upper arm resting on the ground or plinth in front the legs being free for movement. This is useful especially in sling exercises.
- **Sit lying (Fig. 21.30):** The patient lies supine with the knees bent and the lower leg hanging vertically over the end of plinth.
  There is a tendency for lumbar region to extend owing to tension of hip flexors.

HANGING

The body is suspended by grasping over a horizontal bar the forearms being pronated, the arms straight and at least shoulder width apart.

The head is held high and scapular is drawn down and together, so that the neck appears as long as possible.

The trunk and legs hang straight with heels together and the ankles planter flexed.

Muscle work:
- Flexors of lying work strongly to grasp the bar.
- All the muscles round the wrist work strongly to reduce the strain on the joints.
- Flexors of elbow
- Adductors of shoulder
- Depressors, retractors, and medial rotators of scapulae.
- Prevertebral and posterior neck muscles work reciprocally to maintain the position of head and neck.
- Flexors of lumber spine and extensors of hip.
- Adductors of hip work to keep the legs together.
- Extensors of knees may work to maintain full extension.
- Plantar flexors work to point the toes to floor.

Effects and Uses
- Breathing exercises
- Stretching exercises
- To increase muscle strength

Positions Derived from Hanging
- **Fall hanging (Fig. 21.31):**
  - Body is supported in the oblique position by the arms which grasp a horizontal bar and by the feet which rest on the floor.
  - The arms are vertical so that the shoulders fall directly below the hands, while the rest of the body is inclined and straight
  - *Muscle work:* Flexors of fingers grasp the bar and wrist, elbow and shoulder muscle work to reduce tension on these joints
  - Retractors of scapulae
  - Flexors of atlanto-occipital joint and of cervical spine prevent the head from falling backward.
  - Longitudinal and transverse back muscles support the trunk.

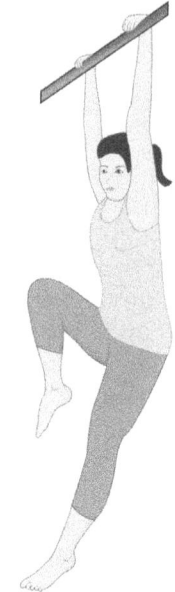

Fig. 21.31: Fallout hanging

  - Extensors of hip keep trunk in alignment and the plantar flexor press the feet to the floor.
- **Prone falling (Fig. 21.32):**
  - The legs are extended in line with the trunk from crook position so that the body is supported on the arms which are vertical and on the toes.
  - *Muscle work:* Extensors of elbows and all muscles of shoulder region was strongly

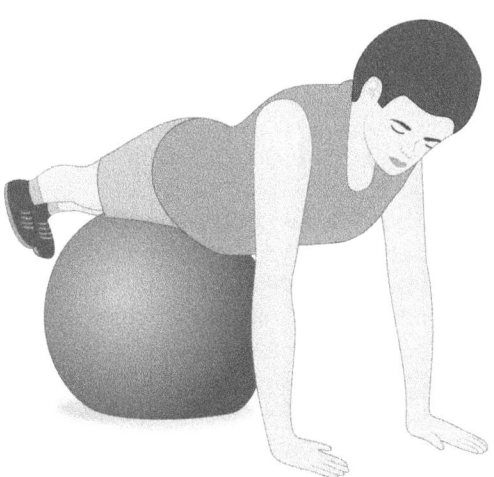

Fig. 21.32: Prone falling

to support the weight of body, while serrates anterior holds the scapulae firmly against the chest wall.
- Neck extensors controlled by the prevertebral muscles maintain the position of head against the pull of gravity.
- Flexors of lumbar spine prevent sagging of the trunk.
- The extensors of knees keep them straight.
- When the foot is fixed in dorsiflexion, the long flexors of the toes work with excellent grip floor.
- **Side falling (Fig. 21.33):** The body may be taken through a quarter turn from prone falling so that the weight is supported on the lateral borders of one foot and one hand. In this case, the muscles on the underside of the body work strongly and balance is difficult.

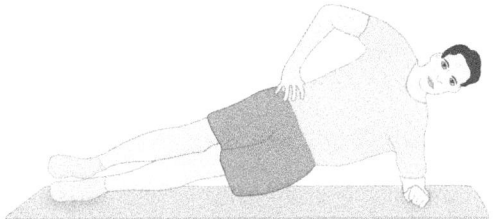

Fig. 21.33: Side falling

Index

Page numbers followed by *f* refer to figure and *t* refer to table.

A

Abdominal depth 255
Abdominal muscles, anterior 186
Abductor digiti minimi 159
Abductor hallucis 159
Abductor pollicis brevis 107
Accidents, potential sources of 311
Acetabular alignment 132
Acetabular anteversion 132
Acetabular fossa 122
Acetabular labrum 122, 123
  uses of 123
Acromial arch 83
Acromioclavicular capsule 86
Acromioclavicular joint 75, 85, 85f, 86f
  disc 86
  external rotation of 87f
  internal rotation of 87f
  ligaments of 86f
Acromioclavicular motions 86
Actin filament 50, 51f
Acute injury 43
Adduction 35, 113
  moment, right 133
Adductor hallucis 159
Adductor longus 128
Adductor magnus 128, 129, 270
Adenosine
  diphosphate 52
  triphosphate 52
Adhesion formation 285
Adhesive capsulitis 82, 83
Aerobic fitness 282
Airways narrow 176
Alveolar duct diameter 176
Amphiarthrosis 30, 178
Anatomical pulley, function of 27
Anesthesia 74
Angle of Wiberg 132, 132f
Angular motion 11, 12
  and spin 11f
Anisotropy 45
Ankle
  and foot paralysis 308
  dorsiflexion 294, 294f
  injuries 276
  interactions of 229, 230f
  knee 251f
  plantarflexion of 22, 230, 247, 294f
  planter flexed 325
  position of 147f
  range 240f
  synergy 201
Ankle and foot complex 154
  joint structure of 154
Ankle and foot orthosis 304, 307
  parts of 308
Ankle joint 299
  axis 15
  complex 157
Ankylosis 286
Annular pulley, thickening of 115
Annulus fibrosis 176, 178, 178f
Anterior tibial
  muscles 269
  translation 142f
Aorta 39
Aponeurotic sleeve 115
Arch
  avoid separation of 161
  integrity of 161
  longitudinal 110f, 111
  thickens, posterior 165
Arch of foot
  longitudinal 161t
  transverse 162t
Arm rests
  adjustable bilateral 315
  dimension of 257, 257f
Armrest-to-armrest width 257
Arteries, walls of 39
Arthritis, type of 36
Arthrokinematic movement 183t
Arthrokinematics 33, 70, 72, 79, 80f, 93, 94f, 96, 105, 114, 127, 145f, 156, 183, 244
  movement 72
Arthrology 66, 99
Arthroscopy 44f
Articular bone 69
Articular cartilage 15, 31, 42, 42f, 43f, 252
  cells of 42
  damage 188
  functions of 31, 42
  mechanical properties of 43
  wear of 44f
Articular congruence 122
Articular disc 31, 65, 65, 68f, 71f, 85f, 104
  inferior surface of 69
  superior surface of 69
Articular eminence 65-67
Articular facets 165
Articular surfaces 37
Articulating angle, type of 260
Articulating structures 179, 187
Articulating surface 67, 75, 76, 85, 88, 91, 94, 122, 155, 156, 159, 160, 190, 192, 193
  orientation of 75
Ascending stair gait 236
Atlanto-axial ligament, posterior 181
Auditory impairments 198
Austin-Moore prosthesis 305
Axilla, prolonged compression of 298
Axillary crutches 298
Axillary pouch 78

B

Back office chair 312f
Back pain 312
Back swing phase 265, 266, 266f
Backrest
  bottom height 257
  center height 257
  dimension of 257
  height 257
  horizontal radius 257
  seat angle 257
  vertical radius 257
  width 257
Backrest-seat angle 260f
Backseat dimension 257f
Backward leaning sitting 253
Backward sitting 253
Baksi's prosthesis 305
Balance beam 273, 274, 274f, 276
Band, posterior 77
Baseball throwing, biomechanics of 264
Bend standing 317f
Bending force 4, 5f
Bending forward 125
Better social skills 282
Biceps 93
  brachii 94
  bulk 286
  femoris 149, 248, 251
  tendon 82
Bilateral stance 133, 137
Biological unit 42
Biomechanical considerations 259

Index

Biphasic creep response 43
Biphasic load relaxation phenomenon 43
Blood vessels 161
Blunt trauma 272
Body
  center of gravity, displacements of 202
  center of mass 268
    control of 228
    equilibrium of 12
    lowering 278f
    posture 260
    stability of 18
    weight transferring through 253
Body segment
  movements of 263
  numbers of 263
Bone 37, 44, 244
  anisotropic behavior of 45, 45f
  architecture of 44
  attachment, types of 40
  compact 132
  failure, causes of 45
  fractures 45
  modeling 45
  remodeling 45
  response 37
  shape 161
  strength, factor affecting 45
Bony block 93
Bony configuration 150, 151
Bottom squat 243
Bow legs 213
Brachial plexus injury 298
Brachialis 94
Brachioradialis 23f, 94
Breathing
  exercises 326
  movement analysis of 260
Bucket handle 173
  movement 261
Bursa 41, 142
Buttocks width 256
Buttress plate 305

C

Calcaneus, eversion of 158f
Calf pain 223
Camper's chiasma 115
Cancellous bone 44, 132
Cane 301
  contralaterally 135
  functions of 301, 302
  gait pattern 302f
  ipsilaterally, use of 134
  types of 302
Capsular fibers, short 69
Capsular pattern 68, 75, 91, 95, 122, 155, 190
Capsule 68, 69, 92, 122
  posterior 79
  rotator interval 78
  tightness
    anterior 93
    posterior 93
Cardiac muscles 48
Carpal bones 99, 101f
  distal row of 99
  proximal row of 99

Carpal instability 108
Carpal tunnel 109f
  syndrome 109, 223
Carpus, translocation of 109
Carrying angle 96, 96f
Cartilage 41
  atrophy of 37
Cartilaginous joint 30
  primary 30
Caster, use of 257
Cavity, superior 71
Cavus foot 212
Cell 39
  body, large 55
Cellular component 39
Center edge 132
  angle 132
Center of gravity, relocation of 17
Central nervous system 165
  structures, safety of 165
Central tendon 115
Cervical
  collar 305
  disc diseases 306
  extensors muscles 210
  orthosis 305
  region 163
  spondylosis 306
Cervical spine 165, 218
  anterior convexity of 209
  intervertebral disc of 166
  kinematics of 168t
  ligaments of 167f, 167t
  muscles of 169t
Cervical vertebra
  midpoint of 15
  structure of 166
Cervicothoracolumbar sacral orthosis 304
Chair base, dimension of 257, 261f
Changeable seat bottom depth 314
Charnley prosthesis 305
Chest
  pain 223
  wall 167
Chondrocyte 41
Chondroitin sulfate chains 42
Chondromalacia patella 276
Chuck grasp 111
Circular motion 10
Clavicular head 88, 90
Clavicular movement, produce 90
Claw toe 208, 208f
Climatic comfort 256, 257
Clinical applications 223
Clinical relevance 129, 132, 233
Closed kinetic chain 11f, 36, 145f, 247
  exercises 247
Coccygeal region 163
Cock-up splint 305, 307
Codman's paradox 79
Colinear force system 5, 6
Collagen 39, 40
  arrangement 42f
  concentration 37
  cross-linking 37
  distribution of 42
  fiber 40, 41, 47
    arrangement of 40
  fibril concentration 47

  molecules 37
  type 1 39
Collagenous tissues, components of 40
Collateral ligamentous testing 114
Collateral ligaments 93, 93, 114, 160
Column, anterior 167
Complex computer programs 239
Complex computerized equipment 237
Complex reflex mechanism 200
Compressive force 4, 39, 302
Computer desk 260
Concave convex rule 33, 34f, 79, 128, 156
Concave proximal phalanx 114
Concentric contraction 55f, 56f, 58
Concentric muscle
  actions 59
  work 242
Concurrent force system 5, 6, 7f, 8f
Condylar blade plate 305
Condyle
  limits rotation of 69
  under disc 70
Congenital stenosis 109
Congruence 67
Connective tissue 39, 49, 151, 222
  function 39
  general properties of 45
  ligaments or 151
  structure 39
  wedge 100
Constant compressive force 181
Continuous passive motion 37
Contractile protein, loss of 61
Contradirectional lumbopelvic
  rhythm 125
Control flexion 181
Convex concave rule 145
Convex inferior facets 165
Coplanar force system 5, 5f
Coracoacromial arch 78
Coronal plane kinetics 270
Cortical bone 44
Counter-clockwise rotation 251
Coupled motions 167
Court dimensions 271, 271f
Coxa valga 131f
Coxa vara 131f
Craniocervical region
  anterior-lateral 189
  muscles of posterior 189
Creep 26
  phenomenon 25, 25f
Crepe bandage 27
Crook lying 324, 324f
Crook sitting 322, 323f
Cross-bridge interaction, generation of 52
Cruciate ligaments, role of 146
Crutch 298
  muscles 299
  walking 135, 223f
Cumulative traumatic syndromes 258
  prevention of 259
Curvilinear motion 10
Cycling 279f
Cylindrical grip 118

D

Daily living, activities of 243

Index

Dance
  and tumbling skills 274
  benefits of 282
  biomechanics of 281
  styles of 280, 281
Data acquisition 239
Data interpretation 239
Deep infrapatellar bursa 143
Deep squat 243
Deep strata 160
Deep tendon reflex 60
Deep tissue injury 216
Deep vein thrombosis 286
Deltoid muscle 80, 88
  consists 6
Depression 84
  elevation 67
Depth pulsating lumbar support 315
Desk job, ergonomics of 310
Dial lock 309
Diamond-shaped structure 186
Diarthrodial subclassification 31
Diarthrodial synovial joints 166
Diarthroses 30
Digastric activity 73
Digastric muscle 73
Digital flexors, tenodesis action of 120
Dip joint's lateral axis 115
Disc
  bulging 188
  extrusion 188
  herniation 188f
    mechanisms of 188
  prolapse 187
    posterolateral 180
  protrusion 188
  sequestration 188
  vertebral body 166
    articulation 166
Dislocation
  region of 286
  types of anterior 83
Displacement, restrains posterior 141
Display monitor 313
Distal articulating surface 67, 75, 122
Distal carpal row 108
Distal phalanx flex 116
Distal transverse arches 110f, 111
Dorsiflexion 156
Double joint system 105
Double support phase 226
Double-layered sheath 40
Dowager's hump 210, 210f
Downhill terrain 252
Downward rotation 84
Driving, ergonomics of 314
Drop lock 309
Dynamic cock up splint 305, 307
Dynamic compression plate 305
Dynamic friction 14
Dynamic posture 197, 198f
Dynamic splint 307
  devices, development of 37
Dynamic stability 67, 76, 78
Dynamic stabilizers 184

E

Ear, external 15

Eccentric concentration 55f
Eccentric contraction 58, 269
Eccentric muscle work 242
Elastic behaviour 26f
Elastic fibers, decrease of 176
Elastic region 46
Elastic structures, stretch of 270
Elasticity 23, 48
  modulus of 24, 46
Elastin fiber 40
Elbow 93, 304
  capsule 92f
  complex 91, 91f
  crutches 298, 299
  extension 94, 94f, 288f
  factors restricting 93
  flexors of 326
  height 255
  injuries 276
  joint, true 91
  pulled 97
  special feature of 96
  turn buckle splint 307
  width, external 256
Elbow flexion 94f, 288, 288f
  biomechanical importance of 302
  factors restricting 93
Elbow flexors 277
  tightness 93
Electro goniometer 284, 285
Elite marathoner 271
Ender's nail 305
Endomysium 49
Energy
  conservation of 19
  cost measurement 238, 242
  types of 19
Epimysium 49
Equilibrium, condition of 18
Erect standing 316f
Erector spinae 184, 215, 248
Ergon 310
Ergonomics 310
  chair 312, 313
  hazards 310
Excessive knee
  extension 140
  hyperextension 147
Exercise 314
  effects of 37
  isoinertial 55
  isokinetic 55
  king of 243
  skeletal 52
  stretching 326
Extended knee 151
Extensor apparatus 115
Extensor assembly 115
Extensor carpi radialis
  brevis 106
  longus 106
Extensor carpi ulnaris 106
Extensor digiti minimi 107
Extensor digitorum
  communis 106
  extends 117
  longus 157
Extensor expansion 115

Extensor hallucis longus 157
Extensor hood 115
Extensor pollicis longus 106
Extracellular matrix 39, 40
  volume of 39
Extrafusal fibers 59
Extreme postural inertia, combination of 278
Eye strain 312

F

Facet joint 178, 179, 182f
  capsule of 179
  orientation of 179
  syndrome 187
Factors resisting
  extension 182
  flexion 182
  rotation 182
  side flexion 182
Factors restricting abduction 79
Fallout hanging 326f
Fallout sitting 324, 324f
Fallout standing 320, 321f
Fascia covers quadriceps muscles 139
Fast twitch 52, 54
  fibers, types of 54
Fatigue resistance 173, 261
Fatigue wear 43
Femoral anterior glide syndrome 251, 252
Femoral condyle 145
  lateral 136
  medial 143
Femoral flexion 123f
Femoral head, stabilizing 129
Femoral neck, stress of 252
Femoroacetabular impingement 130
Femur 140
  angulation of 130
  anterior 142
  osteokinematics, pelvis on 124, 125
Ferguson's angle 187
Fiber
  anterior 129, 130
  length 57
  posterior 128-130
  primarily type II 55
  type II 61
Fibril-forming collagens 39
Fibrocartilage 41
Fibrocartilaginous disc 88
Fibroelastic structure present 176
Fibrous digital sheaths 114
Fibrous sternoclavicular capsule 88
Fibula, lateral malleolus of 155
Fibularis
  brevis 157
  longus 157
  tertius 157
Finger
  extension, mechanism for 115
  extensor mechanism of 114f
  flexion, mechanism for 114
  flexors of 277
First order lever 21, 22
  mechanical advantage for 22
Fixed pulley 27

Index

Fixed support synergies 201
Flat arches 223
Flat back posture 219, 219f
Flat foot 211, 211f, 212f
Flat surface object 294
Flexed knee
   position 252
   posture 208, 209, 209f
Flexible spinal orthosis 306
Flexion 113, 145
   extension 34, 35
   lateral 167, 183
   momentum phase 250
   relaxation phenomenon 213
Flexor digiti minimi 159
Flexor digitorum
   brevis 159, 160
   profundus 107
      tendons of 109
   superficialis 107
      tendons of 109
Flexor halluces
   brevis 159
   longus 156
Flexor muscles 208
Flexor pollicis longus 57
Floor exercise 273, 274, 274f
Fluid film lubrication 43
Fluid goniometer 284, 285
Folding walker 302
Foot
   arches of 160, 161
   bones of 154f
   clearance 237
   drop splint 305
   eversion 294, 295f
      dorsiflexion of 160
   flat 225, 230, 253
      kinematics of 231
      kinetics of 231
   interactions of 229, 230f
   inversion 294, 295f
   medial view of 155f
   muscles, ineffective intrinsic 208
   normal 211f
   number of 257
   parts of 154f
   placement 237, 238t
   pronated 252
   pronation 212f
   rest 313
   structures, protects deep 160
   supination 212f
Force
   classification of 3
   composition of 8
   concepts of 3
   couple, anatomical example of 8f
   measurement of 4
   plate recordings 238
   representation of 3
   system 5, 307
   types of 4
   velocity relationship 58
Forearm 108, 299
   motions, axis of 95f
   pronation of 5, 289f
   supination 5, 289f
      and pronation 95f

Fracture
   calcaneus 308
   conditions, postoperative 286
   unhealed 286
Freedom, degrees of 11, 34, 75, 84, 91, 94, 122, 154, 159, 160, 179, 187
Friction 14
   application of 15
   coefficient of 14
   properties 256
Frontal plane
   deviations 138
   kinematics 232
Frozen shoulder 82, 83
Functional residual capacity 176

G

Gag chains 42
Gait 224
   alterations 222
   antalgic 234
   circumduction 234
   high stepping 235
   kinematics of 231
   kinetics of 231
   laboratory 237, 239f
   pathological 234
   phases of 225f
   scissoring 235
   spatial parameters of 241
   swing phase of 145, 267
   time duration 225f
Gait analysis 232, 239f, 240f
   systems 238
Gait cycle 224, 224f, 226f, 227t, 230f, 267, 268f
   determinants of 229
   kinetic of 233f
Gait patterns 227, 299, 301, 303
   four point 299, 300, 301f
   swing to 301
   three point 299, 300, 300f
   two point 299, 301, 301f
Gastrocnemius 7, 156, 249
   bursa 142, 143
Gastrocnemius muscle 140
   activity of 269
   contraction of 141
Gemellus
   inferior 128, 130
   superior 128, 130
Genu recurvatum 209f
Genu valgum 137, 212, 305
Genu varum 137, 213
Gibbus deformity 210, 210f
Glandular development 222
Glenohumeral rhythm 81
Glenoid fossa 77
Glenoid labrum 76, 76f, 77
Gluteal medius, posterior 252
Gluteus maximus 129, 130, 193, 270
   activation of 232
   attachment of 187
   gait 235
   muscle 149
   weakness of 233f

Gluteus medius 128, 129, 270
   gait 235
Gluteus minimus 128-130
   primary function of 129
Gluteus muscle 207
Glycosaminoglycans 46
Golfer's elbow 96, 97
Golfer's lift 248
Golgi tendon organ 139
Goniometer
   body of 284
   placement 284
   types of universal 284f
Goniometry 283
   principles of 283
Graphical methods 8
Grasping large files 310
Grasping synergies 202
Gravity 15
   center of 6, 16, 197, 229, 244
   dependent 284, 285
   direction of 244
   line of 15, 134, 160, 202, 204f
   segmental center of 17
Greater trochanter bursitis 252
Greater wing 66
Grip
   depends, firmness of 265, 266
   types of 118
Grosse-Kempf nail 305
Ground reaction force 6f, 203, 229, 241
   vector 203
Gutter crutches 298, 299
Gymnastics
   biomechanical analysis of 273
   poses 273f

H

Half kneeling 321f
Hammer toe 208, 208f
Hamstrings tightness 125
Hand
   arches of 110
   complex 110
   external anatomy of 110
   functional position of 111
   grip, measurement of 299
   injuries 276
   muscular function of 120
Hard cervical collar 305
Harrington rod 305
Hartshill rectangle 305
Head
   of talus, plantarflexion of 158f
   stabilization 202
Heel off 226
   kinematics of 231
   kinetics of 232
Heel pad, hysteresis of 25f
Heel strike 225, 230
   kinematics of 231
   kinetics of 231
Hemiplegic gait 235
High intensity sprinting sessions 267
Hinge action 68
Hip 251, 252
   abduction 292, 292f

Index

adduction 293, 293f
adductor 278, 326
   muscles 128
   extension 292, 292f
   extensors 128, 232, 278, 326
   external rotators 130, 234
   fllexion 292f
   hiking force 135
   hyperextension of 251
   internal rotators 129, 234
   joint axis of 210
   keep trunk, extensors of 326
   knee-ankle-foot orthosis 304, 309
   lateral rotation 128, 293f
   medial rotation 128, 293f
   muscles, anterior 207
   orthosis 304
   pain, causes of mechanically
      induced 252
   rotators 234
   segment 121, 121f, 130
   synergy 202
   trabecular pattern of 191f
Hip abductor 234
   mechanism 129
   muscles 129
   weakness 234
Hip flexion 229, 277, 292
   excessive 185
   range 240f
Hip flexor 128, 233
   contracture 252
   significant 129
Hip joint 121, 219, 220f, 232
   anatomy of 121
   angle 129
   axis 15
   compression, total 134
   flexors 128
   forces 133, 134f
   rotation of 128
Hoffa's fat pad 143
Hoffa's pad 139
Hollow cone lies, center of gravity of 16
Hollow hemisphere, center of gravity of 17
Hook grip 118
Hooke's law 24, 26
Hoop stress 178
Human body
   center of gravity of 17
   gravity of 16f
   levers in 22
   segmental weight of 17
Human motion classification 11f
Humeroulnar joint 31, 91, 92f
   articulation of 94f
   axis of 93f
Humerus 92f
   capitulum of 91
   neck of 77
   trochlea of 91
   upper part of 76f
Hyaline articular cartilage 41
Hyaline cartilage 42
Hyaluronic acid 31, 42
Hydrodynamic mechanism 178, 179
Hydrostatic pressure 178
Hyoid bone 66

Hyperextension 114, 147, 289
Hypermobility 153
Hypothetical axis 158
Hysteresis 25, 25f, 47

I

Ideal plumb line alignment 204f, 205f
Iliac crest 192, 252, 317
Iliac spine
   anterior inferior 123
   anterior superior 192, 293
   posterosuperior 190
Iliopsoas 270
Iliotibial band 142, 143f, 151
Iliotibial tract
   irritation 252
   tightening of 252
Illnesses 310
Immobilization, effect of 60
Impingement syndrome 82
Inclination, angle of 130, 130f
Inclinometer 285f
Infrapatellar bursa 143
Infrapatellar fat pad 139, 143
Infraspinatus 78
Injury 60
   chronic 43
   effects of 37
   risk of 272
Innominate 121f
   movements of 191
Inorganic phosphorous 52
Insall burstein prosthesis 305
Inspiration 173
Inspiratory capacity, decrease in 176
Intercarpal articulation 101
Intercondylar tubercles 137
Interdiscal pressures 215
Interfacial wear 43
Interlocking nail 305
Interosseous
   contract simultaneously 116
   intercostal muscles, internal 261
   muscles lines 117
Interphalangeal extension 291
Interphalangeal flexion 291
Interphalangeal joint, proximal 111, 291
Intersegmental attachments 161
Interspinous ligament, functions of 181
Intervertebral disc 166, 167, 176, 179,
   215, 306
   functions of 177
   prolapse 187, 188, 307
Intra-abdominal pressure 176, 246, 248, 306
Intra-articular
   derangement 192
   pressure, negative 76, 122
Intradiscal pressure 259f
Intrafusal fibers 59
Intramedullary nail 305
Ipsidirectional lumbopelvic rhythm 125
Irritability 48
Ischial tuberosity 192
Isolated hamstring contraction 141
Isolated quadriceps contraction 140
Isometric back muscle strength 248
Isometric contraction 55f, 58

Isometric muscle contraction 56
Isotonic contraction 55

J

Jaw
   closing 70
   opening 70
Jogging, characteristics of 271
Joint 37, 75, 154f, 244
   articulation 69
   atlantoaxial 23f, 166t
   atlanto-occipital 166t
   ball-and-socket 33
   carpometacarpal 110, 112
   changes 222
   chondrosternal 172
   classification 29, 29f
      method of 30
   compartments, lateral 101
   condyloid 32
   congruence 137, 151
   costochondral 172
   costotransverse 172, 260
   costovertebra 171, 172f, 260
   derangements, classification of 73
   design 30, 67, 155
   distal interphalangeal 111
   distal tibiofibular 156
   fibrous 30
   fibulotalar 154
   fulcrum-ankle 22
   fulcrum-elbow 23
   function 29, 35
   glenohumeral 11, 66, 75, 83, 85
   gliding 69
   gomphosis 30
   hinge 31, 32f, 69
   humeroradial 32, 91
   immobilization on 37
   interbody 178, 183
   intercarpal 99
   interchondral 172
   interphalangeal 160
   kinematics 143
   less compromised 185
   lower 69
   lubrication 31
   lumbosacral 187, 207
   manubriosternal 171
   metacarpophalangeal 110, 113,
      117, 290
   metatarsophalangeal 159, 160
   motion 33
   nonsynovial 30
   number of 59
   of Luschka 166
   of wrist 99
   pivot 32, 32f
      synovial 94
   plane 32
      synovial 32f
   polycentric knee 309
   position 13
      of individual 239
   range of motion, factors affecting 285
   reaction force 133, 134
   sacrococcygeal 193

scapulothoracic 75, 82, 83
secondary cartilaginous 30
small intercarpal 98
stability 34
stiff hip 185
structure 29, 112
subtalar 155f, 156, 158f
superior radioulnar 91, 93, 94, 95f
surface, proximal 114
surgery, devices after 37
suture 30
symphysis 178
talocrural 154
thumb carpometacarpal 113
tibiotalar 154
transverse tarsal 157, 158, 158f
type of 59, 67, 75, 122
typical synovial 30f
uniaxial hinge 114
upper 69
xiphisternal 171
Joint capsule 31, 77, 77f, 139, 159
 fibrous layer of 139
 inferior 79
 posterior 209
 single 136
 synovial layer of 139
Joint stress 138
 increases 138
Jugular notch of sternum 170

K

Kabaddi 271
Keratan sulfate chains 42
Kicking 276
 ball, stages of 276f
 motion, stages of 276
Kinematic 79, 93, 95, 124, 155, 181, 187, 191, 244, 251, 268
 and kinetics 113, 237, 244
 approach 242
 chain 11
 chain motion, close 11, 79, 93, 96, 156
Kinesthetic sense disturbance 201
Kinetic chain 36
 exercise concept 247
Kinetic energy 19, 270, 270f, 277
Kinetic friction 14
Kirschner wire 305
Knee 229, 304
 and joint diseases 309
 angulation, flexion of 252
 ankle foot orthosis 304, 308
 bent standing 320
 complex 136
 extensors of 326
 flexed 140
 full extension 141
 hyperextension causes 209
 injuries 272, 276
 interactions of 229, 230f
 locking mechanism of 148
 motions 146f
 physiological valgus of 230
 posture, hyperextended 209, 209f
 sitting 321, 322f
 stabilizers of 150

Knee extension 146, 147, 230, 277, 294
 gravitational 207
 seated 145
Knee extensor 277, 278
 act 248
 group 149
Knee flexion 139, 144f, 145f, 146-148, 229, 293, 293f
 contractures 208
Knee flexor
 acts 248
 group 148
Knee joint 136, 136f, 143f, 144f, 147f, 206f, 299
 extension 247
 flexion 247
 function 212
 posterior offset 309
 stability 140
 straight 308
Kneeling 321
 derived positions of 321
Knock knees 212
Knuckle bender 307
Kuntscher nail 305
Kyphosis 210
Kyphotic curves 164
Kyphotic posture 218f
Kyphotic-lordotic posture 218

L

Labral impingement 252
Labral tears 130
Latissimus dorsi 187
 role of 135
Lax stoop standing 320, 320f
Leg
 gait, short 235
 pain 223, 312
 prone lying 325
 standing, single 320f
Levator ani 193
Levator costarum 175
Lever
 analysis of 22
 length used 263
 principle of 22
Ligament 37, 40, 47, 68, 77, 77f, 89, 104, 166, 191f, 246
 acromioclavicular 86
 annular 91-93, 93f, 95
 anterior 112
  cruciate 139, 140, 141f, 142f, 272
  longitudinal 179, 182
 capsular 112
 complex, inferior glenohumeral 77, 79
 coracoacromial 78
 coracoclavicular 86
 coracohumeral 78, 79
 costoclavicular 89
 costotransverse 172
 dorsal radiocarpal 103
 extrinsic 103
  functions of posterior
 longitudinal 180
  heal intrinsic 103
  iliofemoral 123, 123f

 iliolumbar 179, 181, 187, 190
 inferior
  acromioclavicular 86
  pubic 192
 interclavicular 89
 interosseous 190
 interspinous 179, 181
 intertransverse 179, 181, 182
 intra-articular 171
 intrinsic 104
 ischiofemoral 123, 124, 124f
 lateral 112
  collateral 93, 140, 151, 155
  costotransverse 172
 long 104
 lumbosacral 187
 medial collateral 140, 151
 meniscofemoral 141
 middle glenohumeral 77
 palmar ulnocarpal 106
 patella 149
 patellotibial 139
 plantar 160
  calcaneonavicular 211
 posterior 112, 192
  cruciate 139, 141
  intercoccygeal 193
  longitudinal 179, 180
  oblique 141
 pubofemoral 123, 123f
 quadrate 95
 radial collateral 91-93, 103
 radiotriquetral 104
 remodeling of 222
 sacrococcygeal 193
 sacrotuberous 190, 192
 scapholunate 105
 short 104
 sphenomandibular 69
 spring 211
 sternoclavicular 89
 stylomandibular 69
 superior
  acromioclavicular 86
  costotransverse 172
  glenohumeral 77
  pubic 192
 supraspinous 179, 181
 tautness maximum 139
 temporomandibular 69
 tension of 151
 teres 124f
 transverse
  acetabular 123
  carpal 111, 114
 ulnar collateral 91, 92, 104
 volar
  carpal 111
  radiocarpal 104
 weakened 37
 wrist 102
Ligamentous laxity 98
Ligamentous tensile strength
decreases 222
Ligamentum flavum 179, 180
 functions of 181
Ligamentum nuchae 181
Ligamentum teres 123, 124

Index

Limb
  complex 252
  stance, single 132
Linear front-back seat 315
Linear motion 10
Linear strain 23
Lister's tubercle 99
Load application, excessive repetition of 45
Load deformation curve 46f
Load relaxation phenomenon 25, 25f
Location fulcrum 265
Locomotion 224
  types of 224t
Lombard's paradox 245
Long sitting 323f
Long-distance runners, classification of 271
Long-horse vaulting 274f
Longus
  capitus 189
  colli 189
Loose pack position 34, 35, 67, 75, 91, 94, 122, 155
Lordosis 210
Lordotic curves 164
Lordotic posture 218, 218f
Low back
  injuries 276
  pain 223, 307
Low pressure 43f
Low wing standing 317
Lower cervical
  region 165
  spine consists 166
Lower extremity 299
  activities 247
  injuries 275
  kinetic chain, influence of 246
  motion of 230f
  orthosis 307
  transverse rotation of 230f
Lower limb 149f
  orthosis 304
Low-friction surface 42
Lubrication mechanism 43
Lubricative synovial fluid 15
Lumbar extensors 184
Lumbar flexion, excessive 185
Lumbar flexors 184
Lumbar intervertebral disc 178f
Lumbar lateral flexors 184
Lumbar lordosis 253
Lumbar radiculopathy 187, 188
Lumbar region 163
Lumbar roll support 253
Lumbar sacral orthosis 304
Lumbar segment 176
  joints in 178
Lumbar side flexors 319
Lumbar spine 218, 307
  flexor of 278
  stability of 179
Lumbar spondylolisthesis 187, 188
Lumbar spondylosis 187, 188
Lumbar support 253, 315
  adjustable 314
Lumbar vertebra
  ligaments surrounding 180f

midpoint of 15
structure of typical 177f
Lumber spine, flexors of 326
Lumbopelvic rhythm 125, 125f, 184, 185f
  sequence of 185
Lumbosacral angle 187f, 188, 207f
Lumbosacral strain 307
Lung 320, 321f
  capacity 271
Lying down, ergonomics of 315
Lying posture, analysis of 216

M

Macrophage activity 61
Major blood supply 140
Male gymnastics compete 273
Mallet toe 208f
Mandible
  condyle of 65
  elevation 70
  parts of 66f
Mandibular condyle 65f
  sits 65f
Mandibular depression 70, 71f
Mandibular elevation 70, 71f
Mandibular fossa 65f, 66
Mandibular motions 70
Mandibular protrusion 70
Mandibular retrusion 70, 71
Manubriosternum 173
Mass, center of 197, 202
Masseter 72f
Mastication
  attach directly, muscles of 65
  secondary muscles of 73f
Material's stiffness 46
Maxilla 66f
Maximal isometric tension 57
McLaughlin's plate 305
Measurement procedure 286, 298, 299, 302, 303
Mechanical behavior 45
Mechanical functions 44
Mechanical levers 22
Mechanical perturbations 201
Mechanical power analysis 242
Medial meniscus 138
  motion 138
Median nerve 109
Meniscal nutrition 138
Meniscus 138
  homologue 100
  removal of 138
  role of 138
  wedge-shape 147
  weight distribution 138f
Mental functioning 282
Metacarpal ligament, deep transverse 113, 159
Metacarpal rolls, concave surface of 113
Metacarpophalangeal abduction 291
Metacarpophalangeal extension 117, 291
Metacarpophalangeal flexion 117, 290
Metacarpophalangeal joint, destruction of 111
Metatarsal
  base of 160
  break 159, 160

Metatarsophalangeal extension 159, 295
Metatarsophalangeal flexion 295
Midcarpal joint 98, 99
  focuses 101
  lateral axis 101, 102
  structure 101
  surfaces 101
Midstance
  kinematics of 231
  kinetics of 232
Mid-swing
  kinematics of 231
  kinetics of 232
Milwaukee brace 305
Mind 271
Momentum transfer phase 250
Mononucleated cells 61
Moore's pin 305
Mortise 155
Mother's womb 198
Motion
  analysis system 238, 239
  context of 12
  description 266
  excessive 145
  high-velocity 263
  of scapula, frontal plane 84f
  quantification system 239
  repetition of 11, 11f
  repetitive 258
  single 11
  types of 10
Motor system 200
Motor unit 54, 56f
  recruitment of 56
Mouth opening, limitation of 68
Movement
  freedom of 243
  impairment syndrome 251
  restriction of 156
  sinosoid pattern of 228, 229
  timing pattern of 265
  type of 265
Multijoint muscles 58
Multiple muscles, co-contraction of 141
Muscle 68f, 191f
  abdominal 175, 182, 184, 215, 261
  abduction initiator 81
  accessory 261
  action of 174
  adductors 322
  architecture 56, 59
  attachments, location of 59
  biarticular 246
  bulk 285
  classification of 58
  contract 55f
    rhythmically 173
  contraction 54, 205, 272
    types of 55f
  contributing 81t
  dome-shaped 261
  forces, reduction of 134
  hamstrings 149, 269, 270
  influencing 192
  injury 60
  intercostal 174, 175, 261
  involuntary 48

lateral 149
location determines 59
mechanical model of 48, 48f
of mastication, actions of 73t
of ventilation, primary 174, 261
passive tension of 151
piriformis 128, 130
primary 72
recruitment of 174
role 58
sartorius 149
scalene 90, 174, 175, 261
secondary 72
shortening of 54, 55
skeletal 48, 49, 52, 176
smooth 48
soleus 149
soreness, delayed onset 60
spindle reflex 60
sternocleidomastoid 175, 261
strain of 60, 252
strength 282, 326
subclavius 90, 175
suboccipital 189
synergies 201
temporalis 72
themselves 200
tissue 49
tone 282
two-joint 58
types of 48
weakness 309
work 277, 316, 317, 318
Muscle action 55
end of 52
energy for 52
types of 54
Muscle activity 215, 251
bursts of 202
Muscle fiber
action 50
cytoplasm of 49
length 57, 59
types, classification of 54t
Muscle function 48, 57, 133
factors affecting 59
Muscle structure 48
elements of 49
Muscle-tendon unit 47
Muscular attachments 90
Muscular changes 222
Muscular fatigue 315
Muscular imbalance 185, 199
Muscular strength 282
Muscular weakness 286
Musculoskeletal discomfort, reduce 310
Musculoskeletal injuries 248
preventing 282
Myoelectrical signals 239
Myofascial tightness 79
Myofibril 49
Myokinematics 244
Myosin
filament 50, 51f
head 50
tilts 52
Myositis ossificans 286
Myotendinous junction 41

N

Narrowed joint space 188
Nasal septum 40
Natural intercarpal alignment, maintaining 102
Navicular bone, causes depression of 211
Nebulin 50
Neck
muscles, postvertebral 278
pain 223, 312
region 26
Neer's prosthesis 305
Nerve
compression 223
protects 161
Nervous system 286
Neural arch 176
Neural components 200
Neurologic control 174
Neurological conditions 286
Neuromuscular coordination 200
Neuromuscular junction 50, 51f
Neutral equilibrium 18
Neutral zero method 284
Newton's first law 12
Newton's law of
gravity 15
motion 12
Newton's second law 12
Newton's third law 241
of motion 12
Nipples and areolas 222
Noncontractile extensor mechanism 115
Nonholding walker 302
Nonvertebral articulation 166
Nonweight bearing 140, 299
gait pattern 303
Nucleus pulposis 176, 177, 178f
Nurse maid's elbow 96, 97

O

Oblique cord ligament 95
Oblique coronal axis 87
Oblique ligament, elongates anterior 113
Oblique retinacular ligament, fibers of 115
Obliqus capitis
inferior 189
superior 189
Obturator externus 128, 130
Obturator internus 128, 130
Occipital support 306
Olecranon bursitis 97
Olecranon fossa, upper edge of 92
Open kinematic chain 11f
motion 11, 79, 93, 96, 156
Open kinetic chain 36, 146f, 247
Orthosis 304
biomechanical principle of 305
external 304
study of 304
Orthotics 304
Oscillation 11, 11f
Oscillatory movement 20
Osteoarthritis 36, 130, 309
Osteokinematics 33, 70, 79, 93, 95, 103f, 104, 114, 244
Osteophyte formation 188

Osteoporosis 44
passive ROM, region of 286
regional 37
Osteoporotic pain 307
Overarm throwing, kinematics of 264
Oxygen consumption 242

P

Pacinian corpuscles 139
Pain
abdominal 312
location of 258
Painful arc syndrome 82
Painful hip gait 234
Palmar interossei 116
Palmar prehension 119
Palpation 192
Parallel bars 274, 275f
Parallel elastic component 48
Parallel force system 5, 7, 8f
Parallelogram
center of gravity of 16
method 9
Paralysis 306
Parkinson's gait 235, 236f
Partial weight bearing 299
gait pattern 300, 300f, 303
Participating lever 265
Pascal's law 178
Passive finger flexion 120
Passive insufficiency 59f
Passive tension, decreases 116
Patella 27
longitudinal stabilizers of 152
motions of 151
stability, factors affecting 151
tendon 149
Patellar alta 151
Patellar dislocations 276
Patellar height 255
Patellar influence 150
Patellar plicae 139
Patellar shift, lateral 152
Patellar subluxations 276
Patellar tendon, length of 151
Patellar tilt
lateral 152
medial 152
Patellofemoral articular surfaces 151
Patellofemoral joint 151
stability, frontal plane 152
stress 152
Patellofemoral ligament
lateral 139
medial 139
Patellofemoral pain 276
Patellofemoral stabilization, asymmetry of 153
Pectoralis
major 88, 175, 261
minor 175, 261
Pectorals major 90
Peddling techniques 280
Pelvic
girdle 190f
pain 223
motion 191f, 229f

Index

osteokinematics, femoral on 124
rotation 126, 126f, 127, 127f, 229
Pelvic tilt, anterior 209
  excessive posterior 210
  lateral 126, 229
  posterior 232
Pelvis 185
  anterior shift of 185
  lateral shift of 126, 127f
  osteokinematics, femur on 124
  relations to 121
  rotatory mobility of 322
  trabecular pattern of 191f
Pendular goniometer 284, 285, 285f
Pendulum motion 11, 11f
Pennate muscle 57, 57f
Perimysium 49
Peripheral portion 121
Pes cavus 212, 212f
Pes planus 211, 211f, 305
Philadelphia collar 306
Physical confidence 282
Physical discomfort 315
Physical therapy 74
Physiologic valgus 229
Piriformis syndrome 130, 252
Plantar and dorsal interossei 160
Plantar fascia 160
Plantar flexion 294
Plantar flexors 278
  effort-insertion point of 22
  paralysis of 308
Plantar plates 159
Plantar pressure, equal distribution of 160
Plantarflexion 156
Plantaris calf muscles 249
Plastic behavior 26f
Plastic region 26, 47
Player's diet 272
Plica, superior 139
Plunger type lock 309
Poisson's ratio 24
Polygon method 9
Pommel horse 275, 275f
Popliteal muscle shares role 141
Popliteus muscle 149
Portion of sacrum, anterior superior 207
Posterior capsule, ligaments of 141
Postglenoid tubercle 66
Post-traumatic stabilization 306
Postural control 200, 201f
Postural deviations 198f
Postural fault, types of 220t
Postural reflexes 200
Postural stability 200
  and control 200
Postural sway 203
Posture 197
  boards 216
  evaluation of 217
  kinematics of 202
  measurement of 216
Potential energy 19, 270
Power 20
  grip 118, 119f
  phase 279
Practical application of torque 14
Precane training 302

Precrutch training 299
Predominant arthrokinematic 127
Predominant contractile element 181
Prehension, lateral 118
Prepatellar bursa 143
Prepatellar bursitis 153
Pressure
  center of 203, 241
  sore 215f
    decubitus ulcers 215
Prevertebral neck muscles 278
Prewalker training 302
Pronation 289
Pronator quadratus 96
Pronator teres 96
Prone falling 326, 326f
Prone kneeling 321, 322f
Prosthetics 304
Proteoglycan 40, 46
  structure of 43f
Protrusion 67, 71
Proximal articulating surface 67, 75, 88, 122
Proximal body segment, posterior movement of 205
Proximal interphalangeal joint's lateral axis 115
Proximal phalanx 115
  base of 113
  rolls 114
Pterygoid plate
  lateral 66
  medial 66, 72
Pterygoids advance, lateral 72
Pubic symphysis 306
Pubic tubercle 192
Pump handle 173
  movement 261

Q

Quadratus femoris 128, 130
Quadratus lumborum 182
Quadriceps
  function of 150
  gait 235
  muscle 246
    force 28
  tendon 142, 149

R

Radial deviation 102, 103f, 106, 290
  amount of 106
Radial deviators, function of 108
Radial expansion 178
Radial nerve, neuropraxia of 298
Radiocapitate 104
Radiocarpal joint 98-101, 106
  lateral axis 101
Radioulnar joint supination 289
Radius 99
  styloid process of 99
Raising body 278f
Range-of-motion 31, 33, 79, 93, 125, 156, 182, 198, 263, 283
  angles of 78
  exercises 272
  extension 147
  in lower extremity, measuring of 292

in upper extremity, measuring of 287
  larger 81
  total 84
Reaction, normal 14
Reciprocal motion 11, 11f
Reciprocal walker 302
Reciprocally concave-convex 85
Rectus abdominis 175
Rectus capitus
  anterior 189
  lateralis 189
  posterior major 189
Rectus femoris 150f, 269, 270
  low activity of 248
Reflexes, quick 271
Relieve physical discomfort 311
Repetitive movement disorders 312
Respiratory movements 174f
Resultant force 9
Resultant pull 150
Retinaculum, medial and lateral 139, 151
Retrusion 67, 71
Rheumatoid arthritis 36, 109
Rheumatoid changes 306
Rheumatoid disease 111
Rhythmical alternating, series of 224
Rib 170
  false 170
  floating 170
  hump 213
  movement 174f
    generated 260
  parts of 171f
  stabilization of 175
  vertebral 170
  vertebrochondral 170
  vertebrosternal 170
Rib cage
  articulations of 171, 171f
  borders of 170f
  kinematics of 173
  ligaments of 173f
  muscles with 173
Ride sitting 323f
Rolling friction 15
Rotary motion 11
Rotation diminishes, magnitude of 148
Rotation, axis of 261
Rotation-lateral rotation, medial 34, 35
Rotator cuff
  dynamic stability of 78f
  muscle 78
  tendon 78, 82
Ruffini corpuscles 139
Running gait cycle 268f
Running hand touch 272
Ruptured flexor pulley, biomechanics of 120
Rush nail 305

S

Sacral motion 191f
Sacral orthosis 304
Sacral region 163
Sacroiliac corset 306
Sacroiliac joint 125, 189, 192, 207, 306
  dysfunction 192

Index

Sacroiliac ligament, anterior 190
Sacrum
  apex of 193
  counternutation of 185
  movements of 191
  nutation of 185
Saddle joint 32, 32f, 112
  structure 112
Safe lifting, principles of 248
Safety, factor of 25
Sarcolemma 49
Sarcomere 49, 50f
  number of 57
Sarcoplasm 49
Sarcoplasmic reticulum 49, 54
Scapula 84, 218
  lies 80
  parts of 76f
  plane of 80, 80f
  resting position of 83
  retractors of 326
Scapular setting phase 81
Scapulohumeral rhythm 81
Scapulohumeral rhythm, advantages of 81
Scapulothoracic articulation, functions of 83
Scapulothoracic motions, muscles for 81t
Scapulothoracic musculature 85
Scapulothoracic stability 85
Sciatica 223
Scoliosis 213, 213f, 214f
Scorpion kick 272
Seat back incline, adjustable 314
Seat bottom incline, adjustable 314
Seat height, adjustable 314
Seat slope
  adjustable 256
  angle of 260f
Second order lever, mechanical advantage for 22
Seidel nail 305
Self-centering mechanism 67
Semimembranosus 148
Semi-sitting posture 254, 255f
Semitendinosus 148
Sensory
  innervation 106
  perturbation 201
  receptors 59
  system 200
Septic arthritis 309
Shallow alveolar sac 176
Sharpey's fibers 37
Shear force 4, 5f
Shear strain 23
Shock
  absorption 161
  decreased 74
Shoulder
  abduction 287, 287f
    factors restricting 79
    mechanism 81, 82f
  adduction 277, 288
  adductors of 326
  complete abduction of 77
  complex 75, 75f
  dislocation of 82, 83
  extension 287, 287f
    restricted 79

external rotation 80f
flexion 287, 287f
  angle 260
  restricted 79
girdle, rotation of 84f
height 254
horizontal abduction 264
impingement syndrome 82f, 264f
injuries 272, 276
internal rotation 80f
joint 75
  bursa of 79
  lateral rotation 288, 288f
  levels, unequal 213
  medial rotation 288, 288f
  motions 81t
  orthosis 304
  width 256
Sidearm throwing, kinematics of 264
Side-horse vaulting 273, 274f
Simple stretch reflex 60
Sitting
  derived positions of 322
  ergonomics of 314
Sitting posture 213, 253
  analysis of 213
  types of 253, 254f
Sit-to-stand
  concept 249f
  maneuver 250
  phases 250f
Skeletal changes 222
Skeletal muscle
  basic behaviors of 48
  function of 49
  internal structure of 53f
  structure of 49, 49f
Skill requirement 265
Skin
  loss of elasticity of 26
  produces higher degree 26
Skull, parts of 68f
Sliding filament theory 52, 53f
Sliding friction 14
Slight medial rotatory moment 129
Slouched posture 215f
Slumped posture 215
Small bone dimension 45
Smith Peterson nail 305
Soft collar 305
Soft tissue
  approximation 93
  structures 202
  tightness 285
Solid circular cone, center of gravity of 16
Solid hemisphere lies, center of gravity of 17
Sorbo rubber 27
Souter's prosthesis 305
Spastic foot 308
Spatial parameters 228f
Speed
  greater amount of 266
  parameters 227
Sphenoid bone 66, 67f
  spine of 69
Spherical grip 118
Spinal canal stenosis 187, 188

Spinal curvature, lateral 213
Spinal discs 246
Spinal erector's length tension relationship 246
Spinal motion 307
Spinal muscles, posterior 182
Spinal orthosis 304, 305
Spine, normal 211f
Splint, long opponent 307
Spondylosis 286
Sporting activities, movement analysis in 263
Sports runner 271
Spring
  properties of 20
  weight of 20
Squat
  kinematics of 244
  kinetics of 244
  lifting 248
  phases of 243
  technique of 243, 243f
Stable arm 284, 287
Stair climbing
  gait 236
  types of 236, 237
Stair gait
  cycle 237f
  descending 236
Standing job, ergonomics of 315
Standing posture, analysis of 206
Static friction 14
Static isometric muscle action 55
Static posture 197, 198f
Static splint 307
Static stability 76
Steffee plate 305
Steinmann pin 305
Sternal cartilage 40
Sternoclavicular disc 88
Sternoclavicular joint 75, 85, 88, 88f
  capsule 89
  disc of 88f
  ligaments of 89f
  movements of 89f
Sternoclavicular motions 89
Sterno-occipital mandibular immobilizer 306
Sticking region 246
Stiff hip gait 234
Stiff lumbar segment 185
Stoop lifting 248
Strain 23
  hardening 26
  types of 23
Strain-rate sensitivity 47
Stress 25
  compressive 4f
  deprivation 37
  mechanical 310
  strain curve 24, 24f
    application of 24
  units of 23
Stretch standing 318, 318f
Stride sitting 322f
Stride standing 319f
Striking, biomechanics of 265
Student's elbow 96, 97

Index

Subacromial bursa 79, 82
Subacromial bursitis 83
Subdeltoid bursa 79
Submuscular bursa lie 41
Subpopliteal bursa 142
Substitute movements 284
Subtalar joint, ligaments of 156f
Supported limb
　abduction of 127f
　adduction of 127f
Suprahyoid muscle assist 73
Suprapatellar bursa 142
Supraspinous ligament, functions of 181
Swanson prosthesis 305
Sway posture 207
Swayback posture 207, 207f, 219, 219f
Swimming 278, 279f
　strokes 278
Swing limb loading 276
Swing phase 224, 226, 231, 237, 238t
　generation 268
　part of 270
　subdivisions of 226f
Sympathetic nerves 165
Symphysis pubis 192
Synarthroses 30
Synchondrosis 30
Syndesmoses 30
Synergists 58
Synovial fluid 30, 31, 69, 122
Synovial joint
　components of 29
　condylar type of 67
　consists 30
　type of 91
Synovial membrane 30
　failure of 139
Synovial tissue secretes 139
Systematic gait analysis 238
Systemic gait, analysis of 238

T

Talus
　displacement of 211
　forms tenon 155
Talwalkar nail 305
Tarsometatarsal joints 158, 158f
Task factors 258
Technique 273
　demands 281
　employed 238
Temporal bone 65, 66, 67f
　articular eminence of 65f
Temporomandibular joint 65, 65f, 68, 68f-70f
　capsular pattern of 70
　capsule of 65
　dysfunction 74f
　function of 65
　muscles of 73f
　resting position of 70
　structure of 65
Tendon 37, 40, 47
　composition of 41
　determine, length of 41
　hypertrophy 37
　response 37
　structure of 41f

Tennis elbow 96
Tensile force 4, 137
　application of 40
　release of 40
Tensile strength 37
Tensile stress 4f, 210
Tension increases 55
Tensor fascia lata 128-130, 270
　muscle 151
Teres minor 78
Termed coxa vara 130
Therapist hand placement 283
Thick fluid film 43f
Third order lever 21, 23, 23f
　mechanical advantage for 22
Third region 47
Thompson prosthesis 305
Thoracic kyphosis 210
　excessive 211f
Thoracic region 163
Thoracic spine 218
Thoracic vertebra 15, 172f
　parts of 173f
Thoracolumbar fascia 179, 182, 186, 186f, 187
Thoracolumbar sacral orthosis 304
Thoracolumbosacral corset 307
Thorax 167
Three-jaw chucks 119
Throat, base of 66
Throwing and striking 263
Thumb, carpometacarpal joint of 112
Tibia
　beneath femur, posterior shear of 141
　femur flexes on 146
　medial malleolus of 155
　medial rotation of 212
　on femur, resists anterior translation of 140
Tibial condyles, medial and lateral 136
Tibial rotation 144f
　beneath 140
Tibial torsion, lateral 131
Tibialis anterior 157
　action of 7
Tibialis posterior 157
　muscle, lengthening of 211
Tibiofemoral alignment 137
Tibiofemoral angle, medial 137
Tibiofemoral extension 145
Tibiofemoral joint
　factors affecting stability of 150
　function 143
　structure of 136
Tibiofibular ligament, posterior 156
Tilt
　anterior 84, 85, 87, 126
　posterior 84, 85, 87, 126
Tissue structures, specific connective 40
Toe
　out, degree of 242
　standing 318, 319f
　touch 272
　walking gait 235
Toe off 226
　kinematics of 231
　kinetics of 232
　midstance to 230

Torn meniscus 74
Torsion
　angle of 130, 131f
　force 5, 5f
Torticollis 306
Trabecular system 132
Traction external rotation 83
Train naked 273
Translatory motion 10
Translatory movement 69
Transverse abdominis 175
Transverse arch, proximal 111
Transverse arches 161
Transverse plane
　kinematics 269
　motions 84f
Transverse tubules 49
Trapezius, upper 82
Treadmill gait 236
Tremendous upward pressure 73
Trendelenburg gait 235
Triceps brachii 94
Triceps tightness 93
Trick movement 283, 284, 287
Tripod grips 119
Trochanteric bursitis 130
Tropocollagen 40
　structure of 40f
Tropomyosin 50
Troponin 50
　pulls tropomyosin 50
True ribs 170
Trunk extensors, requires co-contractions of 215
Trunk lateral flexion 182f
Trunk left rotation 264
Trunk region, muscles of 189
Trunk-seat angle 260
Two-jaw chuck 119

U

Ulcers, pressure 215
Ulna
　styloid process of 99
　trochlear notch of 91
Ulnar collateral ligament, lateral 91-93
Ulnar deviation 102, 102f, 103f, 106
Ulnar deviators, function of 108
Ulnar direction 113
Ulnar negative variance 100
Ulnar positive variance 100, 101
Ulnar variance
　negative 101
　positive 101
Ulnocarpal complex 104
Uncinate process 165
Underarm throwing, kinematics of 264
Unfavorable acting moments 45
Unilateral stance 133
Upper cervical region 165
Upper extremity 7f, 299
　injuries 276
　orthosis 307
Upper limb orthosis 304
Upper motor neuron lesion 309
Upper trapezius, force of 9f
Uterus 222

Index

V

Valgus 148
Valsalva maneuver 246
 influence of 246
Varum brace 305
Varus 148
Vastus lateralis
 activity of 248
 large 150
 muscle 150
 pull of 150f
Vastus medialis 150f
 large 150
 muscle 150
 oblique 150
Ventilation 176
 accessory muscles of 175
 muscles of 261
Vertebra
 body 165
 inferior 171
 types of 176
Vertebral column 163, 177f, 208, 210, 213
 mobility of 164t
Vertebral curvature 179
Vertebral end plate 176, 178
Vertebral foramen 165
Vertebral trunk, muscles of 189
Vertical anthropometric
 measurement 255f
Video display terminal 312
 users 258
Vinyl hand grips 302
Viscoelasticity 47
Visual distance 260
Visual system 201
Volar intercalated segmental
 instability 108, 109f
Volar plate 113
Volume strain 23

W

Waddling gait 222, 235
Waist angles, unequal 213
Walk standing 319, 319f
Walker
 functions of 302
 types of 302
Walking aids 298
 biomechanical functions of 298
 classification of 298
Walking balance, requirement of 228
Weakness, zone of 133
Weight-bearing 160
 activities 140, 252
 feet and pelvis 126
 forces 137
 gait pattern 303
Weightlifters lift 248
White blood cells 61
Wicket keeping 280
 three phases of 281f
Wing standing 317, 317f
Women's gymnastics composed 273
Work
 injuries 310
 measurement of 19
 surfaces 311
Workbench
 bottom height 258
 dimension of 257
 surface 258
  inclination of 258
 top height 258
Wrist
 and hand complex 98
 arthrokinematics 101
 articulations 101
 complex 98
  structure of 99f
  systems of 99
 comprises 98
 extension 102f, 105, 289, 290f
 flexion 102f, 105, 289, 290f
 flexor
  function of 107
  muscles, active 107
 hand orthosis 304
 joint
  fractures 109
  ligaments of 103f
  structure of 99
 kinematics of 104
 motion, kinematics of 102f
 muscle, functions of 106
 musculature 277
 radial
  deviation 290f
  osteokinematics of 102f
 rotational collapse of 108
 ulnar 290
  and radial deviation of 106
  deviation 290f
Wry neck 306

Y

Yard standing 318, 318f
Yellow elastic fibrocartilage 41
Yield point 26
Young's modulus 24, 46
Younger subjects 202

Z

Z discs 52, 61
Zig-zag fashion 108
Zygapophyseal articulation 166
Zygapophyseal joint 166, 178, 210
 capsule 166
Zygomatic bone 66
 temporal process of 66
Zygomatic process 66

EU GSPR Authorised Reprsentative
Logos Europe, 9 rue Nicolas Poussin
1700, La Rochelle, France
Phone: +33 (0) 6 67 93 73 78
E-mail: contact@logoseurope.eu

www.ingramcontent.com/pod-product-compliance
Ingram Content Group UK Ltd.
Pitfield, Milton Keynes, MK11 3LW, UK
UKHW050456150426

5217IPUK00025B/1712